AS YOUNG AS YOU FEEL

'Age is an issue of mind over matter.
If you don't mind, it doesn't matter.'

Mark Twain, American author

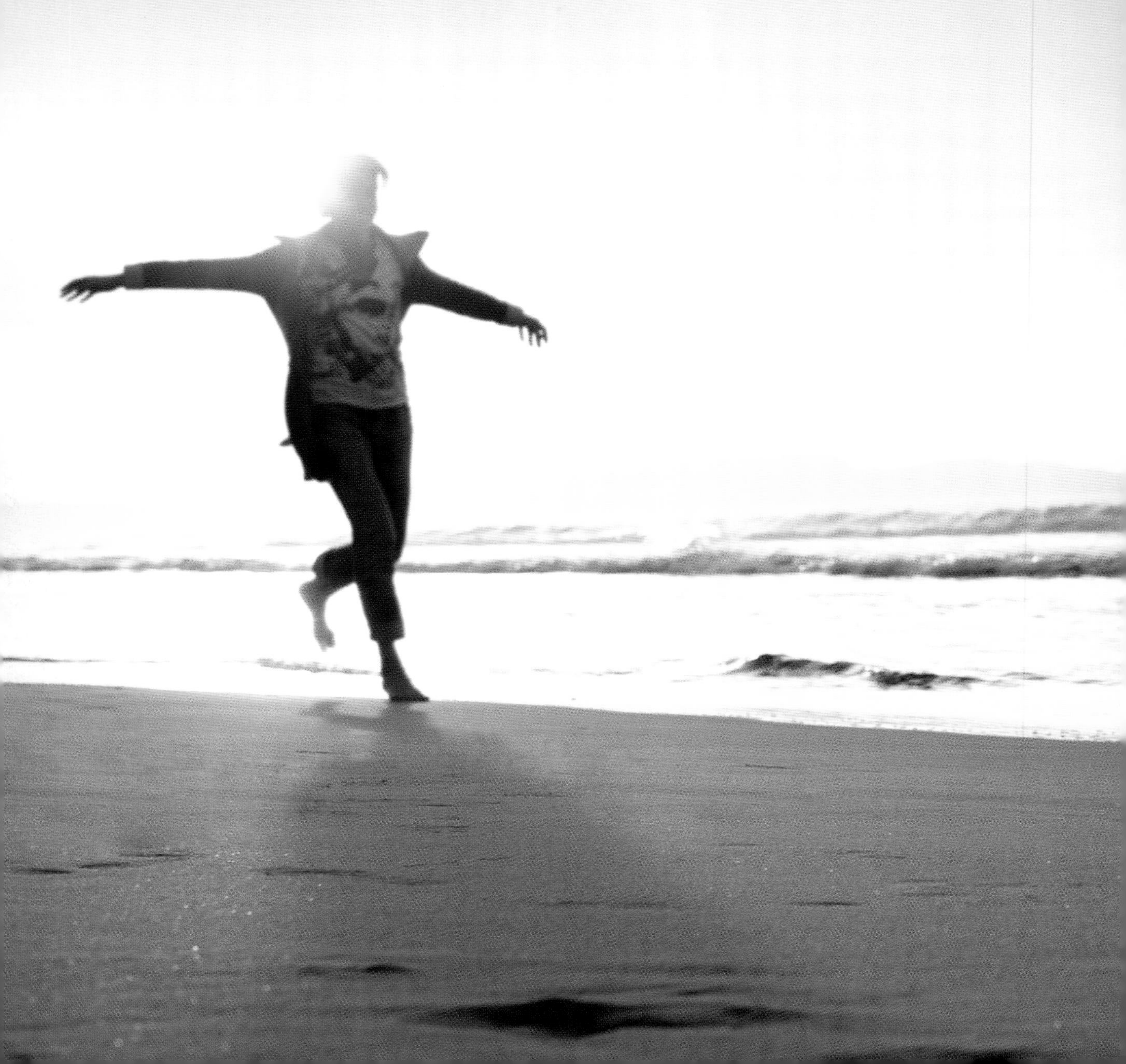

AS YOUNG AS YOU FEEL

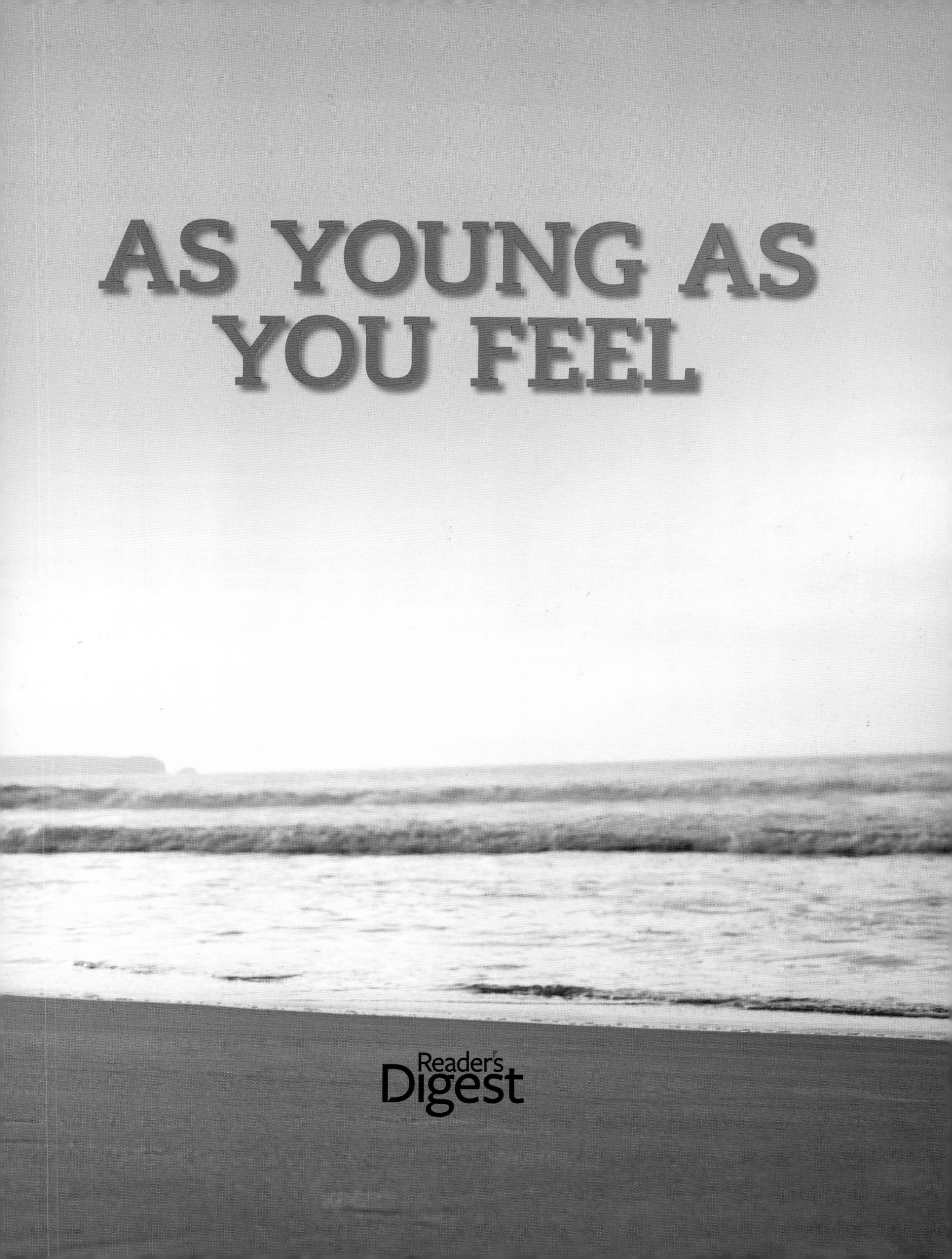

Reader's Digest

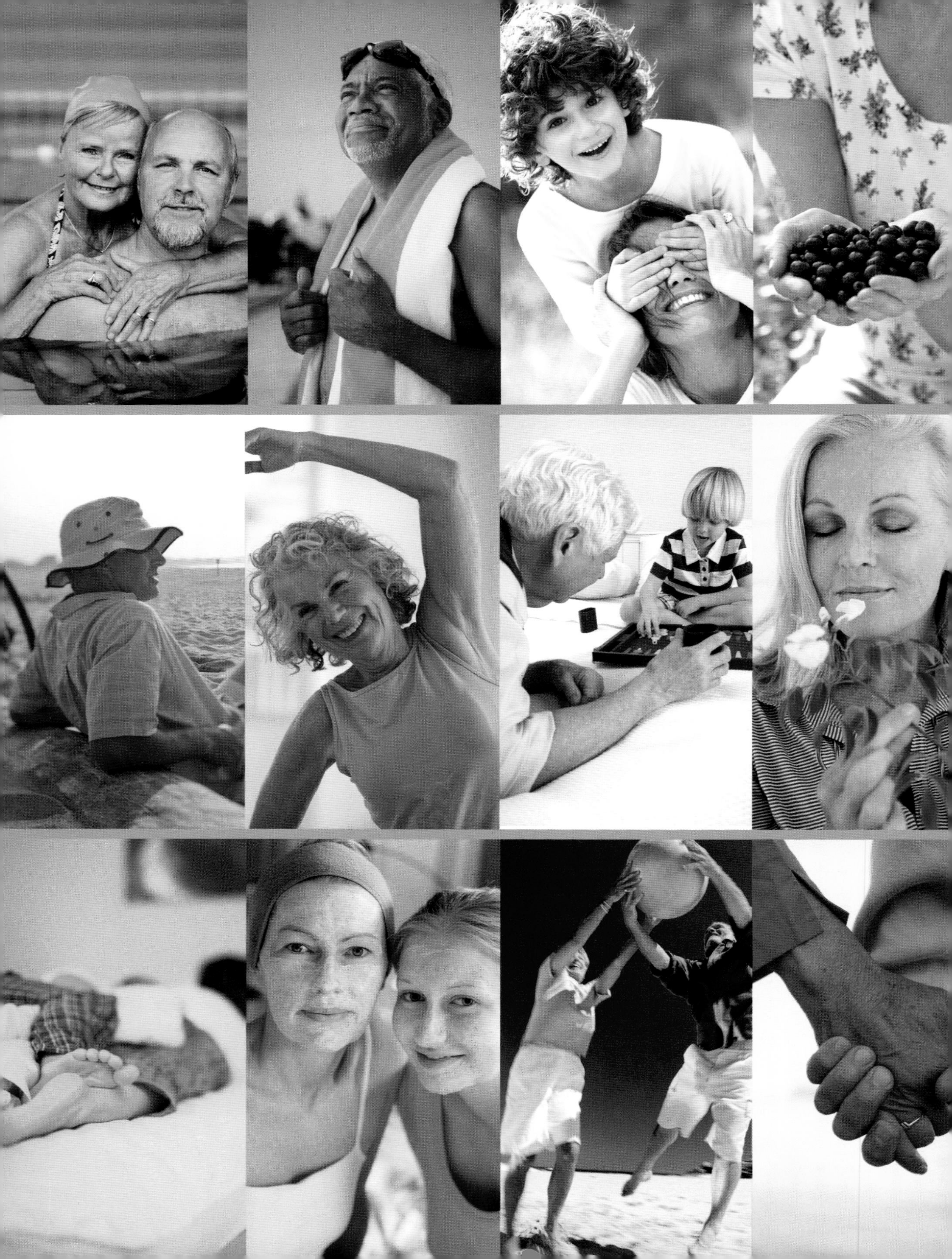

Contents

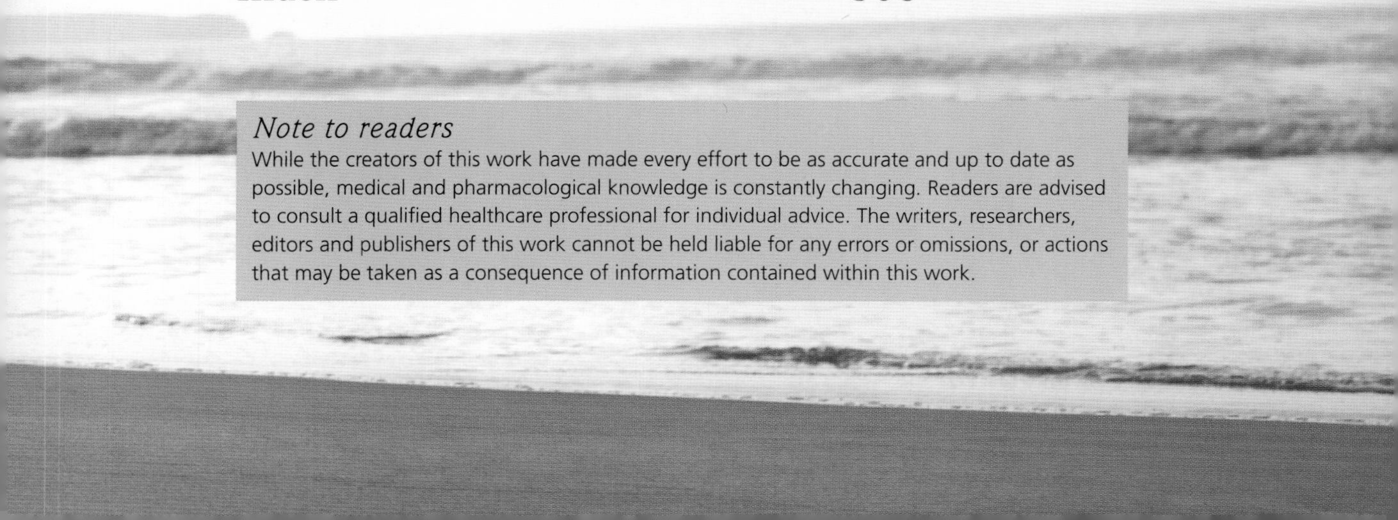

Note to readers

While the creators of this work have made every effort to be as accurate and up to date as possible, medical and pharmacological knowledge is constantly changing. Readers are advised to consult a qualified healthcare professional for individual advice. The writers, researchers, editors and publishers of this work cannot be held liable for any errors or omissions, or actions that may be taken as a consequence of information contained within this work.

GETTING THE BEST out of older age

'Do not regret growing older. It is a privilege denied to many.'

Anon

In so many ways, there's never been a better time to reach 60 and beyond. Surveys suggest that people in this age group are happier and healthier than any preceding generation.

Of course, certain signs of ageing are inevitable. But study after study shows that many of the so-called effects of ageing are not a matter of advancing years but of lifestyle choices – which means we can do something about them.

That's where this book comes in. Unlike most health books, it focuses entirely on what happens after the age of sixty. It embraces the physical, mental and emotional aspects of ageing, showing you what to expect as the years pass – and what you can do about it. The overwhelming message from the experts is that it is never too late to turn back the clock. Whatever your starting point, and whatever your age, scientists have discovered that many aspects of ageing are preventable or reversible.

This book covers all the most important areas of the body – your heart, your lungs, your immune system and more. One chapter is devoted to the older mind – everything from moods to sharpening your memory. Others address key aspects of healthy living: exercise, diet, restful sleep. Finally there is a section on living life to the full. One consistent scientific finding is that laughter, fun and enjoyment are potent health boosters – and they keep you young.

Each chapter explains the changes that are inevitable (surprisingly few), those that are preventable (many more than you'd think), and shows you how to keep body and mind in tip-top condition.

While modern medical science is undoubtedly helping this generation break down the barriers of conventional chronological age, it has also revealed how much lifestyle influences physical and mental wellbeing. This unique book outlines the latest findings and explains clearly all the measures that will help you to stay healthy and feel more youthful in your older years.

Hillary Clinton was 61 when she took office as the 67th US Secretary of State.

Nelson Mandela 'retired from being retired', and at the age of 90 was still contributing to the campaign against AIDS in Africa.

At 78, Jane Goodall was still spending much of her time travelling the world as an advocate for chimpanzees and conservation.

Potato farmer Cliff Young was 61 years old when he won the gruelling Sydney to Melbourne Ultra-Marathon.

Doris Lessing, winner of the Nobel Prize in Literature in 2007, was 88 when she received the highest literary accolade.

At 89, Albert Schweitzer was still tending patients in his hospital in Gabon.

At 90, Pablo Picasso was producing drawings and engravings.

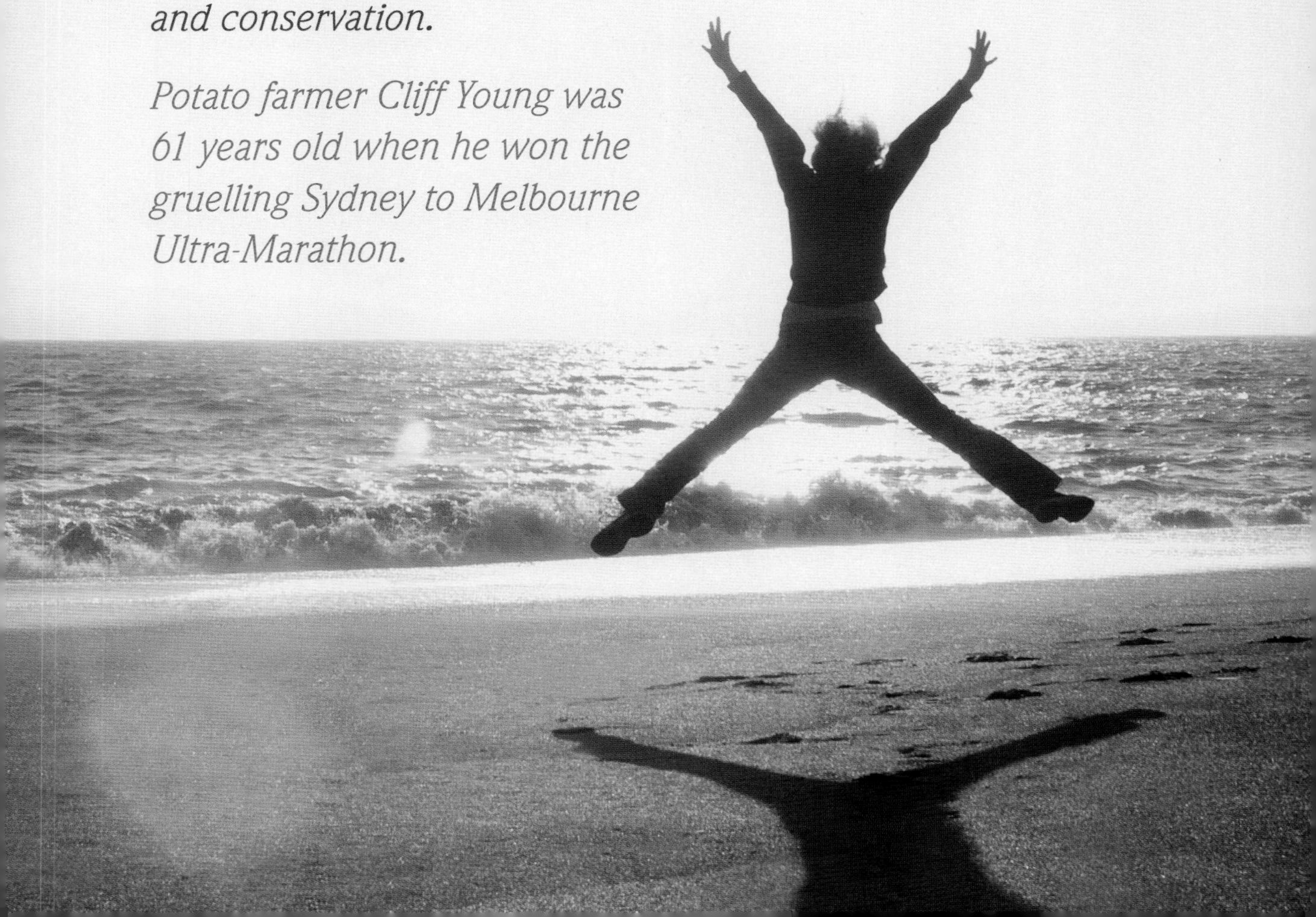

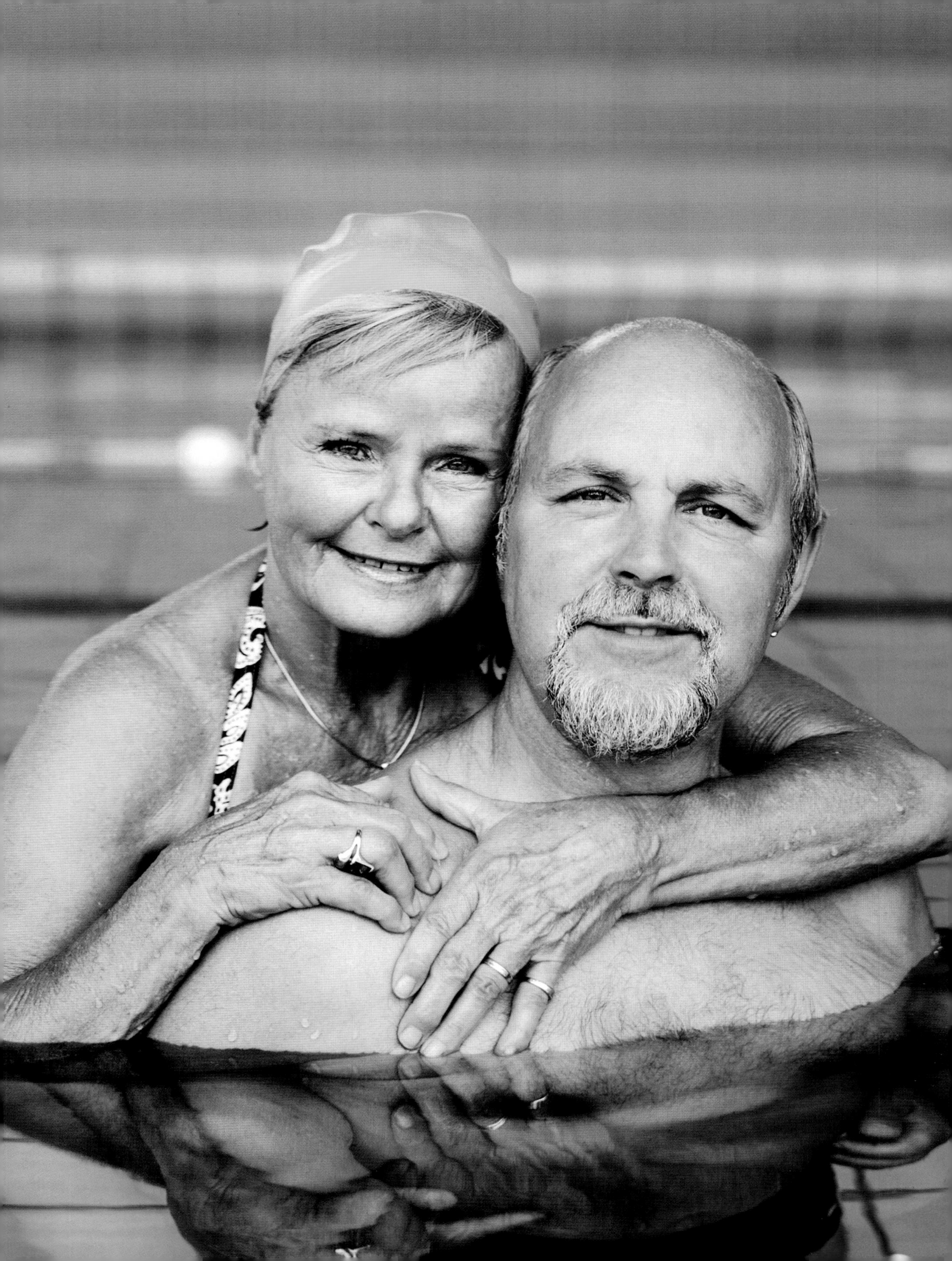

1

Your BODY *your life*

We are living longer. In the past 50 years the likelihood of surviving to 70 and beyond has almost doubled. Thanks to the many discoveries that scientists have made about the ageing process, the chances of leading a full, healthy, enjoyable life are higher than ever. In this chapter you'll begin to find out what these insights mean for you and, more importantly, how to put them into practice – starting now.

By 2050, an incredible 2 billion people will be over 60.

THE SUPER SIXTIES
a time of opportunity

Being over 60 is a cause for celebration, not dismay. Armed with a wealth of scientifically proven strategies, you really can minimise the drawbacks and maximise the benefits of getting older. Why shouldn't this mark the start of a new, exciting phase of life?

Today if you're aged 60 or more, you're in great company. By 2025, there will be an estimated 1.25 billion over-60s. By 2050, there could be as many as 2 billion – almost a quarter of the world's projected population. And this Baby Boomer generation redefined youth, so it's no surprise that now they're redefining the 'third age'.

True, as you'd expect, your body starts to show signs of the time you've spent on this planet, but frailty and ill health are not inevitable. Understanding the physical changes that occur with age and knowing which lifestyle factors can enable you to stay well will help you achieve the goal of long-term health. And better diagnosis and treatments mean that most of us, even if we do develop health problems, can still look forward to living a long and full life.

HOW YOU IMPROVE WITH AGE

There are, in fact, many benefits to getting older. On the physical front, you'll probably catch fewer colds. Your immune system retains a memory of the cold viruses you've been exposed to and pumps out antibodies to fight them off if you encounter them again. If you have allergies, symptoms may ease as the immune system is less reactive. And your skin becomes less oily – so acne ceases to be a problem.

On the mental front, it's equally good news. Your brain power can continue to expand (there's plenty of extra reserve), you get wiser and you become a better decision maker. And you're likely to feel more at ease with yourself. The way you see the world is also important – excitement and optimism will keep you more youthful. Read on to find out how to protect your health and make the most of the decades ahead, starting with what expert research reveals are fifteen steps to loving life.

15 ways to embrace the best of getting older

Modern research is discovering all the ways that you can boost your chances of a longer, healthier, happier life. Here are 15 of the best:

1 FOLLOW YOUR STAR

Setting goals has proven benefits for your health. A US study of older adults found that those with a sense of purpose tended to live longer than those who had none. So plan ahead and enjoy new experiences. Have aims and ambitions. As the singer Leonard Cohen once said on stage: 'I began this tour three years ago; I was 73, just a kid with a crazy dream.'

2 MOVE YOUR BODY

Countless studies show that staying active helps you live a happier, healthier, longer life. If you don't currently exercise, start now: the benefits accrue whatever your age or level of fitness – Texan researchers found that a year of exercise training improved heart function in previously sedentary people over 65. Discover how to fit exercise into your life on pages 130–173.

3 BE HAPPY, DON'T WORRY!

If you were to plot the average person's happiness on a graph, the resulting curve would be smile-shaped. We are happy in our youth, less so in our middle years, then happy again in the latter third of life. A UK survey of 80,000 people found that the 65-to-80 age group enjoyed life most. Older people know how to devote energy to what matters and move on quickly from mistakes. Find new ways to stay happy and beat the blues on pages 191–198.

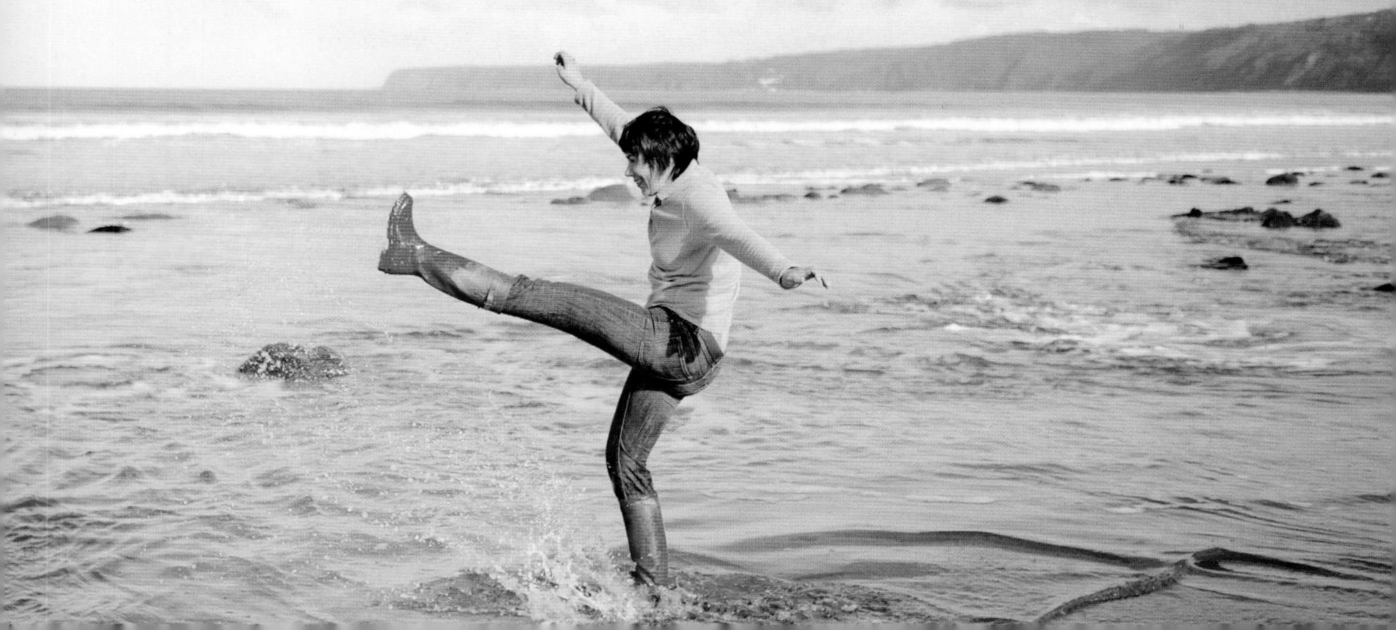

4 WATCH YOUR WAISTLINE

Maintaining a healthy weight is important – but keeping your waist size down is crucial. Fat around the waist is a visible sign of 'visceral fat'– fatty deposits around the internal organs. This fat is dangerous, because it releases inflammatory chemicals linked to a host of diseases from arthritis to diabetes. How do you get rid of it? There's plenty of advice on pages 94–99. Slow and steady weight loss is healthier than crash dieting, and there are many delicious foods to enjoy in a balanced diet. Be sure to exercise, too, to keep yourself strong.

5 KEEP OLD FRIENDS, MAKE NEW ONES

Good relationships are the key to contentment in later life. So said a British survey of 10,000 men and women over the age of 50, and in Loving Life (*see* pages 272–297) there's plenty of information about how to make yours better than ever. Research also shows that the stronger your relationships, the longer you're likely to live. An Australian study of people in their 70s found their chances of living well into the next decade were directly linked to the size of their social network.

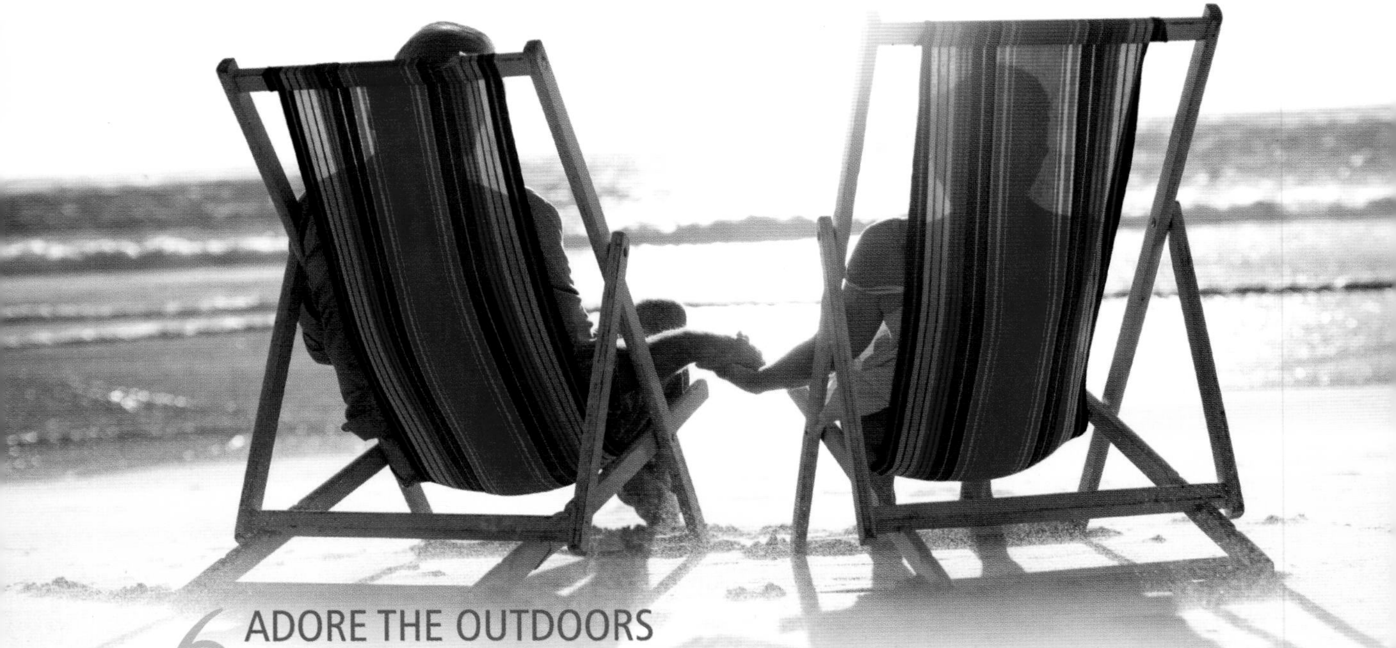

6 ADORE THE OUTDOORS

We've long known that a daily dose of vitamin D, the sunshine vitamin, is important for bone health. Scientists are now discovering that vitamin D deficiency could be a factor in some cancers and in multiple sclerosis. It also helps the immune system function more efficiently. Yet more than half of us don't get enough, even in the summer. Make a point of getting outdoors for a few minutes around midday during the warmer months (*see* page 122). During the shorter days of winter, consider taking a supplement.

7 EAT MORE PLANTS

There are more centenarians on the island of Okinawa, Japan, than anywhere else in the world. And they're less likely to be blighted by the diseases that come with age. What's their secret? It's a lot to do with diet. They actually eat more, kilogram for kilogram, than Westerners, but their food is low in kilojoules – plenty of fresh produce and whole grains, with smaller amounts of high-fat, high-kilojoule foods. Turn to page 76 to start reading about how to eat for a long and healthy life.

8 CARRY ON LOVING

There's no reason why your sex life should peter out – *see* pages 282–285 for ways to keep it fun. A Swedish study found that older couples today have more sex, and better sex, than their predecessors. That's important because an active love life has health benefits – researchers in Bristol concluded that sexual activity had a protective effect. And a Scottish study found that older people who regularly had sex looked up to ten years younger than those who did not.

9 TAKE UP SPANISH ... OR THE TANGO

Swedish researchers found that older people tend to have the same hobbies in later life as in middle age. That's fine, but it's important to challenge your mind with novel activities. The very act of planning them stimulates the release of neurotransmitters, which can decrease with age. New interests can mean meeting new people – also good for you.

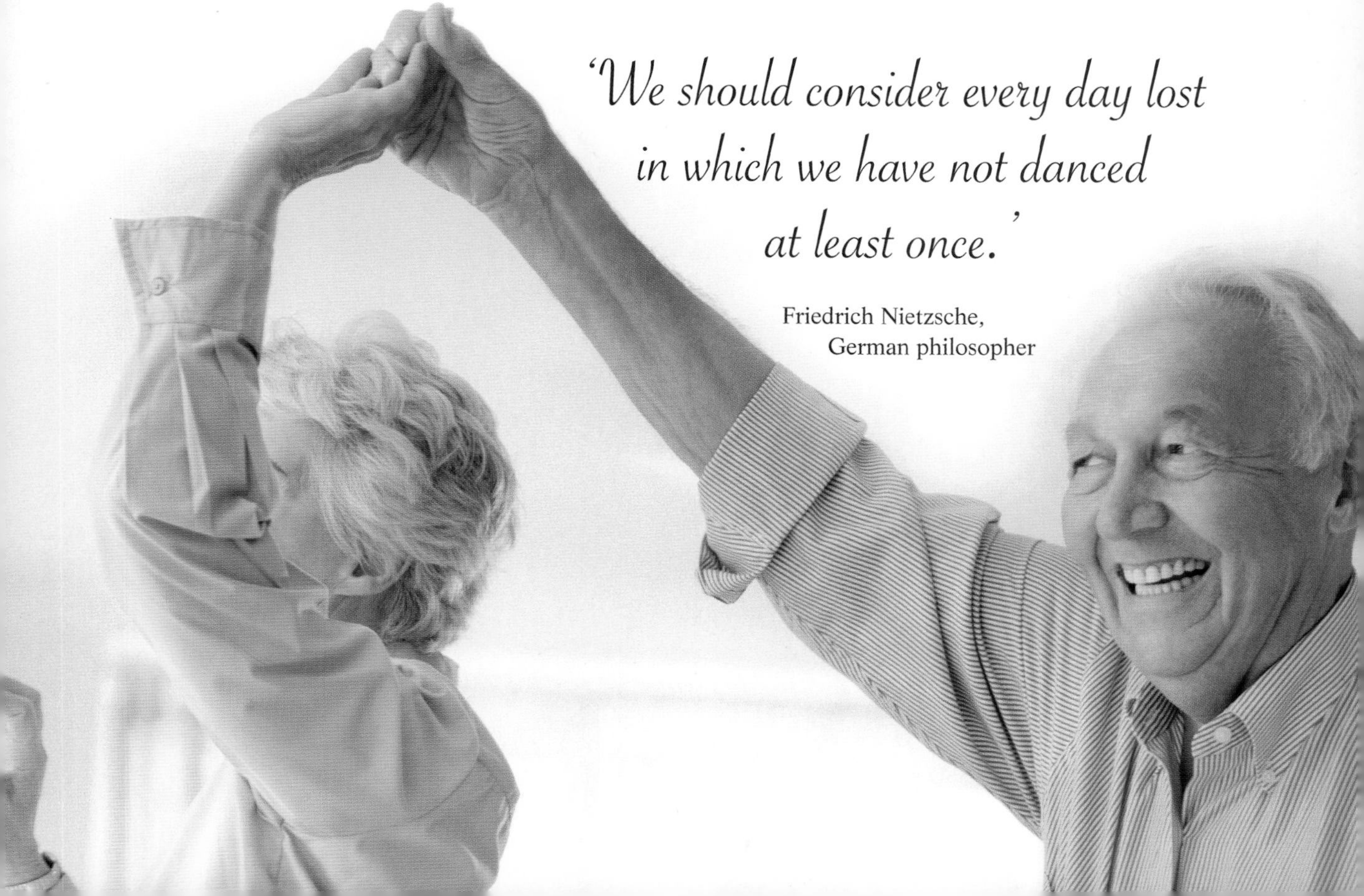

'We should consider every day lost in which we have not danced at least once.'

Friedrich Nietzsche,
German philosopher

10 DRINK WHEN YOU'RE NOT THIRSTY

Your body is 60 to 75 per cent water. But in later years, fluid balance becomes harder to maintain – a result of changes in body composition as well as less efficient kidney function. It's vital to drink enough to avoid dehydration. You can't always rely on thirst or a parched throat to tell you that you need to top up, as the sensation of thirst declines as you get older. So it's a good idea to keep a glass of water beside you to sip regularly.

'The greatest gift of the garden is the restoration of the five senses.'

Hanna Rion, American artist

11 LOOK TO YOUR ROSES

People who garden are more likely to remain fit into old age. If you have a garden to tend, you're probably active for the recommended 30 minutes most days, according to research by the Kansas State University. And a bit of weeding and dead-heading – digging, too, but watch your back – is exactly the kind of gentle physical activity that does you good. Australian researchers found that daily gardening reduced the risk of dementia by 36 per cent in a sample group of over-60s. Gardening is a perfect antidote to stress, and you get a wonderful sense of achievement from growing beautiful roses or tasty vegetables.

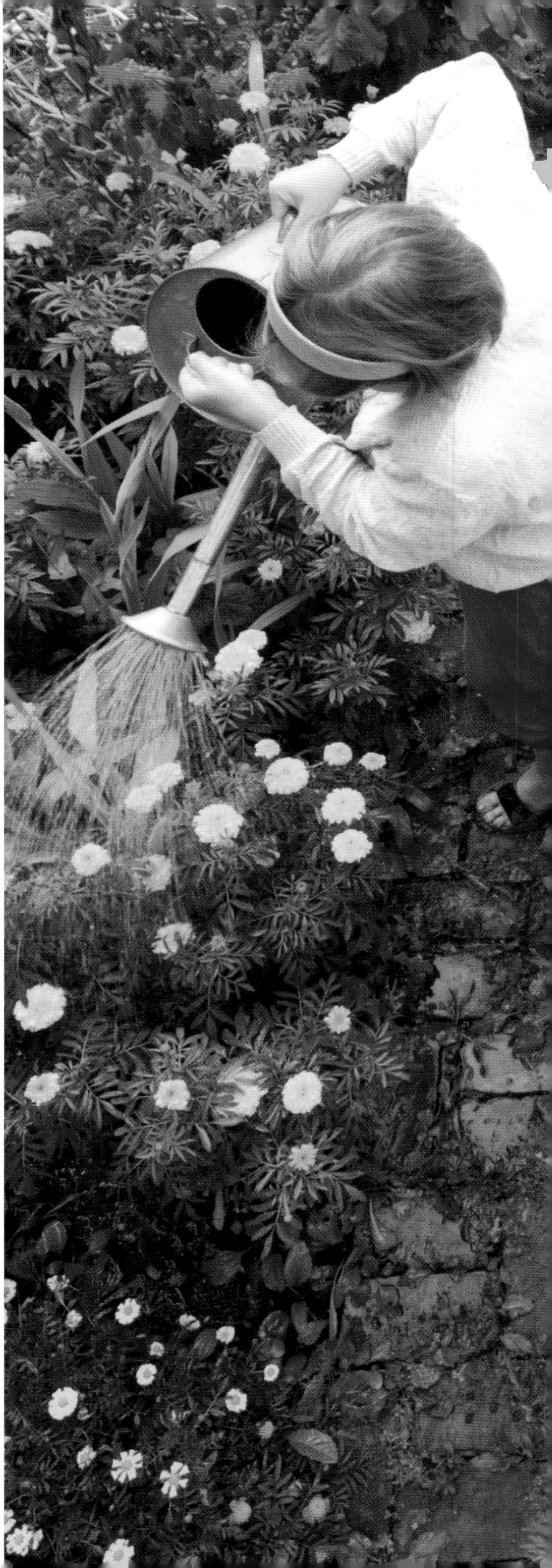

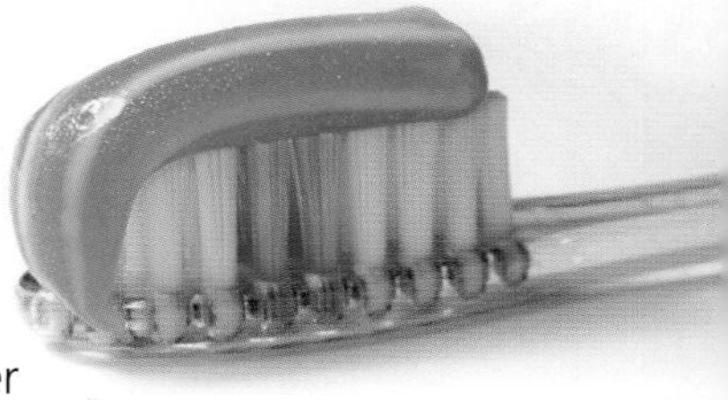

12 BRUSH UP

It's surprising how much dental hygiene matters as you get older. Daily flossing and cleaning twice daily is linked to a healthier old age. Why? Because the bacteria that cause periodontal disease can also cause inflammation elsewhere in the body – and that can contribute to serious problems such as stroke, heart disease and Alzheimer's. Find out more on pages 262–263.

13 KEEP A PET

There's been plenty of research to show that animals can reduce stress in their owners. One study from Miami University in Ohio found that pet owners have greater self-esteem and are more conscientious and less fearful, which all boost mental health. Now it seems pets can help physical health, too – a study by the US National Institutes of Health showed that dog owners have a better chance of being alive one year after a heart attack, regardless of the severity of the attack.

14 DRESS AS YOU PLEASE, DO AS YOU WILL ...

Once you're older you're more likely to do as you like and look the way you want to, without worrying about what other people think. Plenty of older role models – from Helen Mirren to Sean Connery – confirm that you never need to stop being attractive and graceful. There are ideas on enjoying a stylish later life in Looking Good, pages 267–271, which you can, of course, adapt to suit yourself. After all, you've earned the right to be a bit individual, even downright disgraceful. Laugh in the face of people who ask, with a concerned smile, 'Aren't you a bit old for that?'

15 HAVE REGULAR MEDICAL CHECK-UPS

You'll find numerous ways to protect your health throughout this book. The seven below are among the most important, potentially life-saving health checks.

- **Cholesterol test** A blood test is the only way to establish your cholesterol levels (*see* page 42).
- **Blood pressure checks** High blood pressure can damage the heart and make a heart attack more likely. See your doctor for regular check-ups (*see* pages 38–45).
- **Breast screening** Women over 50 should have a mammogram, a type of X-ray (*see* page 126), to check for early signs of breast cancer every two years.
- **Skin checks** Keep an eye on any moles, and report any changes to your doctor (*see* page 257).
- **Eye tests** An optometrist can detect early signs of diabetes and glaucoma as well as sight changes (*see* page 210).
- **Bowel cancer** A bowel cancer screening test every couple of years is important. More than 80 per cent of cases occur in people over 60 (*see* page 127).
- **Cervical smear** This test is used to detect abnormal cells in the cervix early on (*see* page 127).

These tests are especially important as we age. Inevitably, our bodies change – find out more in the following pages. Understanding what is likely to happen puts you in control, helping you to combat and mitigate problems. And it's not all bad news, as you'll discover.

At 60, you can be in better shape than a 30-year-old couch potato.

ALL CHANGE
your body as you age

Your looks and the way your body works both evolve as you get older – and not always for the worse. There's plenty you can do to keep adverse changes to a minimum and maintain your strength and vitality.

Physiological ageing – the changes that happen to your body as time passes – is a complex process. It varies not only from person to person, but also occurs at a different rate within the same individual. So while your sight or hearing may be less than perfect, your heart and lungs can be extremely strong.

A heartening fact is that your body has plenty of spare capacity – what scientists call 'functional reserve'. This means it can work well right into old age. So a healthy, active 60-year-old can be in better shape – inside and out – than a couch potato of 30 who smokes, drinks and eats nothing but junk food. Here's what happens to some key organs and tissues as the years go by.

YOUR BONES, JOINTS AND MUSCLES

You shrink by about a centimetre a decade after the age of 40 as a result of accelerated bone loss (especially in post-menopausal women), reduced synovial fluid (the cushioning in your joints) and loss of muscle tissues and fibres. By the age of 75, you may have as little as half the muscle that you had at 25. Your strength declines by 1 or 2 per cent a year, and your muscle power falls by around 3 to 4 per cent, unless you maintain it. Your feet also become flatter, and you may look scrawnier because tough, fibrous tissue replaces lost muscle.

✓**THE GOOD NEWS** Bones and muscles are living tissues that are constantly broken down and built up throughout our lives. As we get older, the breakdown process accelerates, and we lose bone and muscle mass. But you can slow bone loss through exercise, especially strength or resistance training (using weights),

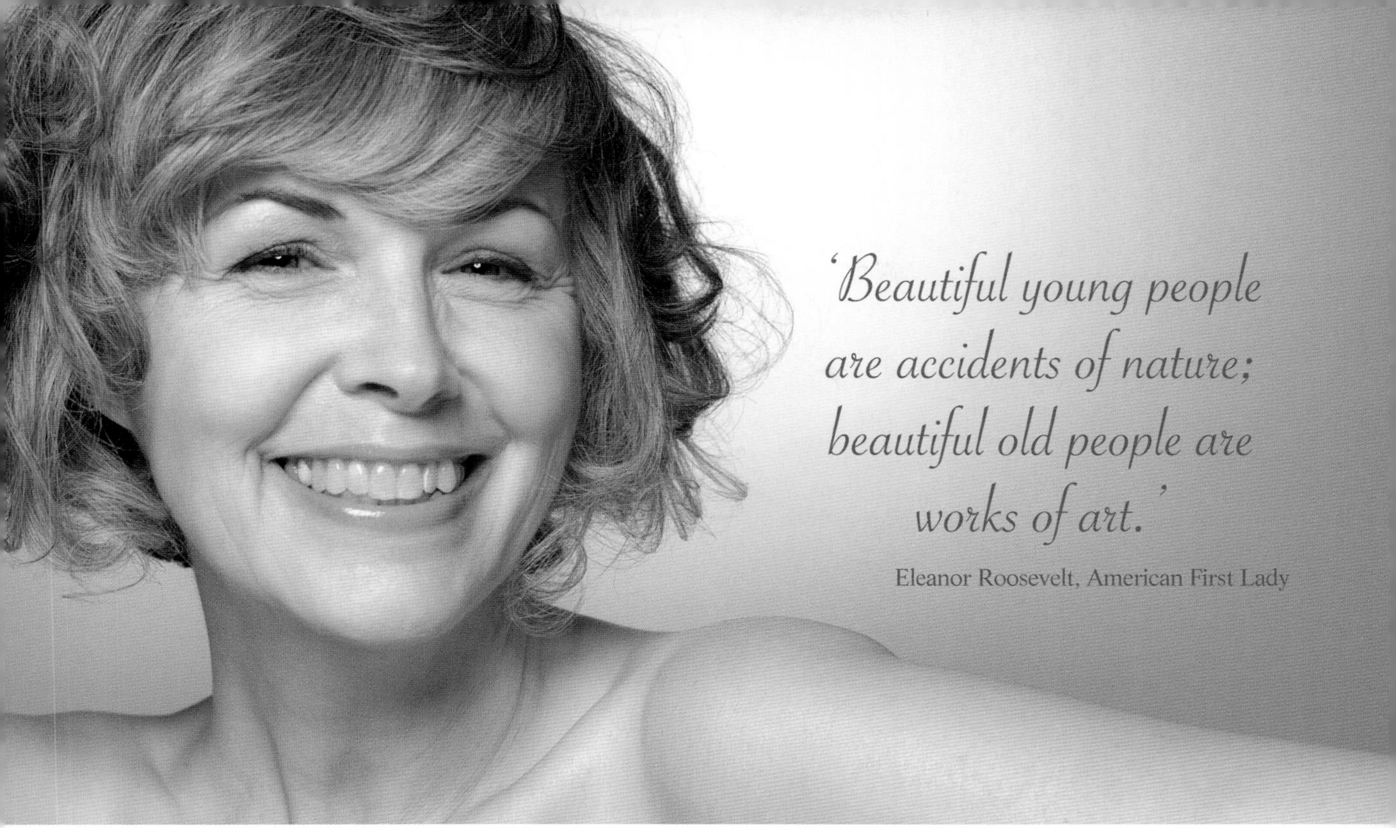

or any activity that loads and stresses the bones – such as hiking, wearing a backpack, skipping, tennis and squash. The same goes for your muscles: though you can't stop muscle cell loss, strength training can minimise shrinkage and improve your strength even into your 80s.

YOUR SHAPE AND SIZE

Fat may gather around your middle – the classic middle-age spread. Even if you weigh the same at 60 as you did at 20, the chances are you're carrying twice as much fat – unless you've always been physically active. Fat around your abdomen could be a sign of insulin resistance, which occurs when your body makes the hormone insulin but cannot use it as efficiently to control blood-glucose levels. This points to a risk of diabetes, heart disease, stroke and some cancers, so it makes sense to have a check-up.

✓**THE GOOD NEWS** Once you hit 60, you tend to lose fat elsewhere. In men, weight loss often sets in a bit early and may be linked to dwindling levels of testosterone hormone. Women may start to lose fat from around 65. Diet and exercise can help you stay shapely.

YOUR HEART AND LUNGS

Your heart shrinks. By the age of 70 it has 30 per cent fewer cells than it had in your youth, and its pumping capacity is reduced. The number of air sacs and capillaries in your lungs diminishes, and your lungs themselves become less elastic. Your maximum aerobic power – the amount of oxygen you take in when you exert yourself – changes, and exercising vigorously makes you more breathless. By the age of 60 the residual air volume – the amount of air left in your lungs after you've breathed out forcefully – is around 35 per cent compared with 20 per cent at the age of 20.

Your liver has to work harder as you age – moderating your alcohol intake is one way to help it.

✓**THE GOOD NEWS** Though you tend to lose heart cells as you age and your heart undergoes many changes, this powerful organ has a remarkable capacity to adapt and keep going. If you exercise well into old age, especially if you regularly do aerobic exercise, you'll be helping your heart to cope with any age-related changes. And refraining from smoking not only benefits your heart – it helps ensure you maintain good lung capacity.

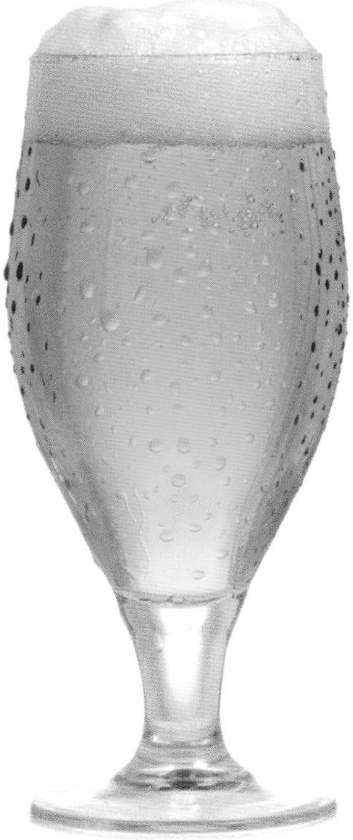

YOUR LIVER AND KIDNEYS

With age, the number of liver cells declines, blood flow decreases, and the enzymes needed for liver function work less efficiently. These changes mean that it can take longer to clear medications and other substances from your system. Meanwhile, your kidneys shrink due to cell loss and poorer circulation, and therefore are not so good at filtering waste products. This can lead to unbalanced water and salt excretion, which may cause dehydration. Poor kidney function can result in high blood pressure, heart disease and stroke, while uncontrolled diabetes can damage kidney function.

✓**THE GOOD NEWS** Your liver has a remarkable capacity for regeneration, all the more so if you moderate your alcohol intake. Your kidneys cannot regenerate in the way that your liver can, but the fact that you have two of them means you have spare capacity. Keeping your blood pressure under control through exercise, diet and, if necessary, prescription medications can help kidney function.

YOUR HAIR AND SKIN

Wrinkles, age spots, dryness and thinning skin are some of the visible signs of the passing years. But much of what used to be thought of as ageing is actually down to skin damage. Changes in your skin can lead to dryness, itching and a greater risk of infections, especially of the mucous membranes in your mouth, urethra, and, in women, vagina. By the age of 50, half of Caucasian people will have grey hair. Hair growth also slows on the head, armpits and pubic region, although it can speed up in the nostrils, ears and eyebrows – especially for men. Loss of oestrogen in women can cause hairs to sprout on the face.

✓**THE GOOD NEWS** Modern skin and hair products help – but the best way to keep your skin smoother and hair glossier is to eat a healthy diet, drink plenty of water and avoid too much sun exposure. And you can always dye greying hair – whatever your sex.

YOUR VOICE

The cartilages of your larynx turn to bone and the laryngeal muscles weaken, which can make your voice quieter and hoarser. Women's voices may become lower, while men's can get higher. One in five people over 65 experience problems with their voice.

✓**THE GOOD NEWS** Age-related voice changes may be minimised by voice training and singing (try reading aloud for 10 minutes a day or singing along to the radio). Or join a choir: you'll have fun and meet new people, and it could be beneficial. Try not to yell or scream, as this strains the vocal cords.

Keep your skin smoother and hair glossier by eating a healthy diet.

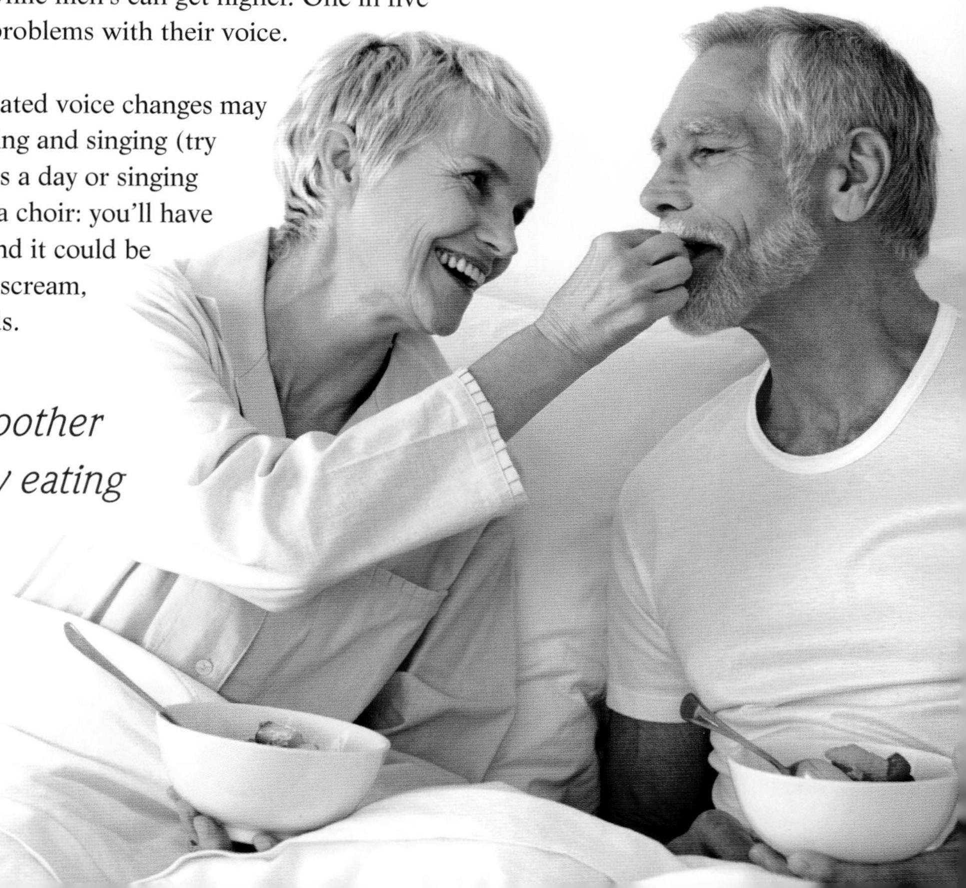

DID **you** KNOW ?

You can improve your maximum aerobic capacity by 10 to 20 per cent until you are at least 70 – an effect equal to losing ten to 20 years off your biological calendar – according to Archie Young, Professor of Geriatric Medicine at the University of Edinburgh. This accounts for the ability of healthy professional athletes to continue setting records, especially in endurance events. Take Canadian Ed Whitlock, who at 73 became the oldest person to run a marathon in under 3 hours.

Doing new and complex tasks can help brain cells to grow at any age.

THE WISER MIND
the brain in maturity

While it's true that the brain, like all your body's organs, changes as the years pass, it's not just about loss. In fact, there are all kinds of major advantages to having an older brain.

'Of all the things I've lost I miss my mind the most,' said the writer Mark Twain. He was joking, of course, but as we get older it's often mental decline that we really fear. There's no doubt that for most people over 60, so-called senior moments – forgetting where you put your glasses, what your pin number is – become more frequent.

Why does this happen? A major reason is that between the ages of 20 and 90 your brain loses 5 to 10 per cent of its volume. And most of this shrinkage takes place in the hippocampus, a key area for memory. There's also a diminishing of the prefrontal cortex, which is the part of the brain responsible for helping you recall information, organise your thoughts and do more than one thing at a time.

In practice, this means that you may find it takes you longer to learn and complete mental tasks than when you were younger, especially if you're interrupted or are trying to multi-task. But simply being aware of these changes means that you can work round them – for example, by giving yourself plenty of time to do things and, if you're attempting something new, not to give up too easily. And, whatever Twain may have thought, the many pluses of the ageing brain can more than compensate for less positive changes.

✓**THE GOOD NEWS** Scientists know that your brain, like your body, has plenty of spare capacity. This means that unless you've suffered damage or illness you can always learn new things. There's also increasing evidence to suggest that, contrary to what we used to believe, the process of forming new brain cells – what scientists

'Cherish all your happy moments: they make a fine cushion for old age.'

Christopher Morley, American journalist

call neurogenesis – carries on throughout your life. The forging of new connections between neurons (called synapses) is also, it seems, an unending phenomenon. This is exciting because it means that – unless you're unfortunate enough to develop a brain disorder such as dementia – you're capable of learning and committing new information to memory for the duration of your life, regardless of your age. What's more, your brain has an amazing capacity – known as plasticity – to reorganise itself, so that even if you suffer damage from, for example, a stroke, it can sometimes reassign jobs to different areas so that recovery of function may eventually be possible.

And your brain's remarkable adaptability means that you can preserve and even improve your brain power through measures such as staying active, reducing stress, eating a healthy

what's **NEW**

HOW THE OLDER BRAIN LEARNS

Making mistakes is part of learning. In fact, it's the best way to consolidate memories as you age. Young children learn by doing something over and over again until they get it right. It used to be thought that such trial-and-error learning taxed older brains, that passive learning – where the correct answer is repeatedly presented – was better. But a 2011 Canadian study that compared learning ability in a group of 20-somethings with a group with an average age of 70 may refute this. It found that the older group learned better when allowed to experiment and make mistakes. So if at first you don't succeed, keep on trying.

Age is no barrier to learning new things …

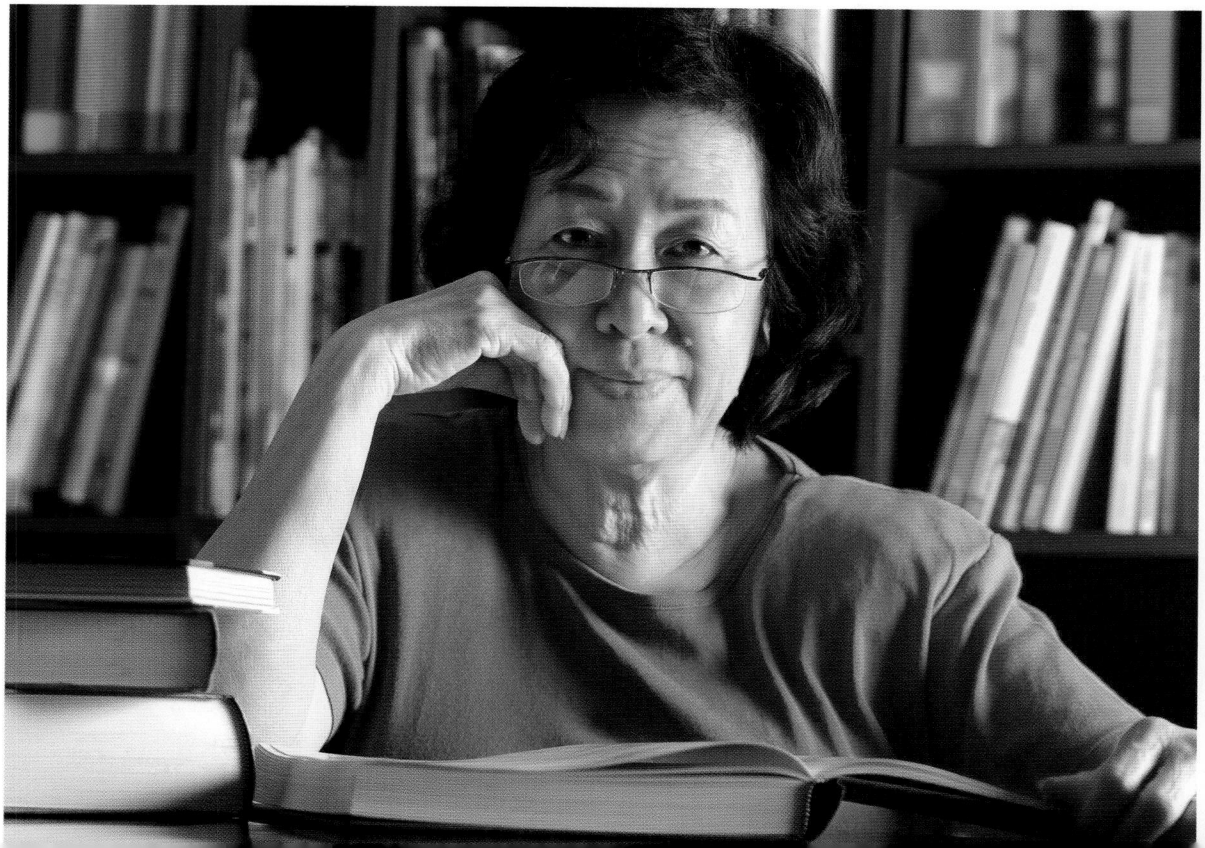

DID **you** KNOW?

Brain power depends on, among other things, the connections formed between your neurons earlier in life. Some researchers even suggest that today's 60-somethings are less likely to show signs of cognitive decline than their great-grandparents because they have been better educated, which established more robust networks of connections early on (this is what experts mean by 'cognitive reserve'). A better diet may play a part, too.

diet and acquiring new skills – for example, learning to play chess or bridge, taking up a new language or a dance such as the tango that involves lots of trial and error. All in the Mind, starting on page 174, gives you the latest thinking on the older brain, and all the ways that you can protect and enhance it in later life.

TALKING SENSES

You are likely to have noticed changes in your sight over the years: most of us, for instance, need reading glasses by the age of 60. Your other senses also diminish in later life, but often the changes can be so gradual that people learn to live with them. And that's a shame because there are plenty of ways that you can prevent problems from occurring or compensate for any age-related changes – both by keeping up with essential health checks and by making simple lifestyle changes (*see* Super Senses, pages 206–235).

As you get older, your sensory organs undergo physical changes and you also experience a general increase in your 'sensory threshold'– that is, you tend to need more sensory stimulation before your body perceives a sensation. Here's a sense-by-sense guide to what to expect in the later years:

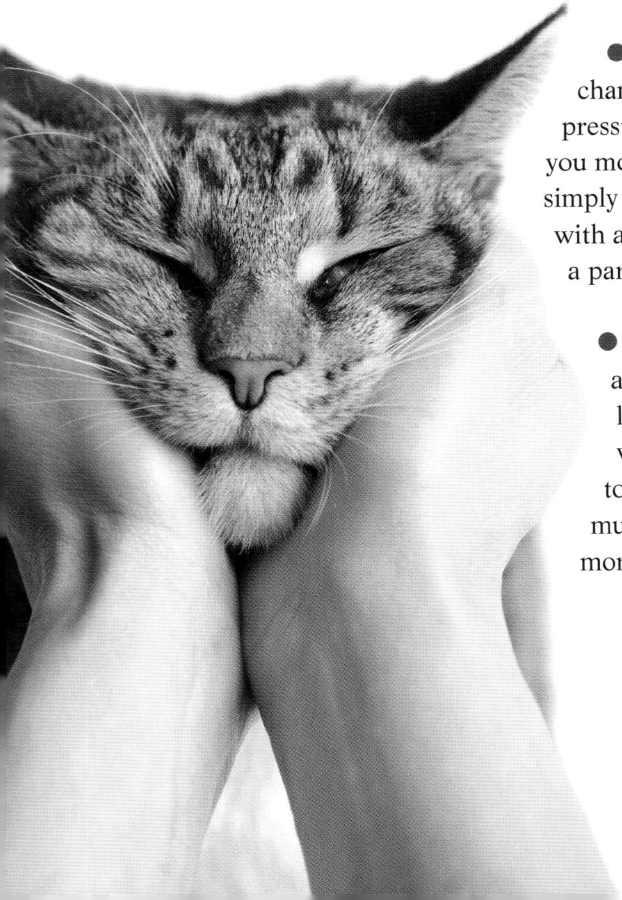

- **TOUCH** You may become less sensitive to – or have a changed perception of – pain, temperature, vibration and pressure. Your skin gets thinner as you age, and this can make you more or less sensitive to touch. Whether these changes are simply down to age or to conditions that become more common with age is still under debate. Poor blood circulation may play a part, as may a deficiency of vitamin B.

- **EYESIGHT** Age-related changes to eyesight (presbyopia) are due to stiffening, thickening and yellowing of the eye lenses. There's also a loss of nerve cells and changes in the way your pupil reacts to light. Most people find it harder to focus on fine print on menus and books, and to see in murky light. Colours appear less bright, and you may be more sensitive to glare, especially when driving at night.

Your sense of touch may become less acute.

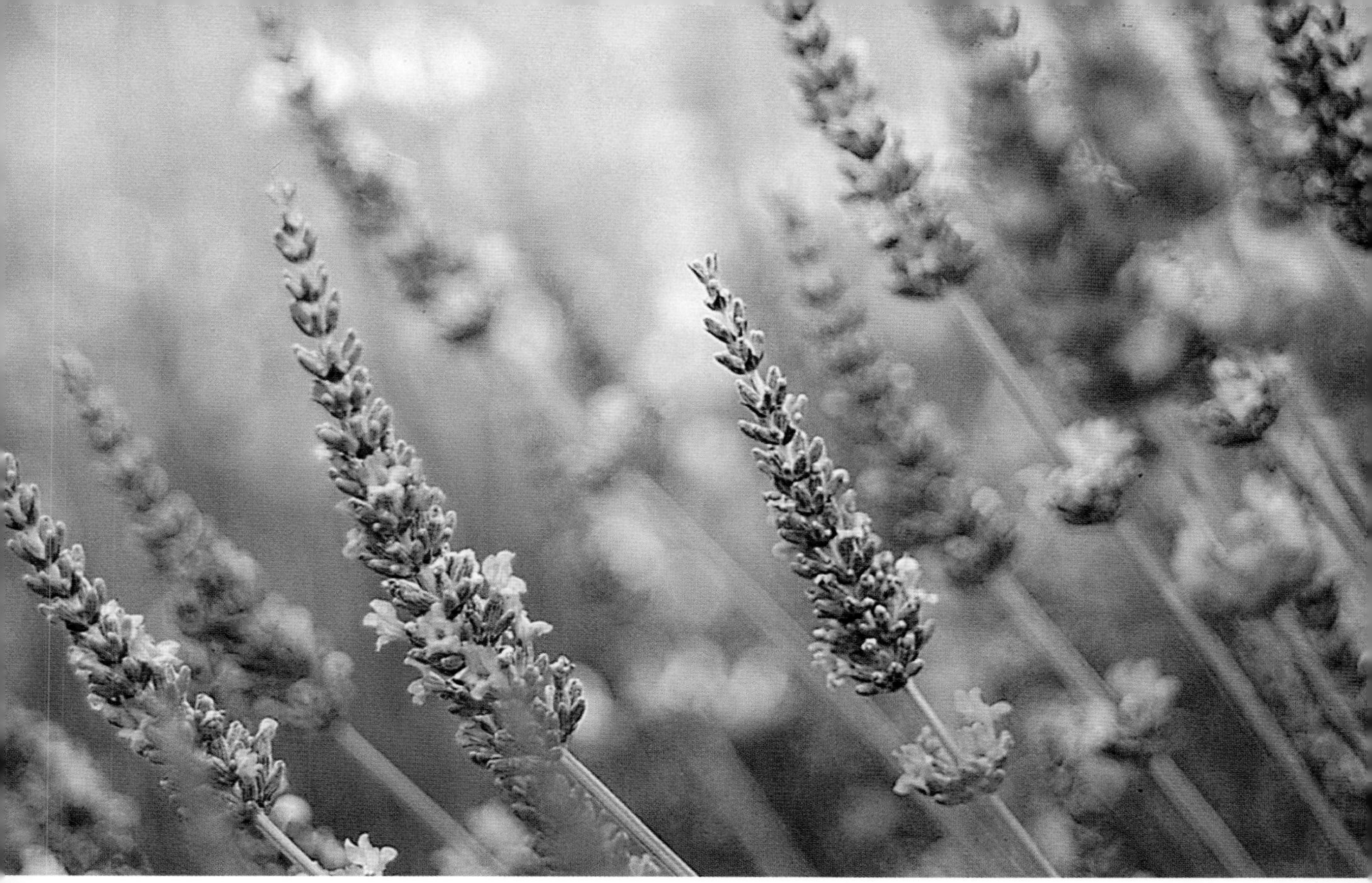

● **HEARING** Age-related hearing loss (presbycusis) is estimated to affect more than a third of adults aged 65 to 75, and up to half of those over 75. It may become harder to understand what people are saying, especially in noisy places. High-pitched sounds are more difficult to decipher and may sometimes be impossible to hear.

● **TASTE** As you get older, your sense of taste gets weaker. This may be partly due to a decline in the number and mass of taste buds, but the biggest cause is a reduced sense of smell.

● **SMELL** Many people find that their sense of smell is less acute after the age of 70. Experts are still debating whether this is due to age, to disease or to controllable lifestyle factors such as smoking.

It may seem that these are things you can't alter, but you can help balance any natural decline by using your senses more consciously. Paying attention to the smells, tastes, sounds, touch sensations and sights you encounter makes you appreciate life's more subtle pleasures. And honing your awareness can, in turn, enhance and refine your senses.

Paying close attention to sights and smells will help to preserve your senses as you age.

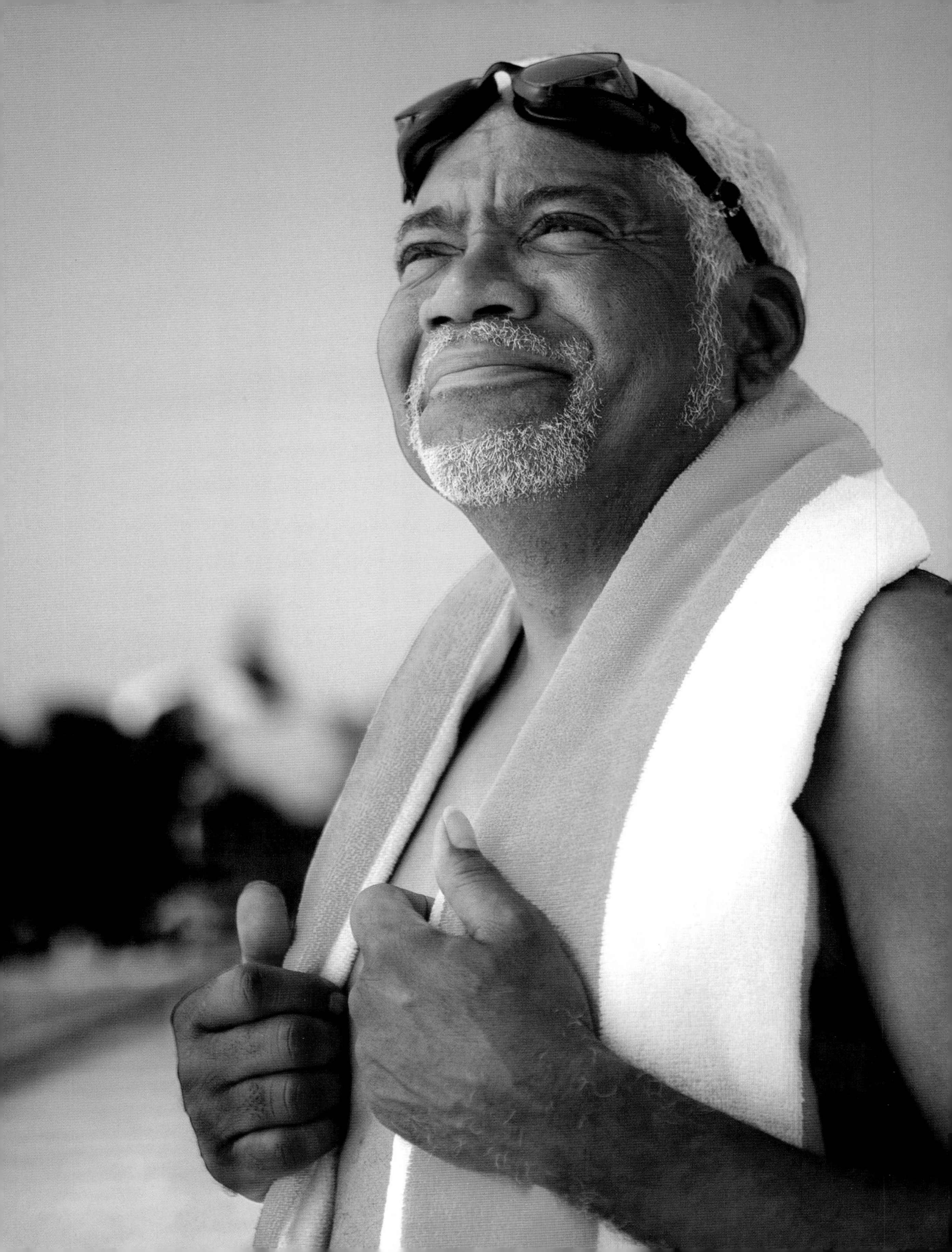

2

Your HEART *matters*

Whether you're fit enough to climb Everest in your 60s or you can barely manage to get up the stairs is very much down to the health of your heart. This astonishing part of the human apparatus is your body's engine or, more specifically, its fuel pump. It has one basic job, which it performs ceaselessly throughout life: to maintain the flow of energy-bearing blood to all of your organs. There is no reason why it should not fulfil this function in a trouble-free way into your seventh, eighth and ninth decade and beyond.

Australian **deaths** from heart attack fell from 21% of all deaths in 2000 to 16% in 2009.

HALE AND HEARTY
your cardiac health

Your heart beats an average of 38 million times a year – mostly without you ever giving it a second thought. But now, as small changes begin to occur, it may be time to start paying a little attention to how this most vital organ works. Your heart matters: take care of it.

Most of today's over-60s have better heart health than any previous generation thanks largely to improved medical care and healthier lifestyles. The improvement has been dramatic – even over the past decade or so. Australian deaths fom heart attacks dropped from 21 per cent of all deaths in 2000 to 16 per cent of all deaths in 2009. Deaths from stroke are also dropping. Your parents' generation may well have lived in fear of heart attacks and strokes as they grew older, but you don't have to. In fact, you can be confident that you can reduce or even eradicate your own risk of serious heart trouble.

YOUR BODY'S DELIVERY SERVICE

Your heart is the dispatcher in your body's own courier service. Located at the hub of your circulatory system, it ensures that essential supplies are delivered to your cells, organs and tissues. It does this by maintaining a constant stream of oxygen-rich, nutrient-bearing blood to your organs. Your blood is a fluid fleet of lorries that carries the vital chemical freight. On the return leg, the blood takes away waste products, transporting them through ever-widening highways of veins, finally reaching the lungs, where carbon dioxide is ejected into the air as you exhale.

The internal engine

Your heart accomplishes its task by keeping the blood constantly on the move. Its mechanism consists of four chambers: the left and right atria (at the top) and the left and right ventricles (below). In the first stage of each heartbeat, your heart wall contracts, propelling blood into your network of arteries and capillaries. From the body's organs and tissues, blood flows through ever-larger veins back to the heart, filling it up as the heart muscle relaxes. The pace at which your heart works is controlled by electrochemical impulses generated within it by so-called pacemaker cells. (The artificial pacemaker that some people with heart troubles have fitted is named after these cells – not the other way round.)

How your heart ages

As you get older, both the heart and circulation undergo several small changes.

- Your heart beats slightly more slowly as your natural pacemaker loses some of its cells.
- The heart muscle itself decreases in size.
- Your main artery becomes thicker and stiffer.
- The volume of blood is slightly reduced as there is less fluid generally in your body.
- Tiny sensors (baroreceptors) that help to keep blood pressure constant when you change position may become less sensitive.

Men experience these changes about a decade earlier than women because the female hormone oestrogen has a protective effect on the heart and arteries. You won't immediately notice a difference when these changes occur, but some symptoms might come to your attention eventually: you may feel dizzy if you stand up from sitting or lying, or your blood pressure may be higher than it used to be. And your heart may be less able to tolerate a sudden increase in workload, for instance, when you go from walking on the flat to climbing uphill.

DID **you** KNOW ?

Flossing your teeth and brushing twice daily is linked to healthier ageing. Why? First, bacteria from the mouth can get into your arteries, causing them to fur up, impeding blood flow. Secondly, your body mounts an immune response to the oral bacteria, causing inflammation, which can lead to narrowed arteries. Gum disease raises your risk of heart disease by 72 per cent and doubles your risk of dying of a heart attack.

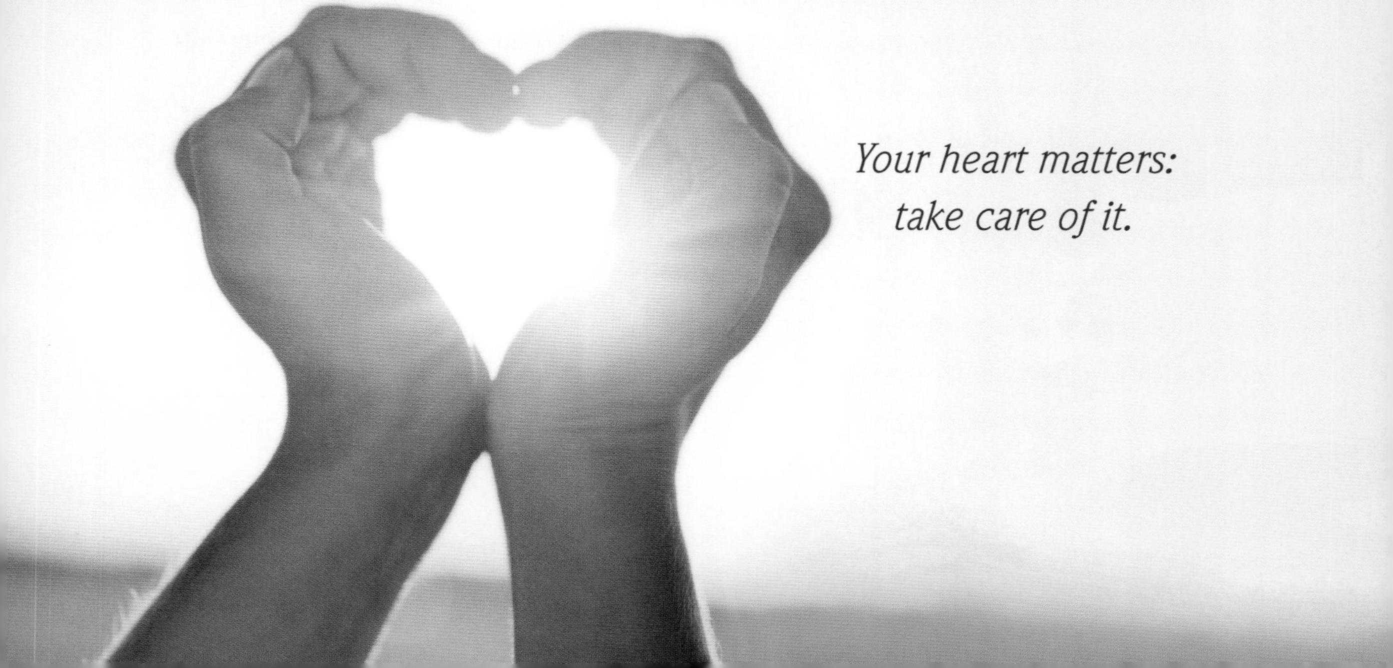

Your heart matters: take care of it.

Get out and walk.
A brisk half-hour walk six days a week will reduce your risk of heart disease by up to 40 per cent.

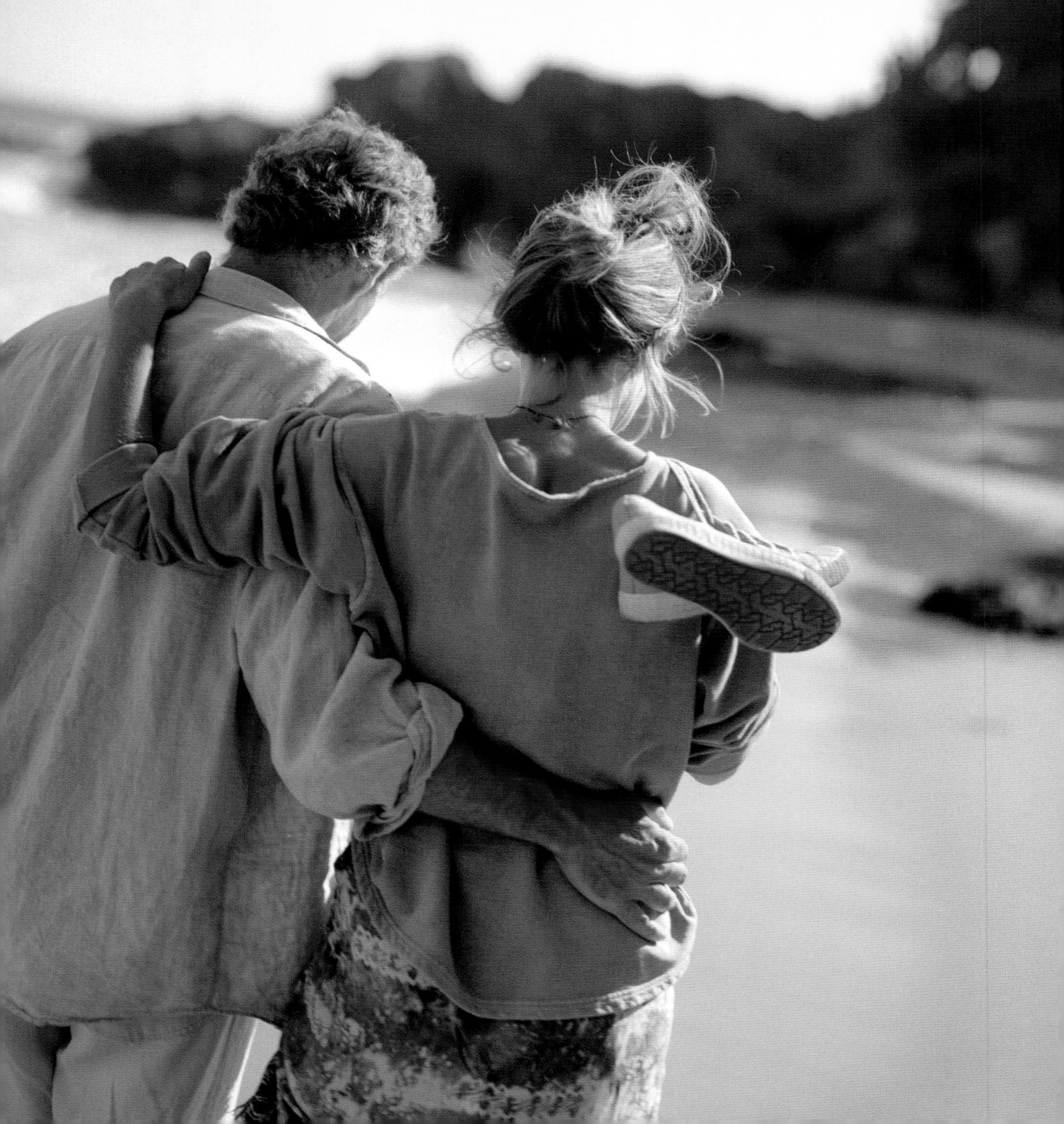

STEPS TO A STRONGER HEART

There's plenty you can do to improve your heart health. First, and most importantly, if you smoke, give up. Why? For starters, it speeds up the hardening and narrowing of your arteries and makes it two to four times more likely that you'll suffer a blood clot than someone who doesn't smoke. Back in 1990, the US Surgeon General published evidence showing that smokers who quit in their 60s experience a better quality of life as well as having a longer life expectancy compared with those who carried on. Since then, scientists have documented specific heart-related benefits. Within just 20 minutes of your last cigarette, your blood pressure and pulse rate decrease. After a year the risk of coronary artery disease is halved, with the risk of a stroke falling to the same as a non-smoker within ten years, whatever your age when you quit.

Action stations

Then take a positive step – literally. Get out and walk. A brisk half-hour constitutional six days a week will reduce your risk of heart disease by up to 40 per cent, according to a major study in which the health and physical activity routines of 72,000 women aged 40 to 65 were monitored over eight years. The study showed the heart health benefits of starting regular exercise even in late middle age. Other studies have found that men benefit in much the same way. And exercise, of course, is the only way to get rid of that stubborn abdominal fat, which tends to accumulate around the waist as we get older. This central fat – the 'apple shape' – is now widely seen as a leading cause of raised blood pressure and cholesterol as well as hardening of the arteries.

Raise a toast to your heart. Enjoy a small glass of wine with dinner.

And you'll certainly stack the odds in your favour if you follow healthy diet guidelines, especially those based on solid evidence. The advice to eat oily fish, for example, isn't new, but Californian researchers have discovered how doing so prevents heart disease. By following 608 people with heart disease for five years, they found that food rich in omega-3 fatty acids slows down the shortening of stretches of DNA, known as telomeres, whose length correlates with heart health and longevity. Another study, by the British Heart Foundation, has shown that the more

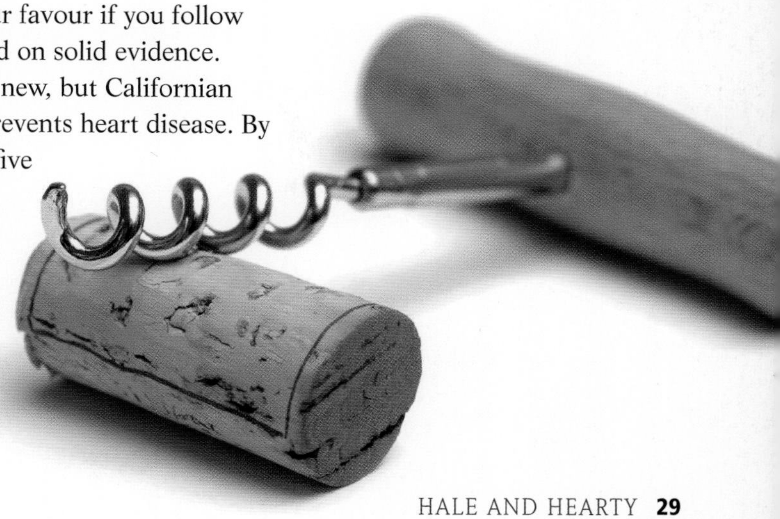

'You don't stop laughing because you grow old. You grow old because you stop laughing.'

Michael Pritchard, US humorist

fruit and vegetables people eat every day, the lower their risk of heart disease. Here are some small – and unashamedly pleasurable – things you can do for the good of your heart:

- **Raise a glass** Enjoy a 125 ml glass of wine with dinner. It will cut your risk of heart disease by 50 per cent, according to Spanish researchers who followed 41,000 people aged up to 69 for ten years.
- **Get intimate** Have sex regularly. Scientists from New England in the US found that men aged 40 to 70 who have sex at least twice a week are 45 per cent less likely to have a heart attack – and that's above and beyond the protection your heart gains from the extra exercise. (Whether the same is true for women has not yet been investigated.)
- **Learn to meditate** You don't have to be religious to give it a go. It's just a way of introducing some stillness into your day. This alone helps you to manage stress levels, and so reduces your risk of coronary artery disease. Doctors aren't certain why stress contributes to heart disease, but there's evidence that if meditation (or yoga) relaxes you, then it could also help reduce your blood pressure.
- **Take time to laugh** Countless studies have shown that laughter is good for your health. In 2010, researchers at the University of Maryland Medical Center studied the reactions of 300 people, half of whom had heart disease, to situations designed to provoke laughter or negative emotions such as anger. They found that the people with heart disease laughed 40 per cent less than the control group, and also exhibited more negative emotions.

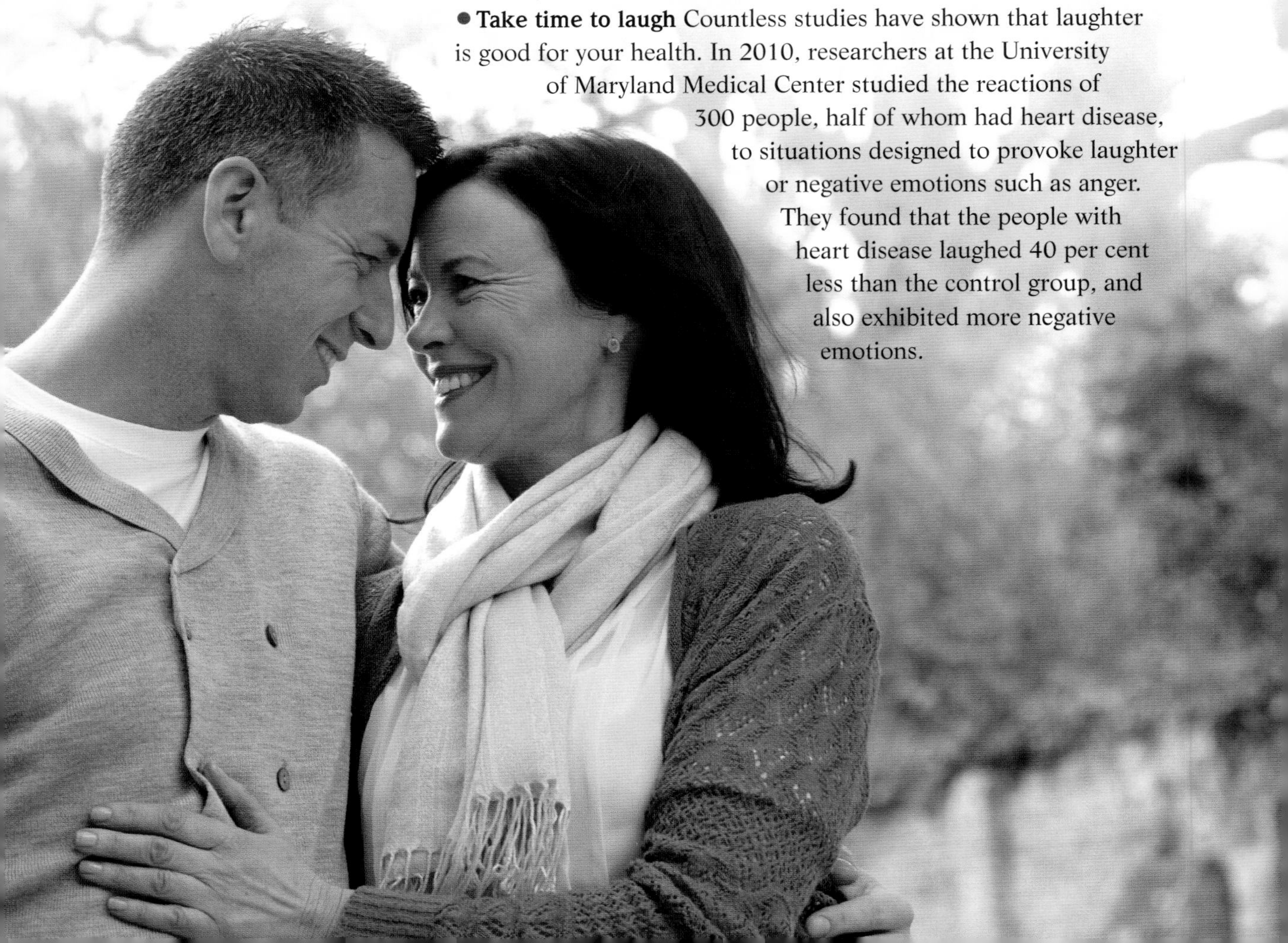

take CARE! Can YOU make a DIFFERENCE?

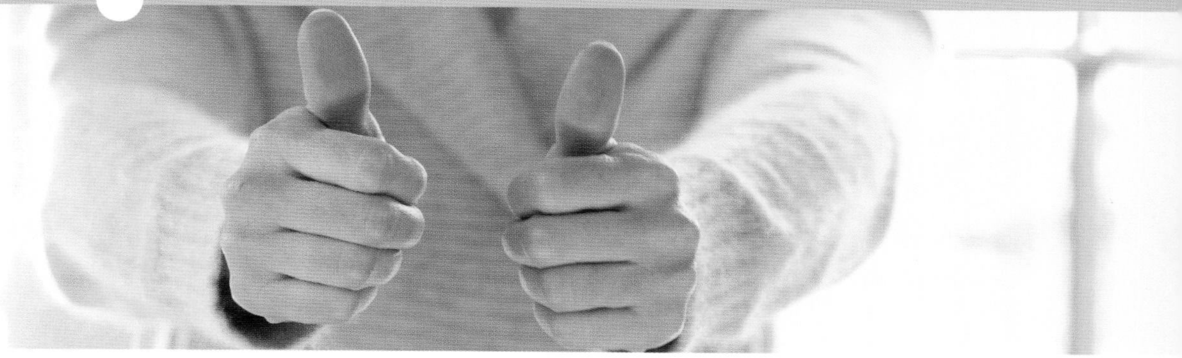

It's true that over-60s are more at risk of heart disease than younger people – but that doesn't mean it's inevitable. The answer to whether you can buck the trend is mostly yes, and that's backed up by a major worldwide research project called the INTERHEART study (*see* page 34). Read on to find out if a healthy lifestyle can reduce your specific risk.

1 One of your parents had an early heart attack. You know that this increases the risk.
YES It's true that a family history of early heart attacks doubles the risk for men, and increases the risk for women by 70 per cent. But you can cut this significantly by tackling other factors such as smoking and high blood pressure. Research published in 2011 by McGill University, Canada, suggests that eating more than five portions of raw fruit and vegetables can lower heart disease risk in people who are genetically predisposed to it by a specific gene – chromosome 9p21. Those who ate high proportions of raw vegetables, fruit and berries had a similar heart attack risk as those without the gene.

2 You know that you should get more exercise, but you're not the sporty sort.
YES Statistics show that even gentle regular exercise can have a dramatic impact on your cholesterol, blood pressure and blood vessel function – as well as on other heart risks such as your weight and stress levels. And it doesn't have to be sport: walk to the shops rather than drive, use the stairs not the lift – it's a start.

3 You have type 2 diabetes and high blood pressure, which increase your heart-disease risk.
YES Eating sensibly, taking regular exercise, and taking your medication regularly can dramatically reduce your risk, so don't delay. Being obese, for example, makes you 80 times more likely to develop diabetes than someone with a healthy weight.

4 You've been through the menopause, which raises the risk of heart disease for women.
MAYBE Women lose the heart-protective effect of oestrogen after the menopause, but the jury's still out over whether taking extra oestrogen in the form of HRT extends that protection, or increases the risk. Having a healthy lifestyle will certainly cut your risk.

5 You have erectile dysfunction and this could be linked to heart disease.
YES A 2010 report found that men aged 40 to 60 with erection problems had a 30 per cent higher risk of dying of a heart attack within three to five years. Do report any such difficulties to your doctor. Not only are there treatments to save your love life, but your doctor can check your risk of heart disease, and help you reduce it.

Quiz How **heart-healthy** are you?

Answering these questions could be your first step to a healthier heart. There are no right answers – but only honest ones count. Pick the answer that's nearest to your own experience.

1 How much do you smoke?

- I have never smoked.
- I smoke 20 a day or more, and I've given up giving up.
- I used to smoke but quit more than a year ago (1 bonus point if it was more than ten years ago).
- I've tried to give up but still smoke occasionally.

2 How would you describe your stress levels?

- I tend to get a bit anxious, but can usually talk things through with friends or family.
- I've learned I can't control everything so now I take things as they come.
- I often get stressed and angry.
- I'm constantly under pressure – there's nothing I can do about it.

3 Do you know your cholesterol levels?

- I have no interest in my cholesterol (or know it's high but tend to ignore it).
- I've had my cholesterol checked. It was reasonably good, but could be better.
- Yes. I know that my total cholesterol is considered good.
- Getting my cholesterol tested is on my to-do list.

4 How well do you sleep?

- I don't sleep too well, so have a lie-in to catch up when I can.
- My sleep pattern varies, but I usually feel that I get enough.
- I sleep soundly each night and wake up feeling refreshed.
- I find it hard to drop off and often wake up in the night, which can make me feel rotten the next day.

5 How much saturated fat do you eat?

- I eat low-fat dairy products and plenty of fresh tuna, salmon, nuts and olive oil – but avoid pastries and animal fats.
- I often eat meat and cheese, but try not to have them every day.
- I enjoy food too much to worry about eating the right kind of fat.
- I eat a little cheese, use olive oil, have meat once/twice a week and salmon at least once a week.

6 How often do you have fun?

- It's hard, but I make time to have fun at least once a week.
- I do something that I enjoy every day.
- I don't have much time to enjoy myself, but I know I should.
- I can't remember the last time I really enjoyed myself.

7 Do you know your own blood pressure measurement?

- Yes, it's in the normal range.
- Yes – it's quite high, but I'm taking advice on how to tackle it.
- I have high blood pressure and have been prescribed pills, but I don't usually take them.
- No, I know I should have it tested but it's not a priority.

8 Is your waist more than 80 cm (women) or 94 cm (men)?

- Yes, quite at lot more, but I plan to join a gym.
- Yes. I can't get into a lot of my old clothes, but I'm not going to start dieting at my age.
- No – and I keep an eye on it.
- Yes, a little more, but I'm already taking steps to get it down.

9 Is your diet rich in fruit and vegetables?

- I try to get seven portions most days, but don't always manage it.
- I eat some fresh fruit and vegetables, but not every day.
- Yes, I love fruit and veg and eat at least seven portions a day.
- No, I don't eat much and never have. I'm not sure it would make much difference to my health now.

10 How much alcohol do you drink?

- I have one or two small glasses of wine/beer in the evening (up to three for men), but not every day of the week.
- I sometimes have more than I should, but not very often (or I don't drink at all).
- I don't drink every day, but I make up for it at weekends.
- I usually drink more than half a bottle of wine (or its equivalent) every day.

11 Do you have diabetes?

- Yes, but I'm not good at controlling it and sometimes forget to take my medicine.
- I'm not overweight, but I've never been checked so I don't know.
- No, and I have no symptoms.
- I have high blood pressure, am a bit overweight and often get very thirsty, so I'm planning to see my doctor for a diabetes check.

12 How active are you?

- I manage a gentle half-hour walk a few times a week, and I'm fairly active at home or in the garden.
- I exercise sporadically. I can go weeks without much activity.
- At my age, I prefer to take things easy and watch TV.
- I exercise at least five times a week for up to an hour. It's a big part of my life.

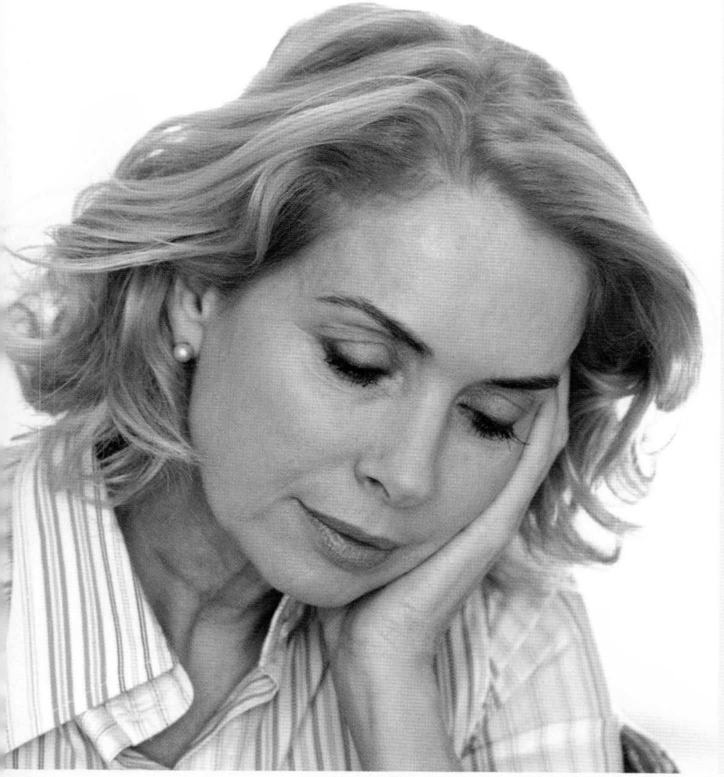

SCORE

Score 0 points for each **red** answer you pick, 1 for each **blue**, 2 for each **green** and 3 points for each **yellow** answer. Add up your total score then read on to find out how well you did.

Over 26: You're doing fine. Keep up the good work for a healthy heart.

17–25: You're doing your best to follow a heart-friendly lifestyle. It's worth putting the extra effort into an even healthier diet and exercise regime.

8–16: As you have some risk factors for heart disease, you need to get your blood pressure and cholesterol checked. Start now by making a doctor's appointment, plan to build exercise into your schedule, and swap fatty and sugary foods for healthy snacks.

7 or less: You're ignoring so many effective and trouble-free ways to maintain heart health. Talk to your doctor about stopping smoking if you need to, and get your blood pressure and cholesterol checked.

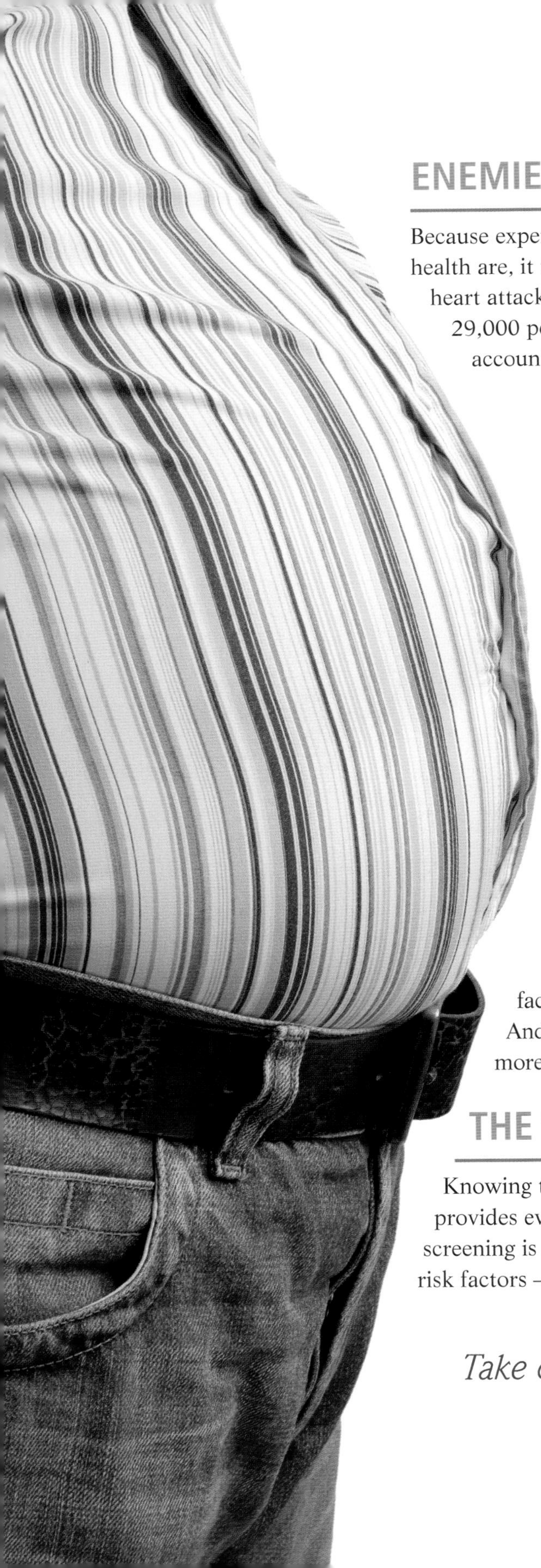

ENEMIES OF THE HEART

Because experts now know exactly what the main risks to heart health are, it is easier than ever to reduce or even avoid the risks of heart attacks and strokes. The 2004 INTERHEART study assessed 29,000 people in 52 countries, and found that just nine factors account for 90 per cent of heart attacks in every ethnic group.

SIX FOES:

- **High cholesterol**
- **High blood pressure**
- **Diabetes**
- **Stress**
- **Obesity**
- **Smoking**

THREE FRIENDS:

Three lifestyle factors help protect your heart (ignoring them has a negative impact):

- **Eating plenty of fruit and vegetables**
- **Taking enough exercise**
- **Moderate alcohol consumption**

What makes the research so exciting is that every factor is lifestyle-related and so mostly within your control. And it's easier to take action later in life, when you have more time and flexibility.

THE WAY FORWARD

Knowing that age is not an inevitable trigger for heart disease provides every incentive for dealing with problems early on. And screening is an essential part of your health toolkit. Two of the key risk factors – high blood pressure and high cholesterol – have been

Take control of your lifestyle and reduce the risk of heart attacks and strokes.

Two key risk factors in heart disease – high blood pressure and high cholesterol – have been dubbed the 'silent killers'.

dubbed the 'silent killers' because they have few, if any, symptoms. One in four older people have undiagnosed high blood pressure, and more than half have undiagnosed high cholesterol.

Regular check-ups are the only way to spot these health issues, and they also offer a chance for your doctor to uncover potentially dangerous conditions such as diabetes early on. A significant development in screening has been the computerised 'cardiovascular risk' calculation. First used in the UK but now widely available, this enables doctors to predict your risk of having a heart attack or stroke within the next ten years by asking just a few simple questions. With these results to hand, they can work with you to tailor a treatment program that encompasses not only lifestyle changes but medication (*see* pages 42–43), too.

With your heart, as with other aspects of your health, there are some risk factors that are out of your control. These include your age, your gender and your family background (that is to say, your genes). But there are plenty of steps you can take to moderate the effect of any factors you were born with: a clutch of potential issues does not mean that you are doomed to have heart trouble. As any card-player will tell you, it's not always the best hand that comes out on top.

LOVE HELPS

You may have some unexpected allies working in your favour. In 2010, researchers at Harvard University found that a satisfying marriage reduces women's risk of cardiovascular disease, while a major study involving over 127,000 American adults concluded that married men are healthier and tend to live longer than those who remained unmarried or who were divorced or widowed. And a decade-long American study published in 2011 of more than 135,000 married or formerly married men aged between 50 and 71 suggests that having children reduces a man's risk of dying from cardiovascular disease by 17 per cent.

In other words, a heart that loves is more likely to be healthy than a heart that doesn't. And isn't that just as it should be?

DID **YOU** KNOW?

More than two-thirds of people over 65 have a low or sedentary level of exercise, and women are the worst culprits, according to the Australian Bureau of Statistics. Yet regular exercise makes a real difference. One American study monitored the exercise patterns and heart health of 12,500 men aged 39 to 88 over the course of 16 years, and found that those who walked farther and climbed up the most flights of stairs were least likely to suffer heart attacks or angina.

EAT TO THE BEAT
food for a healthy heart

Research now makes it clear that some foods are key to heart health in later life. Luckily, those that are best for your cardiac wellbeing happen to be varied and delicious: the colourful cuisine of the Mediterranean.

The Mediterranean diet has long been seen as good for the heart – but researchers had no concrete proof. True, Mediterranean populations from Greece to Portugal had a low risk of heart disease and strokes, but no one could say for sure whether it was the way they eat that made the difference, or whether other factors such as genetics or perhaps the extra sunshine were involved.

Now, however, scientists have authoritative evidence that the best way to maintain heart health in later life is to stick to a Mediterranean diet. The HALE project followed 2300 men and women, aged 70 to 90, from 11 European countries for 12 years and found that those who combined a Mediterranean diet with a healthy lifestyle had more than a 50 per cent lower mortality rate from heart attack and stroke than those who did not.

DID **you** KNOW?

A Cambridge University study found that people who eat one square of dark chocolate a day are less likely to suffer heart disease and strokes. It may be the anti-oxidant flavonoids in cocoa beans that make chocolate heart-friendly. Or people may simply find eating it relaxing, and anything that relaxes the heart is good for it. In other words, a (very) little of what you fancy does you good.

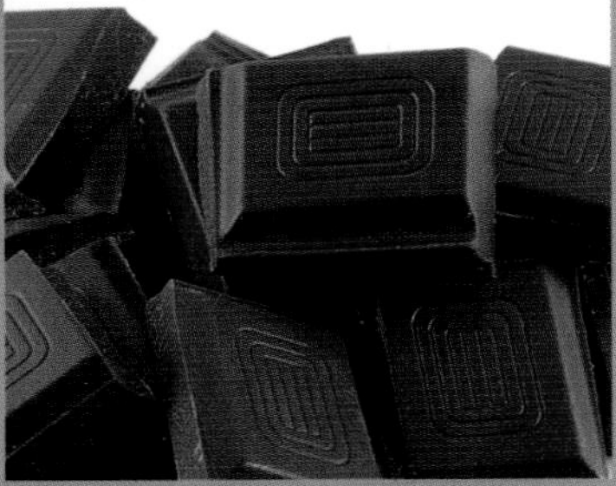

GIVE YOUR HEART A HOLIDAY

The beauty of this healthy diet is that it contains exactly the kind of foods that we fall in love with when holidaying in southern Europe. Meals are rich in monounsaturated fat (olive oil, avocados, nuts), fruit and vegetables, whole grains – all combined with fish, chicken and a moderate intake of alcohol. The wholesome nature of the diet is also a matter of what it leaves out, or uses much more sparingly than in a typical Western diet red meat, refined grains and sugar. And while the Mediterranean diet does aid weight loss, this is not what boosts heart health. A series of studies has shown that the Mediterranean diet is far more effective in reducing bad (LDL) cholesterol (*see* page 42) than simply sticking to a low-fat diet. And it's the best of all food regimes for reducing blood pressure.

9 steps to a **HEART-FRIENDLY DIET**

So, eat like the Greeks and Italians: grilled fish, roasted vegetables, a small glass of wine. Here are some other ways to ensure that what you eat benefits your heart.

1 MAKE SEVEN-A-DAY YOUR MINIMUM Two serves of fruit and five of vegetables, that is. Eat vegetables with a little fat, such as olive oil or oily fish, to help the body absorb fat-soluble vitamins.

2 GO FOR GOOD FATS Aim to get up to 30 per cent of your kilojoules from fat, most of which should come from unsaturated fats – found, for example, in olive oil, oily fish, avocado, and nuts and seeds – which don't raise cholesterol levels.

3 MAKE TIME FOR BREAKFAST A study of 3000 people by Harvard researchers in 2008 found that simply having a good breakfast every day – including whole grains, fruit or healthy protein – cuts the risk of heart attack.

4 CUT DOWN ON SALT Choose low-salt alternatives to the food and drink you normally buy, and avoid processed foods.

5 CUT BACK ON SATURATED FAT, which is highest in full-fat dairy products, fatty meat and ghee (clarified butter used in South Asian cuisine).

6 READ FOOD LABELS Check ingredients when you go shopping to avoid saturated fat in processed food, cakes, biscuits and pastries.

7 GO FOR WHOLE GRAINS Increase your intake of high-fibre whole grains to six serves daily to cut your heart attack risk by 25 per cent.

8 ENJOY CHOLESTEROL-RICH FOODS Eggs, shellfish and offal form part of a balanced diet. They are nutritious and make little difference to your blood cholesterol levels.

9 GET YOUR FIBRE Make sure you're eating plenty of foods high in soluble fibre – they help to reduce LDL cholesterol. Good sources are oats, beans, pulses, lentils, nuts, fruit and vegetables.

Make time for breakfast every day – it may cut the risk of a heart attack.

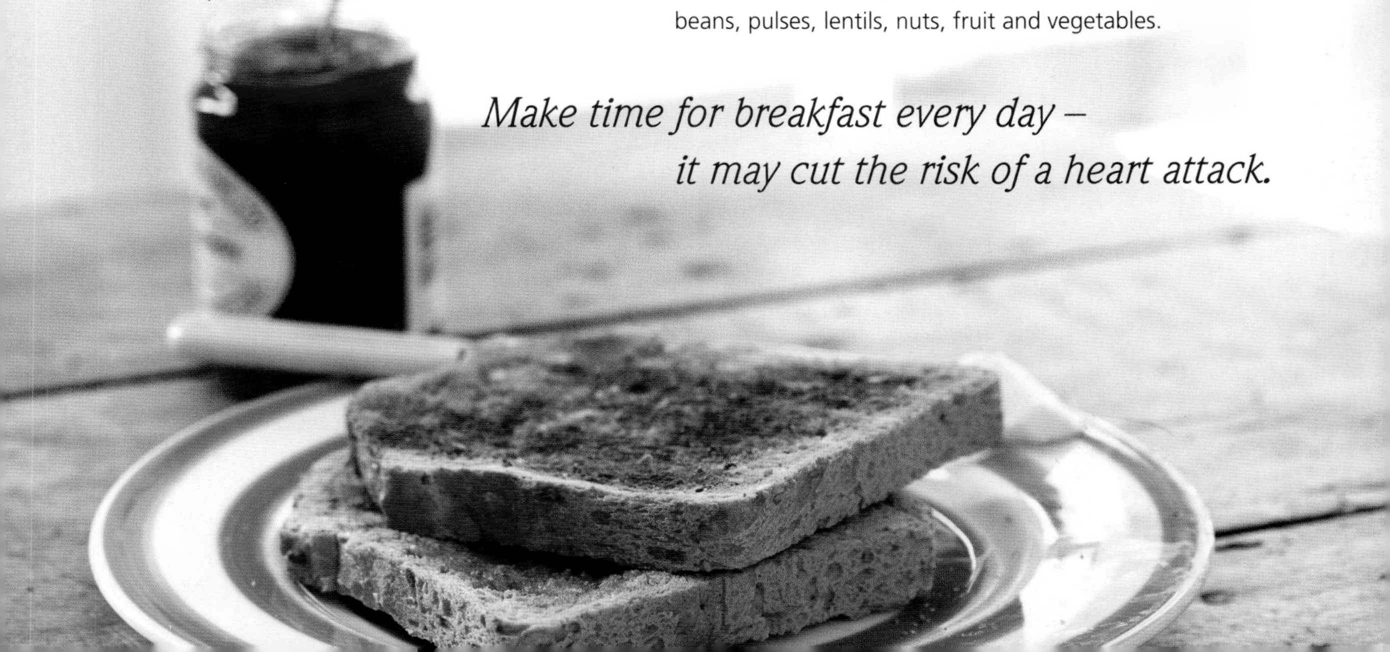

Every kilo of excess weight you lose will reduce your blood pressure.

GO WITH THE FLOW
a good circulation

Your heart, like all pumps, works by generating pressure. It becomes slightly less efficient as your body ages, and may begin to fail – especially if you're inactive or overweight. But regular check-ups can help prevent serious problems.

The changes that occur naturally in your heart as you grow older have a knock-on effect on your blood pressure. Scientists at Johns Hopkins University in the USA carried out MRI (magnetic resonance imaging) scans on 5000 men and women aged 45 to 85. Their experiments demonstrated that the heart muscles take about 2 per cent longer to squeeze and relax every year from the age of 60. Not only that, the amount of blood that's pumped out of the heart falls by about 9 ml, or 2 teaspoonfuls, every year. This is, of course, a tiny fraction of the 5 or more litres that usually circulate in the body.

UNDERSTANDING BLOOD PRESSURE

Your blood pressure (BP) is a measure of how strongly the force of your blood pushes against the walls of your arteries as your heart pumps it around your body. It is a key indicator of health. Too little pressure (low BP) causes feelings of faintness and fatigue and is often a side effect of medication or dehydration.

Of far greater risk to your health, however, is too much pressure – high blood pressure or hypertension. If your BP rises and stays high over time, it can damage your heart and blood vessels as well as your kidneys and other parts of your body. Because high BP usually has no symptoms, it can, if undiagnosed, slowly inflict continuing damage, raising the risk of heart disease and stroke over several years – during which time you may actually be feeling fine.

The risk factors connected with high BP are the same as those linked to the heart in general. Some, such as your age and gender, are unalterable; the lifestyle aspects you can do something about. But a really key thing to know is that high blood pressure is

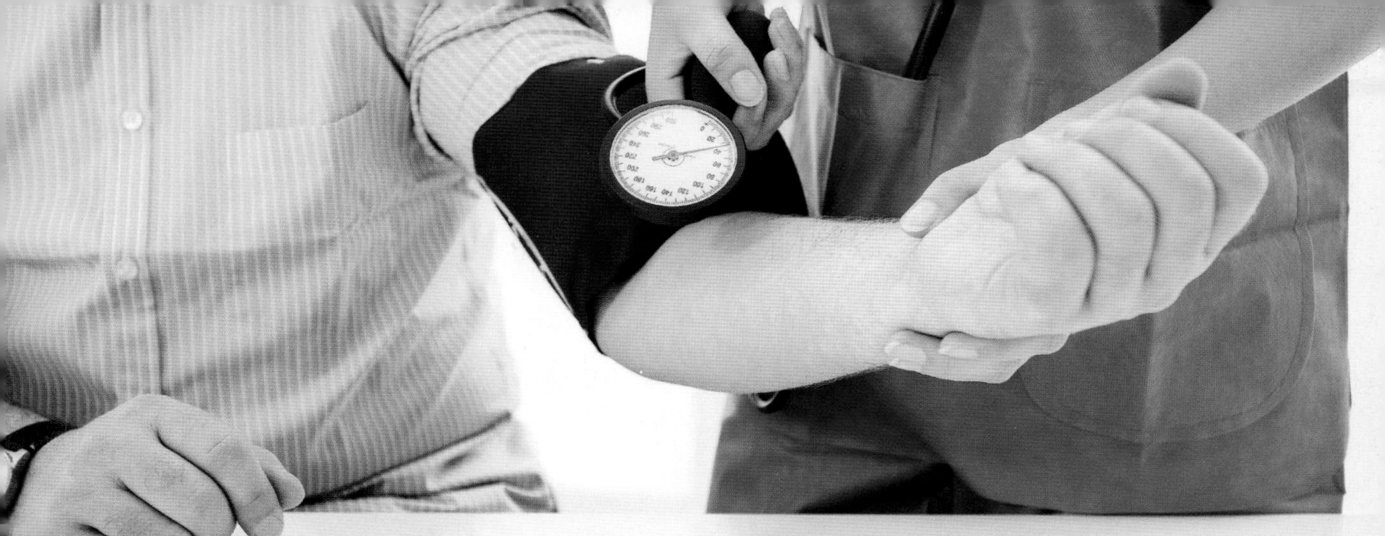

Large numbers of over-60s don't even know they're suffering from this silent and symptomless disorder.

particularly dangerous in combination with a group of other risk factors – especially a large waist size (that apple shape again), glucose intolerance and raised cholesterol. Together this group of health risks, called metabolic syndrome, is known to be responsible for raising the risk of heart disease. Your doctor can effectively treat some of the problems using medication – but some key things you can do are:

- **Lose weight** You should aim to lose between 7 and 10 per cent of your body weight to start with (get your doctor's advice).
- **Cut out sugary fizzy drinks** A US study of 5000 adults found that those who drank at least one soft fizzy drink a day were 44 per cent more likely to develop metabolic syndrome than those who didn't.
- **Get active** Start exercising, slowly at first, building up to regular, moderately vigorous activity for 30 minutes most days of the week.

GETTING TESTED

Millions of people, including large numbers over 60, don't even know they're suffering from dangerously high blood pressure. Because it is – initially – such a silent and symptomless disorder, many never think about having a check-up. Yet there's much that can be done to reduce blood pressure and thereby prevent future heart disease. So having your BP tested regularly is a basic precautionary measure. Have a check-up every two years, or more often if your GP calculates you have an increased risk of heart disease.

Cut out fizzy drinks.

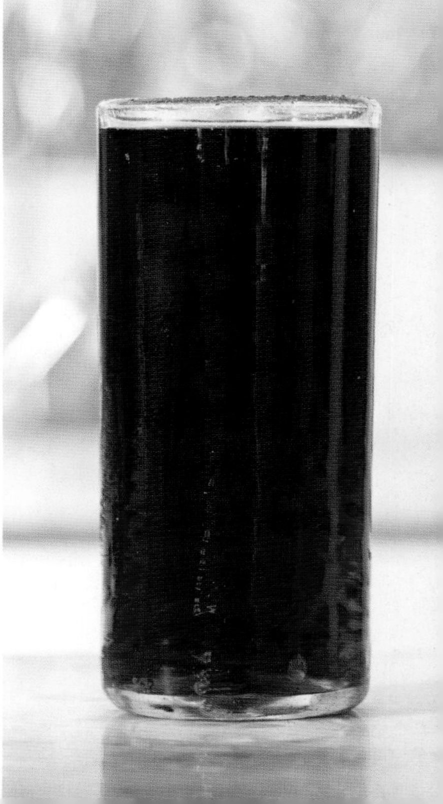

5 steps to reducing HIGH BLOOD PRESSURE

There are plenty of actions you can take to lower high blood pressure.

1 SLIM DOWN Weight gain pushes up your BP – and the reverse is also true. Losing 10 kg can bring about a 20 mmHg or so reduction in your systolic blood pressure (the pressure when your heart beats to pump blood out, *see* page 42). This will increase the efficacy of any medication you're taking.

2 ENJOY HEART-FRIENDLY DRINKS Caffeine causes a surge in blood pressure that is long-lasting in people who are caffeine-sensitive. If you have a home BP monitoring kit (*see* opposite), you can find out if you are susceptible: measure your BP within 30 minutes of drinking a cup of coffee or other caffeine-rich drink. If it goes up significantly, you should avoid coffee in future. As for alcohol, small amounts can potentially lower your BP by 2 to 4 mmHg. That protective effect is lost if you drink too much, though.

3 AVOID SMOKE The nicotine in tobacco products raises your blood pressure by 10 mmHg or more for up to an hour after you smoke – and the same seems to be true if you inhale secondhand smoke. If that happens frequently, your BP may remain constantly high, so make your home smoke-free.

4 EXERCISE EVERY DAY Regular exercise – aim for 30 minutes most days – is good for you, whether you have high blood pressure or not. But here is one more reason to do it: daily physical activity can reduce your systolic BP by up to 9 mmHg. If you have a condition known as pre-hypertension (up to 139/89 mmHg), exercise will help you avoid developing full-blown high blood pressure.

5 CUT DOWN ON SALT Even a small reduction in your salt intake – adults should eat no more than 6 g a day – can reduce your systolic blood pressure by up to 8 mmHg. To cut down, read food labels and choose low-salt alternatives to the food and drinks you normally buy (those with 0.3 g or less of salt per 100 g), and avoid processed foods.

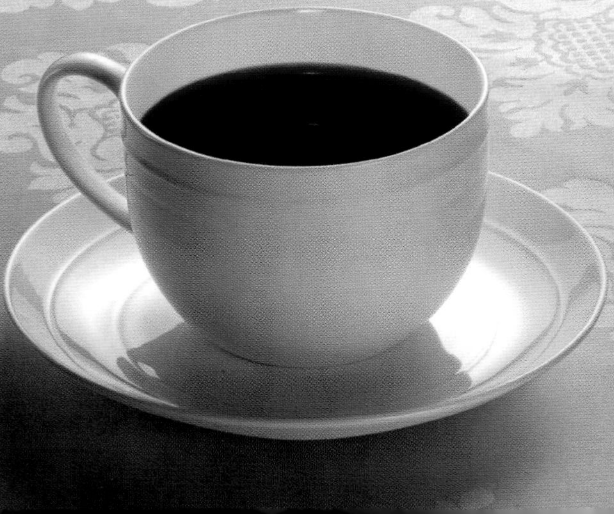

Check to see if you're caffeine-sensitive – caffeine can cause a surge in blood pressure that is long-lasting.

Your blood pressure naturally rises and falls throughout the day. Physical exertion causes it to rise, and so can stressful events – such as a visit to the doctor. One in four people diagnosed with high BP may simply be experiencing a temporary rise caused by the prospect of being medically examined, a phenomenon known as 'white-coat hypertension'. Doctors are very aware of it, and increasingly recommend extra checks outside the surgery to ensure the results are not distorted by waiting-room nerves. There are various ways to check your blood pressure, as follows:

Avoid processed foods if you need to reduce your salt intake.

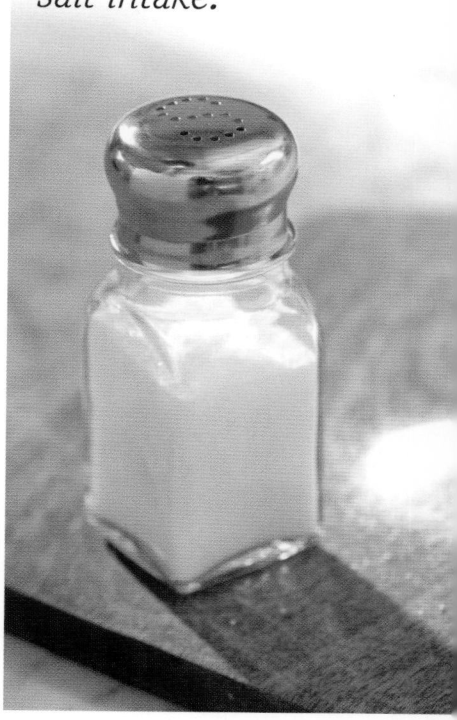

CHECK 1 **AT THE CLINIC**

The doctor or nurse will put a cuff-like monitoring device on your upper arm. If the measurement shows that your blood pressure is 140/90 mmHg or above, your doctor or nurse should measure it twice more in the clinic, at intervals of a few minutes. (*See* page 42 for an explanation of what these figures mean.) If the lowest of these is 140/90 mmHg or above, you may be offered ambulatory blood pressure monitoring.

CHECK 2 **AMBULATORY BLOOD PRESSURE MONITORING**

This monitor, available from your doctor's surgery, also takes the form of a cuff, worn for 24 hours. It measures your blood pressure twice an hour during normal waking hours. Your final BP reading is based on an average of at least 14 of these measurements.

CHECK 3 **HOME BLOOD PRESSURE MONITORING**

If ambulatory blood pressure is too uncomfortable or inconvenient for you, your doctor may recommend a home blood pressure monitoring device, hired or purchased from a chemist or online. Automatic monitors are best, and it's important to ensure you have the right size of cuff: they are sold in three different sizes – standard, large or extra large – based on the girth of the middle area of your upper arm. You should use the device twice a day, once in the morning and once in the evening while you are sitting down. Interestingly, researchers in Finland found that when 2000 men and women aged up to 74 years old tested their own BP at home, the readings were much more accurate than those taken in the doctor's surgery. The research suggested that people who use home monitors are able to maintain healthier BP levels and also feel more in control of their health.

focus ON ... Your BLOOD PRESSURE and CHOLESTEROL results

Two sets of numbers can tell you how healthy your heart is, and reflect the effect your lifestyle is having on your body. Knowing your numbers (and what they mean) is an important way of taking charge of your health – and may nudge you into making some heart-friendly changes to your routine. These measurements are also essential information for your doctor in assessing your medication needs.

UNDER PRESSURE Your blood pressure (BP) number is made up of two measurements: systolic blood pressure, which is taken when your heart is beating and pumping blood; and diastolic blood pressure, taken when your heart is filling up with blood between beats. Both are measured in millimetres of mercury, which is written as mmHg. The result is recorded as systolic BP over diastolic BP – for example, 120/80.

For people over 50, the systolic pressure (in other words, the top number in a BP reading) gives the most accurate diagnosis of high BP. Systolic blood pressure increases with age, while diastolic BP (the bottom number) increases until the age of 55 or so, after which it starts to decline. You're at risk if your systolic blood pressure is 140 mmHg or above, and the risk of heart disease and stroke increases with each 2 mmHg rise.

WHAT'S YOUR CHOLESTEROL? Your cholesterol number is made up of a total cholesterol measurement and numbers for:

- **Low-density lipoprotein (LDL)** This is the molecule that carries cholesterol from your liver to other cells in the body. It's dubbed 'bad' cholesterol: too much causes a harmful build-up in the arteries.
- **High-density lipoprotein (HDL)** is 'good' cholesterol. It carries excess cholesterol out of your blood to your liver, where it's broken down.
- **Triglycerides** are produced by your liver, and found in dairy products, meat and cooking oils.

For most people, healthy levels are regarded as a total cholesterol of 5.5 mmol/L or less, along with an LDL cholesterol of 3.5 mmol/L or less. However, if your doctor assesses that you are at risk of cardiovascular disease, these levels may be lowered to 4 and 2 mmol/L respectively.

TAKING THE MEDICINE

It can feel unfair, but your blood pressure reading may remain high even though you're doing all the right things, such as eating healthily and getting plenty of exercise. If this is the case, you will probably need medication. Blood pressure medicines today are highly effective, but do watch out for any unwanted symptoms and report them to your doctor. You may suffer adverse effects if there's an interaction between the different medicines you're taking, for instance. If so, your doctor should be able to identify the problem and eradicate or reduce any side effects by swapping brands or doses of one or more of your prescriptions.

Once you've discovered the right medication, you may need to continue with it for the rest of your life – though your doctor will want to see you at regular intervals to check your prescription is still right for you. Controlling high blood pressure is not always straightforward; you may have to take more than one medication.

A typical medication regimen

You begin with one agent. You and your doctor will pick the medication that suits you best from the following choices:

- **An ACE inhibitor** This blocks your body's ability to produce the chemical known as angiotensin II, which can cause the blood vessels to narrow and blood pressure to rise if it gets into the bloodstream.
- **A calcium channel blocker** This lowers blood pressure by blocking the effects of calcium on the blood vessels, thereby helping the blood vessel walls to relax and widen, making it easier for blood to flow through.
- **A thiazide or thiazide-like diuretic (a 'water tablet')** This reduces high blood pressure by flushing out salt and unwanted fluid in the urine.

You start with a low dose. If this doesn't do the trick, the next step is to add a second medication. If necessary, a third medication can be added. After that, doses can be increased.

The right prescription is only the first step – you have to take the pills. That might sound obvious, but a 2011 study by pharmaceutical company Daiichi Sankyo UK found that a fifth of older people fail to take prescribed medications for high blood pressure within a year (that's better than younger people, though, more than half of whom give up). One in ten say that the number of medications they have makes it hard to follow the doctor's instructions. Here are some tips to help.

Fill up a medicine box divided into days to ensure you don't miss a dose.

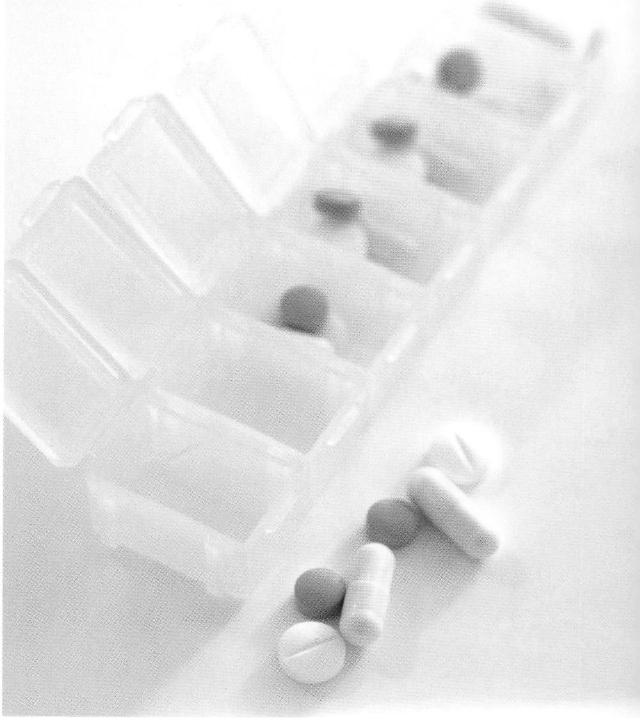

- Fill up a medicine box divided into days and times, available from pharmacists, to ensure you don't miss or repeat a dose.
- Make medication part of your routine; take your pills before brushing your teeth at night or with your morning cup of tea. Use Post-it notes or an alarm on your mobile phone to remind you.
- Keep your medicines in the same, easy-to-reach place – but obviously out of reach of children.
- If you live with someone, let him or her know when you should take your medication – that way there's someone else to remind you if you do forget.

And take heart from the fact that advances in pharmacology may soon reduce the number of pills you have to take. Some blood pressure pills are two-in-one, and 'polypills' with multiple agents may soon be available.

ARRHYTHMIA

Sometimes the beating action of the heart loses its regular, rhythmic pattern for a moment or for longer periods. Palpitations – pounding, fluttering or irregular heartbeats – are the most common symptom. They are usually not serious but simply the result of anxiety, over-exertion or even of drinking a cup of strong coffee.

If you experience palpitations regularly, you can't pin down any obvious cause or you have other symptoms, then see your doctor. It's possible that they could be caused by an abnormal rhythm or cardiac arrhythmia, a troublesome group of disorders that are more common in older people and which can cause cardiac arrest.

The heart of someone with arrhythmia beats at the wrong rate. There are two basic types: bradycardia, where the heart rate is too slow, usually less than 60 beats per minute; or tachycardia, where the heart beats too fast, usually more than 100 beats per minute.

what's NEW

A DEFIBRILLATOR IN YOUR BODY

Medication has long been the main treatment for dangerous tachycardia (abnormally fast heartbeat). But a small device called an implantable cardioverter-defibrillator (ICD) is taking over as the most effective therapy for the majority of people with the condition.

The ICD is a miniature version of emergency room-style defibrillator paddles. It's about the size of a pack of cards, and can be fitted inside the chest cavity. It works by monitoring the heart and providing electrical pulses or shocks to slow it down if it begins to race out of control.

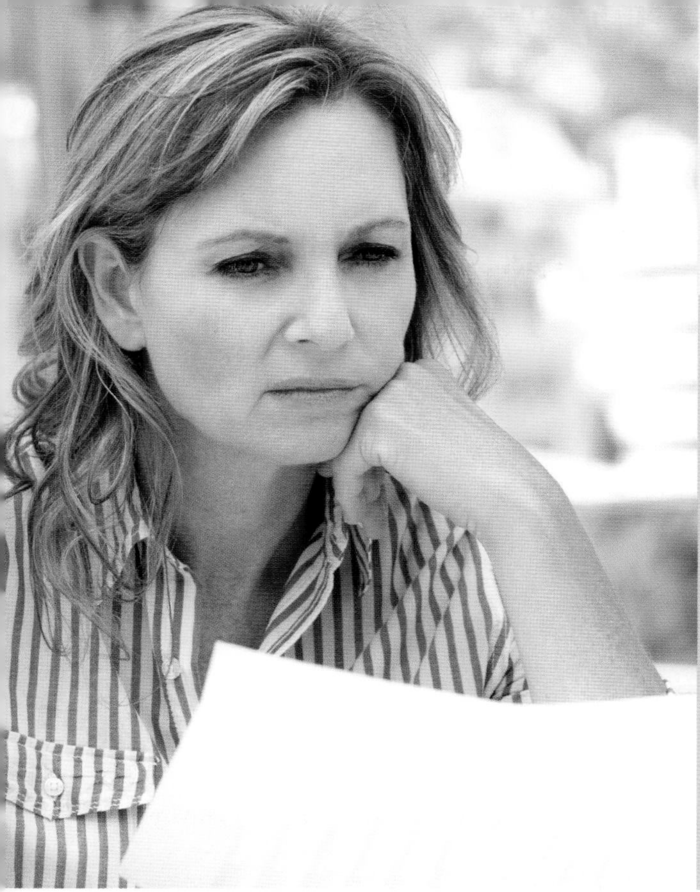

it's a MYTH …

… that HIGH BLOOD PRESSURE is a MALE issue

Some doctors still see men as the main target for heart disease–related advice and symptom checks. But researchers at Johns Hopkins University in Baltimore, USA, have found that it's just as important for older women to control their blood pressure. Women are much more likely to die from coronary artery disease than breast cancer – with their risk of heart attacks increasing by 8 per cent a year. Diabetes and high cholesterol are both greater risk factors for women over 65 than for men of the same age.

High blood pressure is not just a male issue. Women are much more likely to die from coronary artery disease than breast cancer.

Getting diagnosed

Arrhythmias are caused by electrical faults in the heart – either in its upper chambers (atria) or the lower chambers (ventricles). They can be hard to diagnose, but fainting should be seen as a sign of a dangerously abnormal heart rhythm. Other symptoms, such as skipped or irregular beats, dizziness and light-headedness, can be hard to distinguish from 'normal' palpitations.

For an accurate diagnosis, the irregular rhythm needs to be captured on an ECG (electrocardiogram). Sometimes your ECG may be recorded while you do an exercise test. To demonstrate some irregular rhythms you may need monitoring for 24 hours or more – an ambulatory ECG. You are fitted with a monitor that records electrical signals over 24 hours. Event monitors are similar and can be worn for longer periods. They record only abnormal rhythms or palpitations.

focus ON ... ASPIRIN and STATINS

Top performers in the heart-health pharmacy are aspirins and statins. A major international study, published in 2011, shows that a polypill containing aspirin *and* statin could in the future halve the chances of those at risk of having a heart attack or stroke.

● **ASPIRIN** In the 1980s aspirin became an essential medication for anyone with coronary artery disease, angina or atherosclerosis, or after a heart attack. Scientists unveiled a study showing that a daily dose of the humble headache pill inhibits the build-up of plaque in the blood vessels and halts clot formation (thus preventing heart attacks and strokes). Taking a low dose of aspirin every day (75 mg) does the job and keeps the risk of side effects to a minimum. But you should take it only on the advice of your doctor: the risks can outweigh the benefits in healthy people, according to a study published in 2012.

● **STATINS,** the most widely prescribed medicines in the world, block the production of 'bad cholesterol' by the liver, also enabling more cholesterol to be removed from the bloodstream. Studies show that they reduce the risk of heart attacks by 60 per cent and stroke by 17 per cent. They are most effective when taken by people with cardiovascular disease – and are also prescribed for high cholesterol. They can have side effects, especially muscle aches. The risk of these increases with age and dose, but changing statins may resolve the problem. It's worth persevering if they are prescribed, although your liver function should be monitored while taking them.

The most common abnormal heart rhythm is atrial fibrillation (*see* page 49). Sufferers say that it feels as if they have a squirrel running around inside their chest. It becomes more common with age, with one in ten people over 75 affected, especially if they have other conditions such as high blood pressure or atherosclerosis. The rhythm gets its name because the muscles of the atria fibrillate or quiver, instead of having a coordinated contraction. This occurs when abnormal electrical impulses suddenly begin firing into the atria of the heart, overriding the heart's natural pacemaker, which causes the upper chambers to contract chaotically and out of coordination with the ventricles.

Atrial fibrillation often remains undiagnosed, but if you suspect you have it, it's important to see a doctor and get it treated because it increases your risk of a stroke by up to seven times.

A TROUBLED HEART
treating disorders

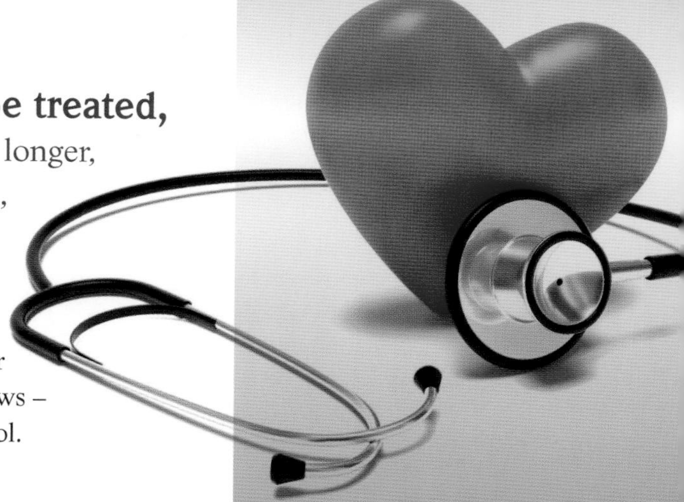

Almost every heart problem can be treated, which means more and more of us can live longer, fuller lives with ongoing cardiac conditions, or after crises such as a heart attack.

Plumbing problems are among the most common conditions affecting the heart as you age. These occur when the arteries – the pipeworks in which blood flows – become clogged with fatty material such as cholesterol.

WHAT CAN GO WRONG

As deposits gradually form, the space through which blood can pass gradually narrows – known as **atheroma**. Age is a major risk factor: the older you become, the more likely you are to develop the associated disorder **atherosclerosis**, which is more commonly known as 'hardening of the arteries'. This is caused by fatty deposits building up to form solid structures called plaques. Over the years, the build-up leads to narrowing and hardening of the arteries, until blood flow is impeded and you develop noticeable symptoms (such as pain), especially during exercise when blood flow needs to increase. Blockages can also occur when blood clots form in the narrowed arteries or plaque breaks off from the artery wall (an embolus).

Such blockages can trigger a serious health crisis: a **heart attack**, if the clot blocks one of the coronary arteries supplying the heart; a **stroke** if the blood supply to the brain is blocked; or **peripheral arterial disease** if the arteries supplying the legs are narrowed. Plaques may also cause a weakening bulge or ballooning in the wall of an artery, leading to an **aneurysm** that can break open or rupture, resulting in life-threatening bleeding. An **abdominal aortic aneurysm**, or 'Triple A', is a condition that mainly affects men over 65, and is largely symptomless.

The damage caused by atherosclerosis may not be reversible, but the risk of a dangerous clot forming can be dramatically reduced

what's NEW

STEM CELLS FOR ANGINA Injecting stem cells directly into the heart can reduce the number of chest pain episodes in angina patients and enable them to become more active, a study has found. A new method, trialled on 167 patients in the USA, involves injecting patients with a particular type of stem cell harvested from their own bone marrow. Treated patients were able to tolerate an exercise test for twice as long as before treatment. 'It translates as going from being able to watch television to being able to walk at a normal pace or going from being able to walk slowly to being able to ride a bike,' said lead researcher, Professor Douglas Losordo.

by the simple measure of taking a low-dose aspirin or another anti-platelet medication – though this should never be done without first talking to a doctor. Following a healthy-heart lifestyle and taking medication to reduce high blood pressure and blood cholesterol can slow down the damage.

- **ANGINA** is linked to atherosclerosis and is characterised by disagreeable pain in the chest. It occurs when the heart fails to get the extra oxygen it needs – as when arteries become hardened or clogged up, or damaged by a heart attack. Episodes of angina are triggered by the four Es – Exercise, Eating, Emotional stress and Exposure to cold. Attacks last just a few minutes, and respond to rest or a medicine called nitroglycerin. A common treatment is to insert a stent – a small tube – that opens up the clogged artery. This relatively minor surgery is effective alongside long-term medication.

- **PERIPHERAL ARTERIAL DISEASE** is easily overlooked. It affects nearly one in ten people over 60 and one in five over 70. It's caused by a build-up of fatty deposits in the arteries, restricting blood supply to the leg muscles. The main symptom is painful cramping after walking, so it's important to recognise that leg pain is not a normal part of ageing. Researchers have shown that the best way to reduce pain is to exercise regularly, ideally by joining a group exercise session designed for people with cardiovascular disease. Medication might include statins and drugs to reduce blood pressure. Some people need surgery to unblock the artery.

- **HEART FAILURE** is more serious but there's much that can be done to control it once you've been diagnosed. It occurs when the heart muscle has become too weak or stiff to pump enough blood out of the heart to the organs and tissues: the main causes are clogged arteries along with high blood pressure or damage to the heart valves as a result of a heart attack, or valve disease. It starts slowly, with symptoms that include breathlessness, extreme tiredness, dizziness

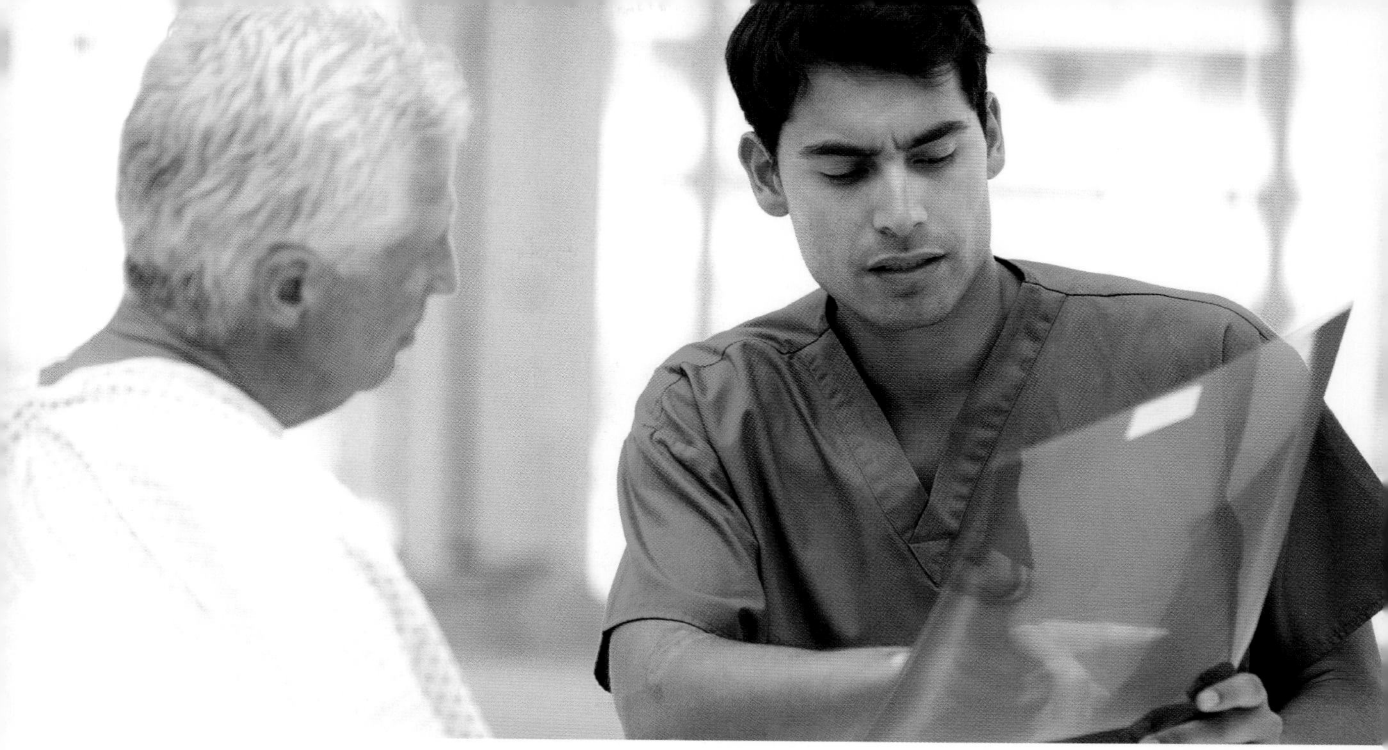

It may take time – but heart failure can be controlled, and many people can continue to lead a normal life.

and weakness, along with swelling in the legs, ankles and feet. It is most common in older men: the average age of diagnosis is 76. You will need a referral for X-rays/echocardiogram tests; treatments vary from medication to surgery, and you may need a pacemaker or defibrillator to stop life-threatening abnormal rhythms. It may take time – but heart failure can be controlled, and many people can continue to lead a normal life.

● **ATRIAL FIBRILLATION** is more likely if you have high blood pressure or coronary artery disease (*see also* page 46). It occurs when an electrical fault causes chaotic electrical activity in the upper chambers of the heart. One successful therapy is catheter ablation: thin soft wires (catheters) are guided through a vein into the heart, where they record electrical activity in order to trace the fault. High-frequency radio waves are then transmitted through one of the catheters to destroy the tissue that's sending out the troublesome signals. It's usually done when you're awake (though it may be performed under sedation or a general anaesthetic).

DID **you** KNOW ?

As you get older, you're more likely to develop anaemia, which occurs when depleted levels of red blood cells struggle to carry oxygen around your body. Symptoms may include weakness, dizziness, breathlessness, palpitations and looking very pale. Don't assume anaemia is due to a lack of iron, and that supplements will fix the problem. In later life, it can be associated with heart disease or other serious illnesses, including bowel cancer, and symptoms should always be checked by your doctor.

IS IT A HEART ATTACK?

Many more people survive a heart attack nowadays than in the past thanks to crucial factors such as more effective medical treatment. Heart attacks occur when the supply of blood to the heart is suddenly blocked, often in people with atherosclerosis (*see* pages 47–48). They are most common in older people, and men are more at risk than women, though the gap between the genders narrows with age.

A severe, squeezing pain in the centre of the chest is the best-known symptom. But you could experience something quite different: a pain in the back or shoulder, mild discomfort in the chest or stomach (like bad indigestion), accompanied by shortness of breath, light-headedness, jaw and arm pain, nausea, sweating and especially anxiety.

Getting help

It's crucial to call the emergency services immediately if you think you (or someone else) might be having a heart attack. 'It's the only option when you have a heart attack because the second the artery blocks, which is the cause of the heart attack, heart muscle cells start to die,' says Professor Peter Weissberg, medical director of the British Heart Foundation. The longer it takes to get the artery open – either with clot-busting medication or an operation – the more heart muscle dies and the more permanent damage that occurs because the heart can't repair itself. Not only that, a blocked artery can disturb the normal electrical pulses that regulate your heartbeat, increasing the risk of a rhythm disturbance that could lead to a cardiac arrest. If this happens and medical

If you think you might be having a heart attack, don't delay. Call the emergency services …

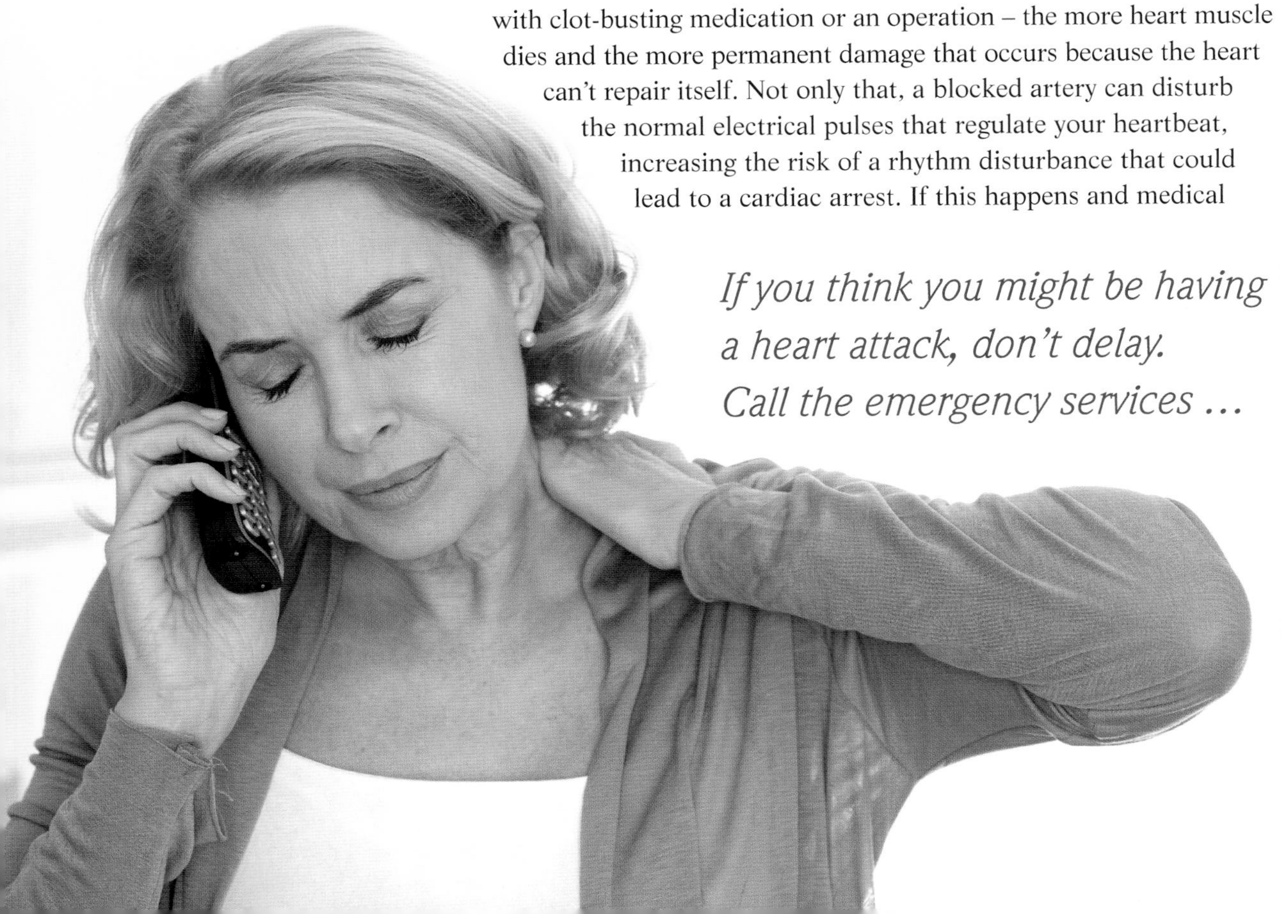

take CARE! If someone has a **HEART ATTACK**

● **IF YOU KNOW** the person is not allergic to aspirin, give him or her a 300 mg tablet – to chew – while waiting for the ambulance. This is potentially life-saving as it could prevent a clot from worsening.

● **IF THE PERSON HAS HAD A CARDIAC ARREST** and has lost consciousness, you may be able to save their life by performing cardiopulmonary resuscitation (CPR). This involves administering chest compressions in the centre of the chest no less than 5 cm deep at a rate of at least 100 per minute in order to create artificial circulation by manually pumping blood through the heart.

● **GET THE RIGHT RHYTHM** One problem with resuscitation is getting the rhythm right. Doing chest compressions to the beat of the Bee Gees' fortuitously titled hit 'Staying Alive' can help. The song has just the right number of beats (103) per minute to create artificial circulation. Tests on University of Illinois medical students performing resuscitation on dummies showed that the music helped them to keep the rate of compression steady. It's worth knowing – a *Lancet* study found that patients were 22 per cent more likely to survive if given hands-on compression only (without mouth-to-mouth breathing).

help gets to you in time, a defibrillator can be used to put an electric shock across your chest and restore a normal rhythm, which may save your life.

Immediate treatment for a heart attack aims to restore circulation to the heart muscle as fast as possible. Clot-busting medications may be given on arrival at the hospital, or, as with angina (*see* page 48), an operation (coronary angioplasty) may be performed to widen the blocked artery, often with a small tube called a stent left in place to keep the vessel open. Sometimes angioplasty is not possible, and coronary artery bypass graft surgery – to bypass the blocked artery with a vessel taken from elsewhere in the body – may be needed.

GETTING CHECKED OUT

If you have heart problems, a range of modern tests can be used to ensure that you get the right treatment. These include:

● **ECG (electrocardiogram)** This gives a recording of the electrical activity of the heart. Electrodes are positioned on the chest, wrists and ankles to show what's happening in the heart and circulation. An ECG helps identify abnormalities or damage (*see also* page 45).

If you have heart problems, a range of modern tests can be used to ensure that you get the right treatment.

BE **prepared** ... Living with a **PACEMAKER**

A pacemaker can improve your quality of life – and may prevent cardiac arrest. It takes time to get used to, but that is a small price to pay for a potential life-saver.

You may need to have a pacemaker fitted if:

- **You have a particular type of heart block that makes it beat too slowly.**
- **You have heart failure.**
- **Your heart beats too fast.**

A pacemaker is an artificial substitute for the natural pacemaker inside your heart. It works by sending electrical impulses to your heart to produce the beat. Most work only when they are needed.

Pacemakers are much smaller than they used to be: about the size of a matchbox. They can be fitted just under your collarbone with a lead to your heart through a vein. Your pacemaker will probably feel a bit heavy at first, but it won't take long for you to stop noticing it. It's fitted under a local anaesthetic, and most patients have their pacemaker checked several times in the first year, then once a year thereafter. The battery will need to be changed every seven years or so (a simple procedure).

A pacemaker shouldn't affect your life unduly, but there are a few precautions you should take:

- When using a mobile phone, don't put it near the pacemaker (for example, in a breast pocket). Use the opposite ear, or a headset.
- Tell airport security that you have one. You can go through the security device, but do so quickly.
- Do not have an MRI scan (strong magnets are used, which can interfere with the pacemaker).

- **Exercise ECG** Also known as a stress or tolerance test, this is a variation on the ECG, recording the activity of the heart as you make it work harder by walking or running on a treadmill.
- **Angiogram** This provides an X-ray picture so doctors can assess the damage or the extent of narrowing in the arteries. Under local anaesthetic, a cardiac catheter is inserted into the heart via an artery. Dye is injected into the blood vessels, then an X-ray is taken.
- **Echocardiogram** This machine uses sound waves to map information about the structure of the heart. It shows up the size of the heart and how well the muscle and valves are working.
- **Magnetic resonance imaging (MRI)** The patient lies inside a large chamber with a scanner, which uses a magnetic field to produce detailed images of the heart and blood vessels. It is used if other tests are inconclusive and for those who can't have a stress test.
- **Cardiac computed tomography (cardiac CT)** This uses a special X-ray machine to take very detailed pictures of the heart and is used like an MRI scan.

AFTER A HEART OPERATION

Whether you've had a stent fitted or a bypass operation, recovery after heart surgery can be a challenge. Some people get back to normal very quickly: the explorer Ranulph Fiennes, for example, was jogging just two weeks after his double-bypass operation. And he ran a marathon within three months. But everybody recovers at different rates. The key point is not to think of yourself as being on borrowed time after having a heart operation. Plenty of people live happily and healthily for decades afterwards.

At first, though, you will feel tired and weak. If your heart has been damaged, some symptoms may be lasting – but many won't. You're bound to be sensitive to twinges in the chest area, but these are not necessarily a sign that anything is wrong. You will also need to be philosophical about the consequences of heart surgery. Post-op tests take time, and meanwhile you will face restrictions on what you can do; you will worry about complications; you will spend time waiting in hospitals. Don't let these things get to you: they will all pass.

Know your goals

As your strength returns, set yourself physical targets and try to extend them a little every day (with your doctor's approval). Walking is a flexible way of exercising. Six weeks after your operation, start walking for an hour or so – at a pace that makes you slightly out of breath, but still able to talk. Do this as often as you can.

You can usually drive four weeks after a heart op (ask your doctor for advice and tell your car insurance company), and your sex life can be resumed soon after (four to six weeks) – in the long term, sex is an excellent form of heart-healthy exercise. Recovery is not just a physical matter, of course. Your confidence may be sapped for a while, but with time you may well discover a renewed self-belief and zest for life.

You can have sex within four to six weeks of having a heart attack or cardiac surgery – in the long term, it's an excellent form of heart-healthy exercise.

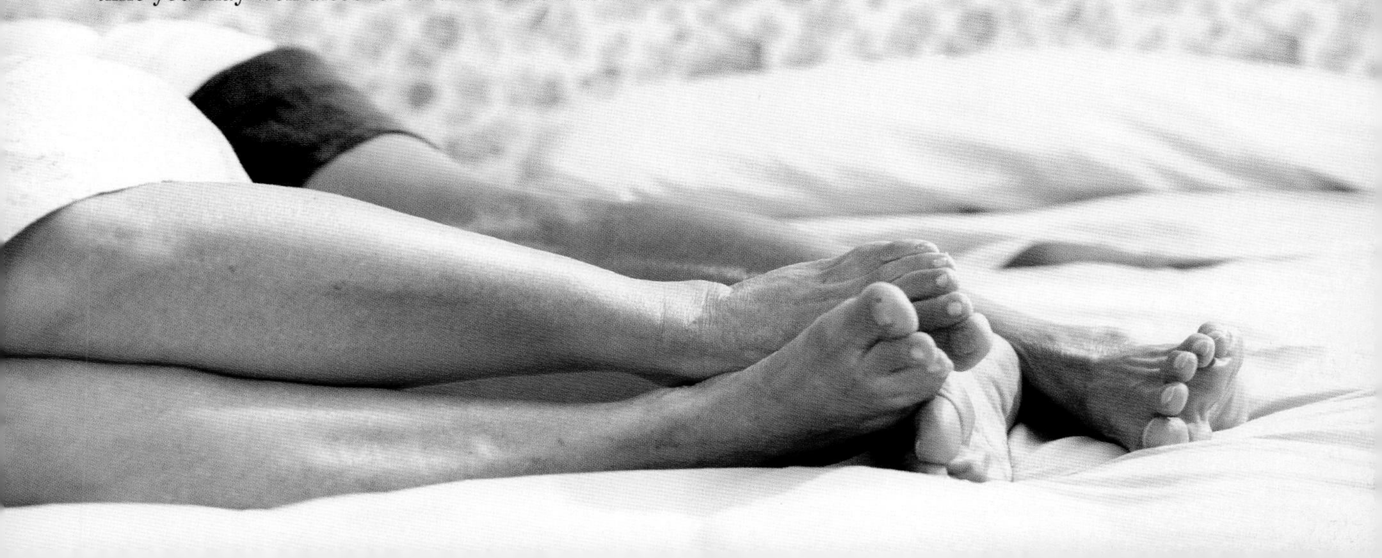

Music can help recovery after a stroke: take much-loved CDs to stroke patients.

STROKES
new developments

Seven out of ten strokes occur in over-65s. But while a stroke is one of the most frightening health events, there's a growing pile of good news about the potential for recovery.

The same health problems that affect normal blood flow and cause heart disease can also trigger strokes. They are much more common in people with hardening of the arteries, high blood pressure and cholesterol, in smokers and in those with diabetes.

A stroke occurs when the blood supply to the brain is cut off. Four out of five strokes are classed as ischaemic, which means that they're caused by a blood clot. The clot can develop either in the artery that supplies the brain (a cerebral thrombosis), or it may have travelled to the brain from elsewhere in the body (a cerebral embolism). The other main type of stroke is called a haemorrhagic stroke: a blood vessel inside or on the brain bursts and bleeds into the brain.

If you experience temporary stroke symptoms (*see* box opposite), lasting less than 24 hours, you may have had a 'transitory ischaemic attack' (TIA). It's easy to dismiss this: it happened, you got better. But a TIA is a clear indication that you're at risk of having a stroke within days or weeks – or at any time in the next five years. So treat it as the warning it is, and make sure you get specialist assessment, including a CT (computed tomography) scan of the brain and a special ultrasound scan called a carotid duplex that looks at major blood vessels in the neck to enable your medical team to decide on preventive action.

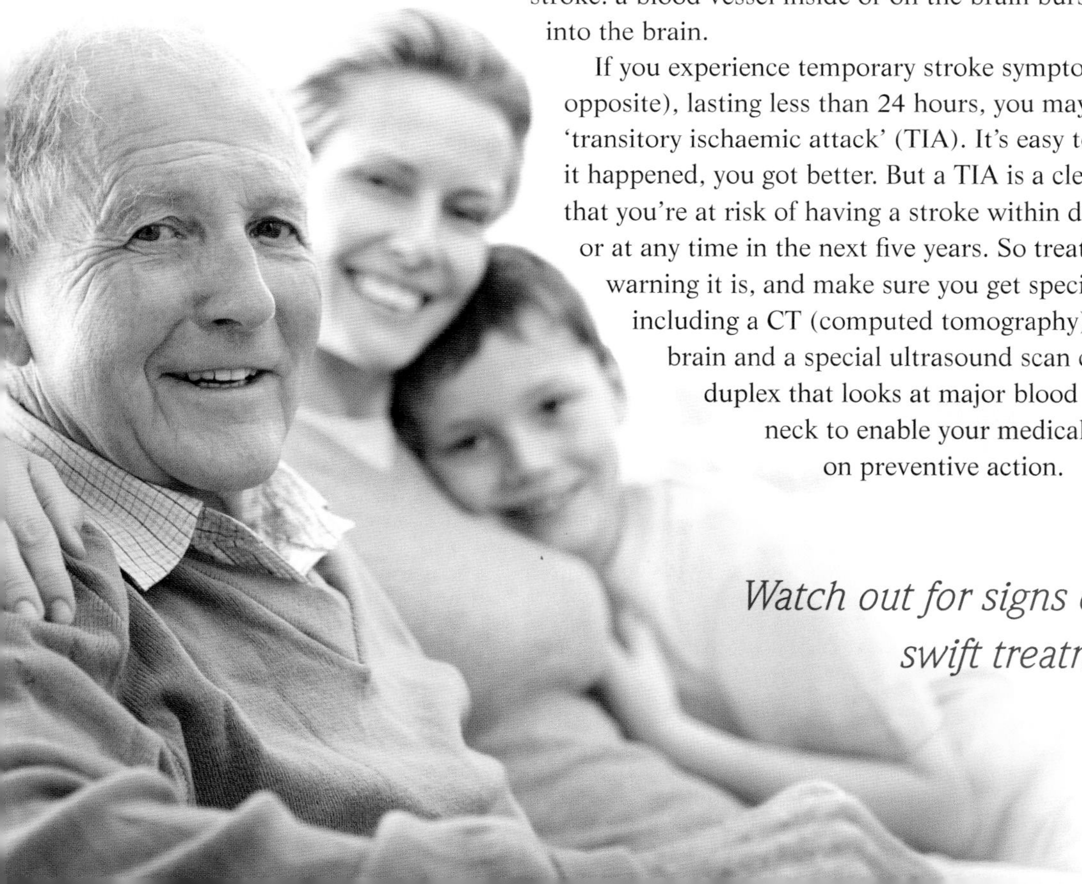

Watch out for signs of a stroke – swift treatment is vital.

AFTER A STROKE

If you do have a stroke, there's much that can be done to help minimise the effects:

● **SWIFT TREATMENT** Get to hospital as soon as you can. If you are having a TIA, your symptoms may be wearing off but it is important to find out why it happened and start treatment to reduce the risk of a real stroke. If you aren't getting better, you are probably having a stroke. The first step is an urgent CT scan to determine whether this is ischaemic or haemorrhagic. If it is ischaemic, many neurologists recommend a clot-busting medication that they hope will dramatically improve the chance of recovery. The catch? The medication must be given within six hours of the onset of symptoms (and the sooner the better), and many emergency department doctors believe it does more harm than good.

● **WORK THE BODY** More than half of those affected have mobility problems or balance and coordination difficulties. And one in three suffer spasticity – tight or stiff muscles that can make moving the arms and legs difficult and painful. Fortunately, there are good treatments, including muscle-relaxing medications. Regular, specialist physiotherapy and occupational therapy can also make a big difference, especially if started soon after the stroke.

● **AIDING RECOVERY** People who've had a stroke may suffer weakness or paralysis on one side, as well as problems with talking, memory, thinking and problem solving. Here, too, scientists have been finding ways to help. Listening to your favourite music has been found to improve brain-function recovery dramatically, according to research carried out at Helsinki University – taking some much-loved CDs to the hospital could be the best gift you can offer. And don't underestimate how much friends and family can help: physiotherapy and speech therapy are far more successful if therapists can teach family members the stimulating techniques.

take CARE ! STROKE

The Stroke Association in the UK has developed the **FAST** test to recognise when a stroke has occurred.

If you think someone has had a stroke, check for the following symptoms, then act fast.

FACIAL WEAKNESS Can the person smile? Has his or her mouth or eye drooped?

ARM WEAKNESS Can the person raise both arms?

SPEECH PROBLEMS Can the person speak clearly and understand what you say?

If the answer to one or more of these is **NO**, it's:

TIME TO CALL AN AMBULANCE

Hospital care can improve their chances of a good outcome.

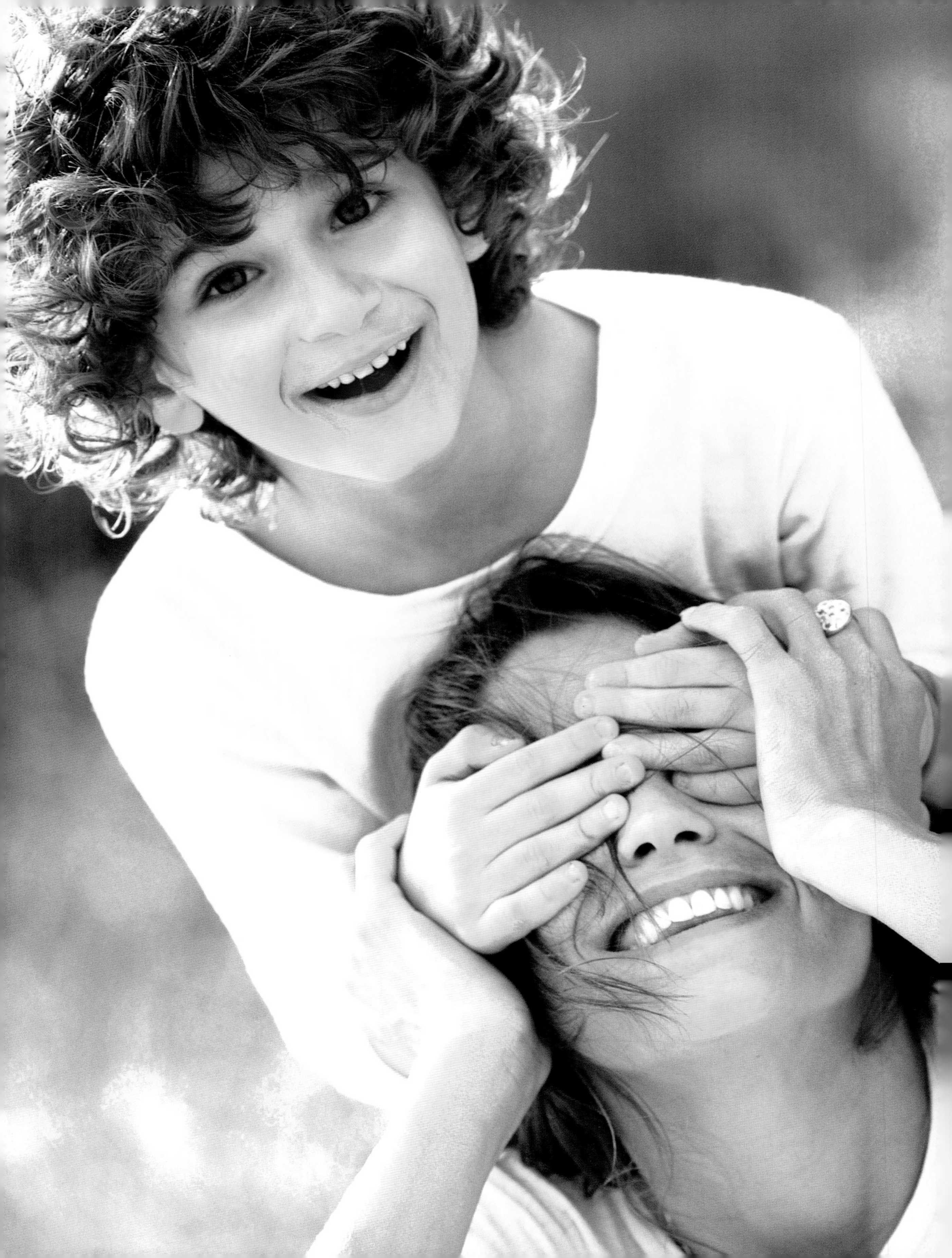

3

BREATHE *freely*

Uniquely within your body, breathing is entirely automatic most of the time, yet is completely under your control whenever you want it to be. You can choose to breathe faster or slower, or to hold your breath, on a whim. This is amazing (you can't command your heart or any other internal organ in this way) and also very useful. It means that you can take charge of the work of your lungs. So it is within your power to ensure that your breathing remains strong and healthy, even as the changes of later life begin to kick in.

Exercise and weight control can almost halve the decline in oxygen uptake that occurs with age.

LUNG POWER
take in the air

Throughout life, the health of your lungs is key to your general wellbeing. Consciously developing good breathing techniques will help you to preserve your lung power and avoid potential health problems as you age.

Every part of your body needs oxygen to survive, and it is your lungs' job to harvest this precious gas from the atmosphere – which it does 20,000 times a day, or 600 million times in a lifetime. The oxygen from the air that you breathe in is transferred to the red cells in your bloodstream, which carry it around your body. Your brain constantly receives signals about the amount of oxygen you need, and sends messages along your nerves to your breathing muscles to ensure your lungs gather adequate supplies.

Keeping guard

Your lungs are more than a set of bellows. They are also a complex defence system, a filter against germs and other foreign materials. First, the cilia – tiny hairs in the bronchi (the large airways) – help waft unwanted materials up to your mouth; mucus produced in the walls of your airways helps keep them clean and lubricated; and cells in the lungs themselves contain enzymes that mop up invading germs.

HOW YOUR LUNGS AGE

Like other body systems, your lungs change with age, although exercise and deep breathing can keep them working well. As you get older, they become stiffer, your respiratory muscle strength and endurance diminish, and your chest wall becomes more rigid. Your total lung capacity – the maximum amount your lungs can hold – remains fairly constant throughout life. But there is a decrease in the volume of air you can forcibly exhale (your vital capacity).

This is because the so-called residual volume – the amount of air left in your lungs after you breathe out fully – increases: at the age of 20, residual volume makes up 20 per cent of the total lung capacity;

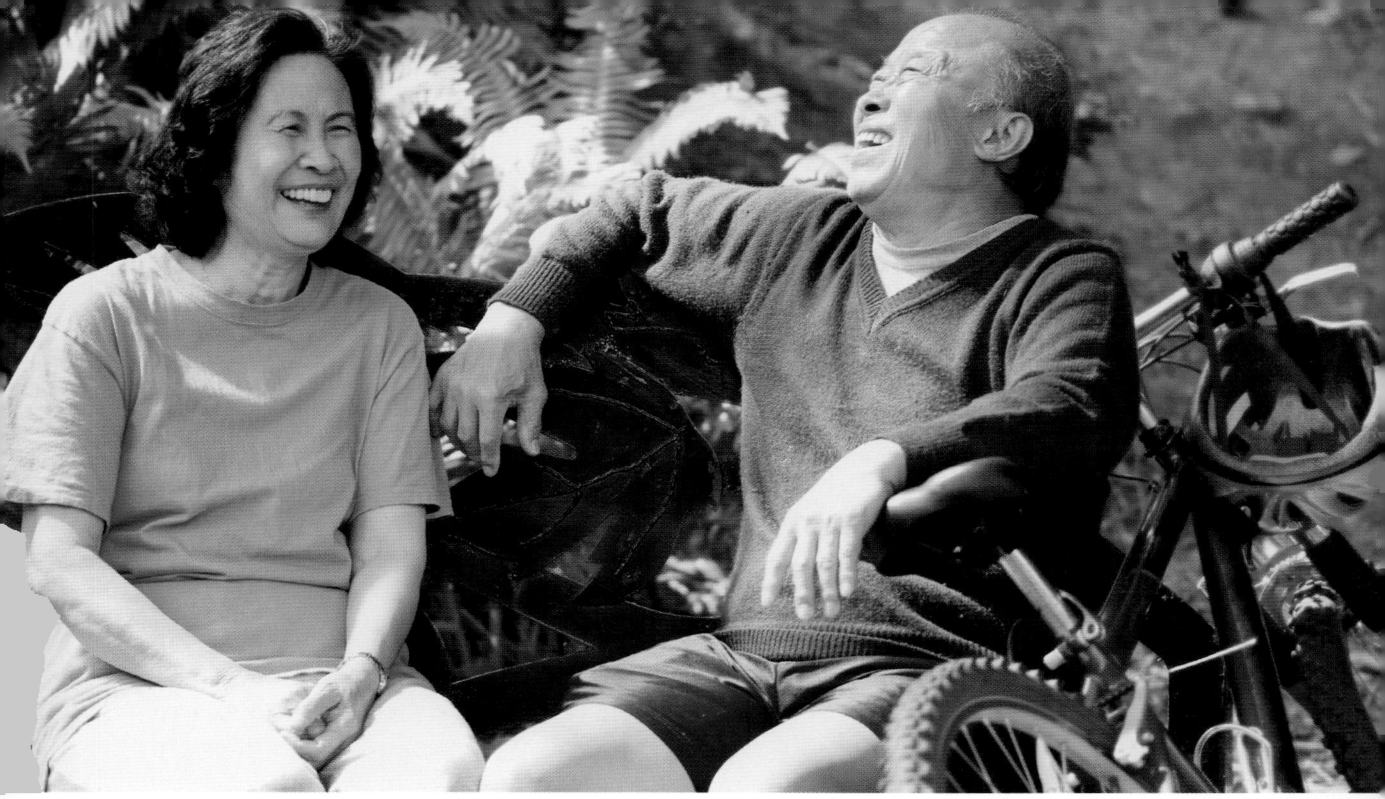

Preserve your lung power by exercising in fresh air.

at 60, it is nearer 35 per cent. Consequently, your reserve lung capacity – the space left for fresh air – is reduced, because more stale air remains in your lungs after you breathe out.

The good news is that most of the normal respiratory changes that come with age don't have much adverse effect on lung function in healthy older adults. But a smaller reserve lung capacity does mean that you may not take in as much oxygen as you did when you were younger. You won't normally notice this change during ordinary activities, but you may become breathless when exerting yourself (or if at higher altitudes). Decreased lung capacity can also affect your concentration and memory, and make you more tired in general. It can even increase your risk of heart attacks and other debilitating health problems.

DID you KNOW?

Deep breathing can aid weight loss. How? It triggers the relaxation response in the body, helping to stop the release of cortisol, and this encourages your body to burn fat. By way of a bonus, deep breathing strengthens the abdominal muscles, too.

Breath of life

You don't have to become an opera singer to achieve good lung capacity and breath control but it's worth ensuring that you exercise your lungs and breathe effectively as this is key to an active, healthy life in later years. Long-term studies show that pulmonary function – how well your lungs operate – is a good gauge of your general health.

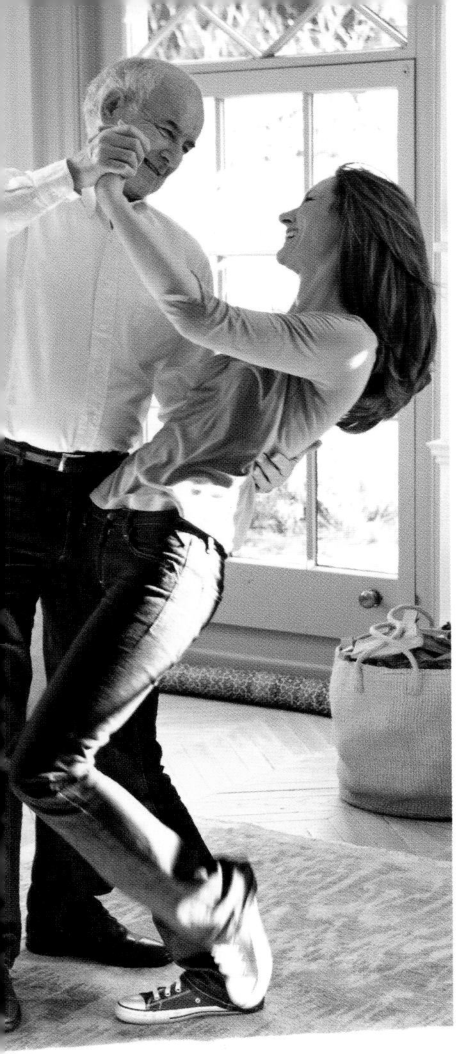

Avoid high-impact exercises – opt for low-impact activities such as dancing instead.

ENERGISE YOUR BREATHING

If you find that you get breathless easily, lifestyle factors are more likely to be responsible than ageing. We tend to be more sedentary as we get older and our breathing becomes lazy. We often put on weight, too. This is a common cause of breathlessness because carrying too much fat puts extra strain on the lungs, making it more difficult for them to work properly. These are things you can do something about. Below are four of the most effective ways to improve your breathing:

● **WORK THE LUNGS** Exercise helps maintain the elasticity of your lung walls, while increasing lung power, so oxygen enters your lungs more rapidly and carbon dioxide leaves more quickly. Endurance exercises – activities that increase your heart and breathing rate for a continuous period – can produce significant rises in lung capacity in older people who have previously been sedentary. You don't need to push yourself hard – in fact, it may be wise to avoid high-impact exercises such as jogging, which put strain on the muscles and joints, and opt for low-impact activities instead. Try walking, cycling, swimming and dancing (anything from ballroom to Zumba). Choose something you enjoy, and aim for at least 30 minutes most days.

● **FOCUS ON THE BREATH** Yoga breathwork lengthens each inhalation and exhalation, strengthens the lungs and is deeply calming. Do this quick exercise at least once a day – it doesn't matter when or where – to help train yourself to breathe well.

- Sit or lie comfortably; place one hand on your chest, the other on your stomach.
- Breathe in through your nose, counting slowly to three. Feel your abdomen expand. Focus on breathing with your diaphragm.
- Breathe out through pursed lips to a count of six, feeling your abdomen relax, and then repeat.

● **STAND TALL** Poor posture can cramp your lung capacity, so keep checking you are sitting up straight and walking tall. Anxiety, which makes the shoulders rigid and the whole body tense, can result in shallow, restricted breathing. Practising simple yoga can improve your posture, increase your flexibility and strength and allow your lungs to work freely again. A 2011 study at King's College London

Work it out INNER POWER

The Chinese art of chi kung is a gentle way to work on your posture and it has a big impact on your lung function. A study at Arizona State University found that both chi kung and tai chi helped older people to improve cardiopulmonary fitness as well as bone health, balance and confidence in their physical abilities. Try this simple breathing exercise, which you can practise a few times a day.

1 Stand with your legs hip-width apart, feet facing forwards. Keep your shoulders relaxed and your arms by your sides.

2 Bend at the knees slightly, just so that your legs are not rigidly straight.

3 Keep your spine straight and in a neutral position, maintaining its normal curves.

4 As you inhale, slowly lift your arms up in front of your chest with your hands facing downwards. Keep your fingers and hands relaxed as you lift.

5 When you reach the end of your inhalation, breathe out through your nose and lower your arms at the same time. Do six to eight breaths. Pause, then repeat once more.

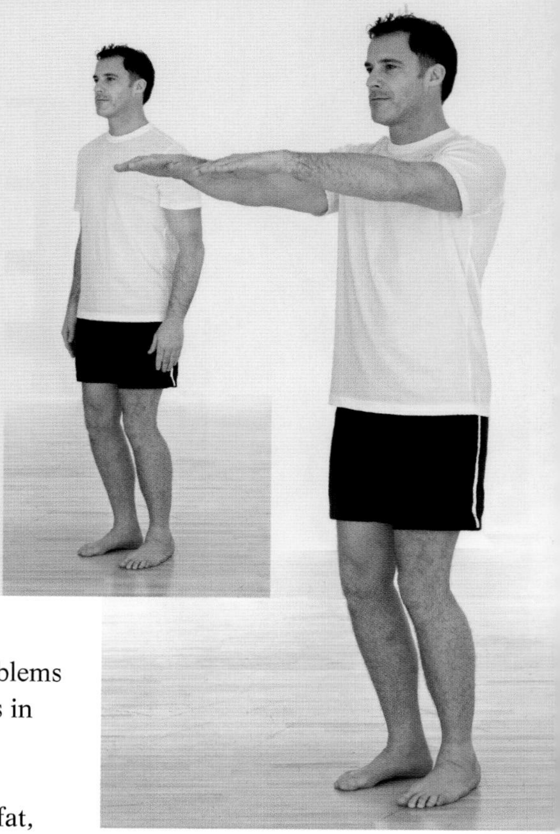

found that women in their 60s with breathing and mobility problems who did yoga classes and dance therapy reported improvements in their physical problems and enhanced wellbeing.

● **BE A HEALTHY WEIGHT** If you're carrying too much body fat, some of that may be pressing on your lungs, which can constrict your breathing. And if you suffer from obstructive sleep apnoea, a condition that causes interrupted breathing as you sleep, that could be weight-related, too. Fat accumulates in the tissues in the neck and at the back of the throat, and when you lie down, these tissues can collapse, blocking the airways. It can be harder to lose weight as you get older – *see* page 98 or ask your family doctor to help assess your current diet and levels of physical activity, and set realistic goals.

7 ways to AGE-PROOF YOUR LUNGS

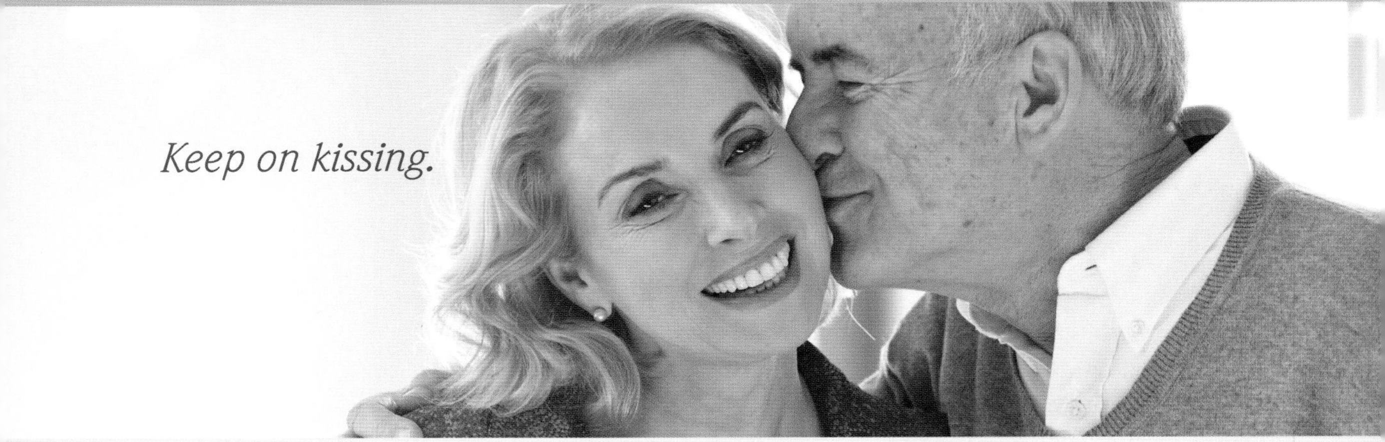

Keep on kissing.

Pulmonary fitness There are lots of ways to keep your lungs in peak condition as you get older. Here are some simple things you can do:

1 WATER, WATER Drinking water is important for lung health. Lungs lose water during exhalation. Keeping yourself well hydrated helps keep any mucus and secretions thin, making them easier to cough up.

2 KEEP ON KISSING As well as its other benefits – lowering blood pressure and cholesterol, regulating heartbeat – kissing makes you breathe more deeply. After kissing, your lungs work harder.

3 GET A FLU JAB If you're over 65 – or have diabetes, asthma, or heart or lung disease – be sure to have your annual flu jab, which is free for these groups in Australia.

4 STOP SITTING Cut your TV time, and break up the amount of time you spend sitting down. Instead of sitting for hours on end, take short walks around the garden or neighbourhood.

5 HUM ALONG Humming can help increase your oxygen intake. Sit on a chair, hands at your side. Take a deep breath. Then, as you expel the air, start humming a single note. As you tire, pull your stomach muscles in, hold for as long as possible and continue humming.

6 EAT WELL Avoid heavy meals – feeling full can make it harder to breathe – and eat a few small meals a day rather than one or two large ones; eating in a slow, relaxed manner will also help. Include plenty of fruit and vegetables in your diet to help keep infections at bay.

7 BREATHE CLEAN AIR Giving up smoking is obviously a key way to help your lungs (*see* page 65), and you should also avoid smoky atmospheres. Smoke that you breathe in from someone else's cigarette contains carbon monoxide, formaldehyde and other dangerous substances. So make your home a completely smoke-free zone.

FIGHT THE FUMES

It's not news that fresh air is good for you. The oxygenating benefits of sea air, in particular, have been known for centuries. But it pays to be aware of pollutants in the air, both outdoors and inside, especially since many of them are invisible and odourless.

City air is more polluted than the air in the countryside, of course, and many urban pollutants are caused by road transport. These include nitrogen dioxide, which can irritate the lining of the airways and cause coughing and breathlessness, and particulate matter (PM) – airborne dirt – from diesel engines and other sources. At high levels, PM makes existing breathing problems worse, and also raises the risk of heart attack and strokes in vulnerable people. Volatile organic compounds (VOCs), produced by motor fuel, contain chemicals such as benzene, which can cause lung cancer if inhaled over a long period. The carbon monoxide in exhaust fumes obstructs the transportation of oxygen in the blood, causing problems for those with pre-existing heart and lung disease (as confirmed by a 2008 study at the University of Crete). And finally ozone, produced by the action of sunlight on nitrogen dioxide and VOCs, irritates even healthy airways.

What can you do about it? Well, one good thing about being older is that you're less likely to be tied to the 9-to-5 work routine. Make the most of this freedom and steer clear of rush-hour fumes. And plan your route to avoid heavy traffic as much as possible.

DID you KNOW?

Walking is known to be one of the best forms of exercise, but try to walk faster if you can. Analysis of nine studies, published in the *Journal of the American Medical Association* in 2011, showed that among men and women aged 75 years, those who walked fastest increased their chances of living for ten more years by as much as 91 per cent.

AIR YOUR HOME

Low-level pollutants can be harmful when trapped in insulated, centrally heated, double-glazed homes. There's much you can do to combat this. For a start, fling open the windows to let in fresh air – and let out old, stale air. Do it even in winter: just 10 minutes makes

Avoid exhaust fumes; take your walks on leafy lanes.

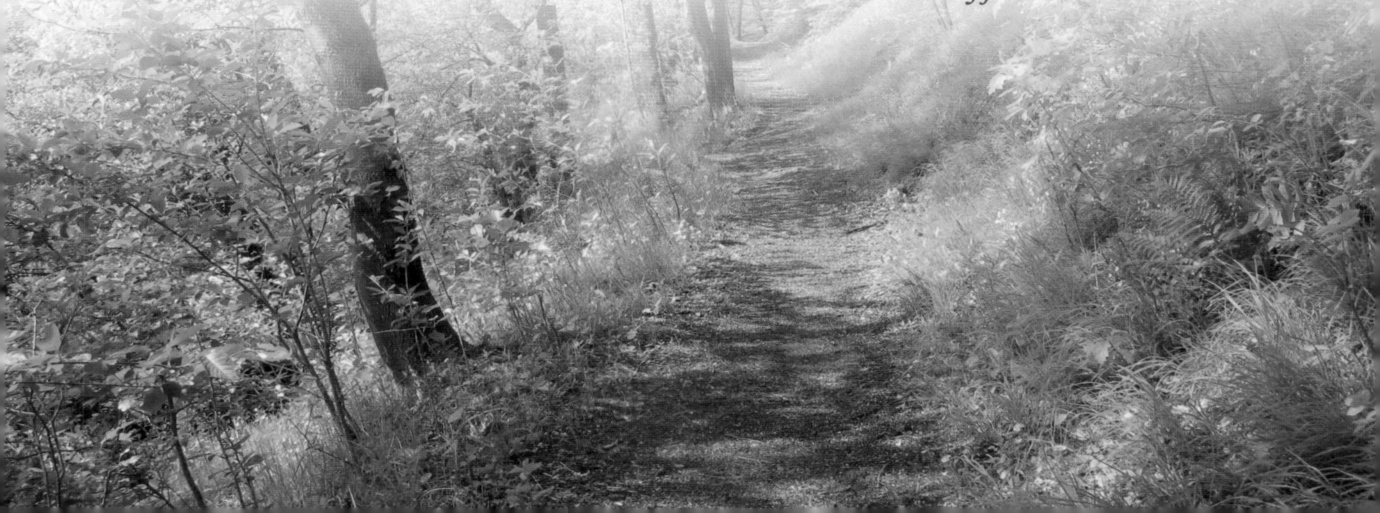

it's a **MYTH ...**

... that long-term **LUNG PROBLEMS** rule out **EXERCISE**

People with lung problems often worry that exercise will harm them by making them more breathless. In fact, gentle exercise helps both your health and your mood. Consult your doctor first for a personal action plan and gradually build up the amount of exercise you take each day. Over time, this can improve your breathing, boost your immune system and help your self-confidence. It also helps break the vicious cycle whereby you feel breathless so you do less, which in turn means your breathing muscles become weaker, which makes you more breathless, and so on.

a difference. If you have pets, keep them out of the bedroom, and dust and vacuum regularly to reduce animal dander in the atmosphere. Here are some other good ways to improve your air quality:

- **Be appliance-safe** Make sure your cooking and heating appliances are professionally installed, regularly serviced and have a vent to the outside. Gas or propane can produce harmful amounts of nitrogen dioxide and carbon monoxide.
- **Read labels** Opt for non-toxic household products: the chemicals in some aerosols, cleaning products, pesticides, paints and solvents can irritate the eyes, nose and throat, and cause dizziness, nausea or allergic reactions. Be sure to dispose of old, toxic products safely.
- **Tackle mould and mildew** Eliminate damp. Don't leave bathroom surfaces wet as it encourages mould to grow. Use exhaust fans vented to the outside to prevent condensation.
- **Be green-fingered** Houseplants can purify your air, by helping to remove airborne contaminants, as well as absorbing carbon dioxide, emitting oxygen and controlling humidity. Try the peace lily, spider plant, English ivy or heartleaf Philodendron.
- **Minimise mites** Wash bedding often. This cuts down on fast-breeding house-dust mites (they love warm, humid areas). Try special mattresses and pillowcases, which stop mites getting through. In Australia, the most important trigger for year-round allergies is house dust mite faeces.
- **Get asbestos advice** Lagging on any pipes, tanks or boilers may contain asbestos if it is more than 25 years old. Asbestos is also sometimes found in roofing, flooring and insulation boarding. Contact your local council for advice on getting rid of it – do not try to do it yourself. If it isn't damaged, it's often best to leave it as it is. Take care not to drill into it, sand it or cut it.

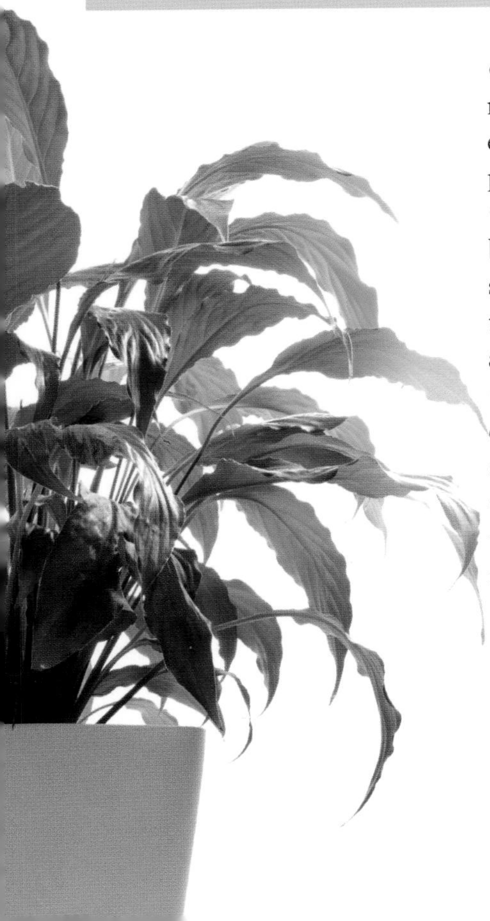

Peace lilies help to purify the air in your home.

STUB IT OUT

It's never too late to stop smoking. If you quit at 60, you can add three years to your life. And your life is more likely to be lived in a state of good health. Stop smoking, and you'll reduce your chance of furred-up arteries and blood vessel blockages, making heart disease, stroke and dementia all less likely. You'll suffer less from coughing and phlegm, which may clear up altogether. Your skin will benefit too: it will look less sallow and be less inclined to wrinkle.

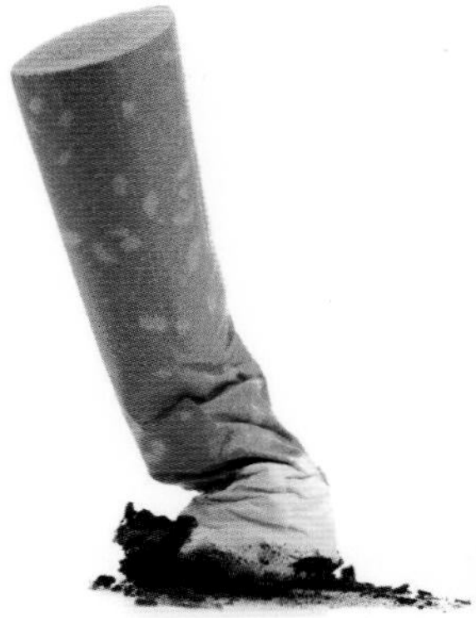

If you quit smoking at 60, you can add three years to your life.

How to do it

Yes, there's a huge hurdle to surmount, but plenty of help is at hand: ask your doctor about local stop-smoking services (*see* Resources for useful organisations that can help). And take heart from the fact that older smokers are more likely to quit for good than younger people. Not everyone will go about quitting the same way – our temperaments are all different – but here are some tips known to have worked:

- **Name the day** Set a firm date for stopping, and stick with it.
- **Enlist support** Tell everyone what you are doing, so you have people to keep you going when you feel like caving in.
- **Change your routine** Keep away from places and situations where you are likely to be tempted. Get rid of anything that reminds you of tobacco, and clean any clothes that smell of smoke.
- **Drink plenty of water** This is important not only for good hydration, but to counteract a dry mouth.
- **Take up a new hobby** Choose one that involves using your hands, to give them something to do other than hold a cigarette.
- **Take one day at a time** Give yourself a 'treat' for each tobacco-free day that you manage.

To help minimise withdrawal symptoms, nicotine replacement therapy – in the form of patches, gum, lozenges, microtabs, nasal sprays or inhalers – provides a daily dose of nicotine that is tailored to the amount of tobacco you've been smoking. The prescription medications bupropion and varenicline dampen down cravings. Herbal preparations, dummy cigarettes, mouthwashes, as well as hypnotherapy and acupuncture, are alternative approaches.
If quitting feels hard, take comfort from the fact that your risk of sudden heart attack decreases the next day. The day after that, your sense of taste and smell begin to return. Two weeks on, your brain

focus ON ... ASTHMA

If you develop breathlessness or a wheeze, however old you are, there is a significant chance you have asthma. See your GP fast. Some people are diagnosed with asthma for the first time later in life.

More than 90 per cent of people who die from asthma are aged over 45, and the number of adults being diagnosed is increasing. The number-one trigger in older people is the common cold. Irritants such as cigarette smoke, household chemical sprays and fragrances can also play a part, although some 70 per cent of 'late-onset' asthma does not have an allergic basis.

It can be difficult to detect asthma in later years because some symptoms – cough, wheezing, shortage of breath – are similar to those of COPD (*see* pages 70–73) and heart disease. If you've had asthma all your life, you may find it affects you differently now. Shortness of breath may be your only symptom.

Help yourself

- **REVIEW TREATMENTS** A 2011 study at Aberdeen University found a non-steroid tablet (a leukotriene receptor antagonist) was an effective alternative to steroid inhalers for warding off attacks.
- **HAVE THE JAB** Older people are at risk from chest problems – don't miss your annual flu vaccination. If you're over 65 or using steroid tablets, consider a one-off pneumococcal jab.
- **KEEP EXERCISING** Exercise can trigger attacks but is beneficial if your asthma is controlled. Swimming helps, too, because of the warm humid air (avoid cold, heavily chlorinated pools).

adjusts to the absence of nicotine, so any cravings start to fade. Between three weeks and three months later, your circulation and capacity for exercise improve, and lung congestion and phlegm reduce. Over the six months after that your lungs become better able to launch a defence against infection, and your energy levels increase.

The health advantages of quitting do not end there. One year after your last puff of a cigarette, your heart attack risk will have dropped to half that of a smoker. After ten years, your lung cancer risk is half that of a smoker. After 15 years, your heart will have forgiven you entirely: your heart attack risk is similar to that of someone who has never smoked.

CAN YOU BANISH colds and flu?

Wash your hands: cold germs can live on surfaces for two days or more.

If you're over 60, the good news is that you're far less likely to succumb to a cold virus because your immune system has seen most of them before. And there's plenty you can do to steer clear of new respiratory bugs against which you have no natural defences.

Of the many effective strategies to help you avoid colds and flu, handwashing is the simplest and best. Wash your hands regularly – at least five times a day, and always after going to the lavatory and before preparing food, as well as after shaking hands. Do it with soap and water – hot or cold, it doesn't matter – and for a full 20 seconds, to remove viruses. That's roughly the length of time it takes to sing or hum 'Happy Birthday' twice. Dry your hands thoroughly with a paper towel, and carry antibacterial handwash with you when you go out.

Another easy precaution is to use an antibacterial cleaner to wipe door handles, switches, phones, bathroom taps and remote controls, regularly, and especially if anyone in your home has a cold. These much-touched surfaces can harbour cold viruses for many hours – a study by the University of Virginia found that volunteers could pick up the virus two days after surfaces were contaminated.

Avoid overcrowded spaces as much as possible, by choosing when and where to shop. If you can, travel outside school holidays, so as not to encounter many children. Children are the world's germ brokers, and school playgrounds the great trading floors of new and untried bugs.

Try to travel outside school holidays: children often spread new, untried bugs.

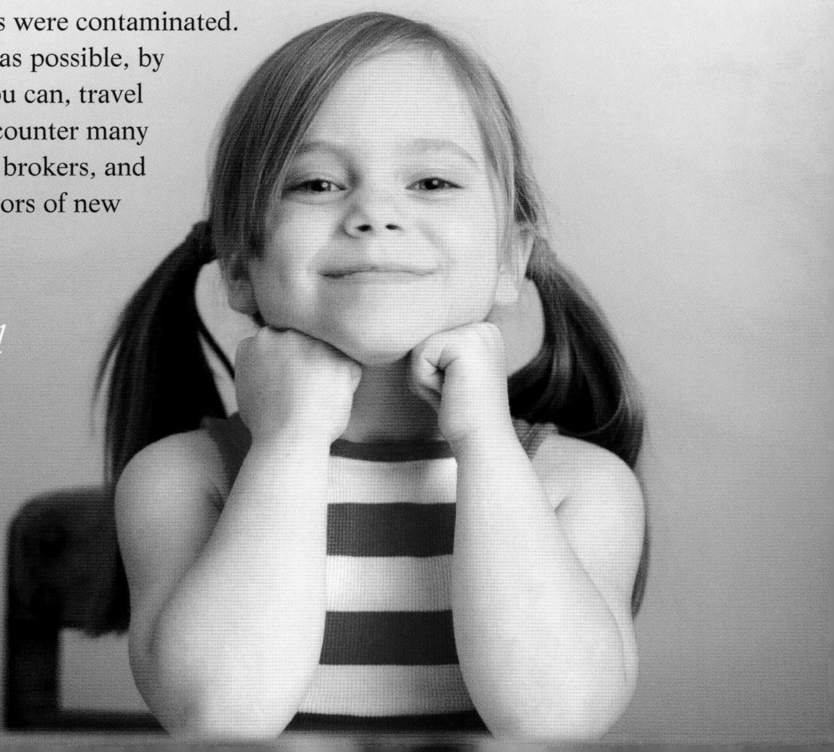

it's a MYTH ...

... that getting COLD OR WET gives you a cold

Only a virus can cause a cold. If you are already carrying the virus in your nose, however, becoming cold might weaken your defences and allow the symptoms to develop. In one study at Cardiff University, people who chilled their feet for 20 minutes were twice as likely to develop a cold as those who did not. This suggests that people can carry viruses in the nose with no symptoms, but that becoming chilled causes the blood vessels in the nose to constrict, affecting your nose's defence system and making it easier for the virus to replicate. The virus also has a protective shell that makes it better able to survive in colder temperatures.

MORE THAN A COLD

It's unwise to dismiss problematic respiratory symptoms as 'only a cold'. As you get older, serious complications are more likely to occur, especially if you have existing lung problems. Never leave anything to chance: your doctor is there to advise you.

The following are signs that you may have flu, rather than a cold:

- Flu tends to hit quite suddenly and severely.
- You simply cannot keep going (whereas with a cold, you can usually function).
- You have a bad headache.
- You have a fever, are sweating and chilled, and ache all over.

Flu is nasty, and it's wise to see a doctor if you have flu-like symptoms and are over 65, or if you have a long-term health condition such as diabetes or a heart, lung, kidney or immune system problem. Your doctor may wish to give you an antiviral medicine to lessen the symptoms.

Even a common cold can lead to a condition such as sinusitis, or a chest infection – where your lungs become affected by a virus or by bacteria, either in the larger airways (leading to bronchitis) or the smaller air sacs (pneumonia – *see* box opposite). A build-up of pus and fluid (mucus), and swelling in the airways, combine to make breathing difficult.

Common symptoms of chest infection include:

- Fast or difficult breathing.
- Coughing up brown or green phlegm.
- Fever (sweating, shivering, feeling chilled).
- Chest pain.

If you're over 65 or have lung or immune system problems, see your doctor promptly if you suspect you have a chest infection. He or she may arrange investigations such as a chest X-ray, a phlegm sample and blood tests. Most chest infections are caused by a virus, so your own immune system should be able to deal with it provided you look after yourself. But if you have a bacterial chest infection, you'll usually be prescribed antibiotics.

focus ON ... PNEUMONIA

Anyone can contract pneumonia, even young, fit people, but it is four times more common – and often much more serious – in over-65s.

Pneumonia causes the air sacs and smaller bronchial tubes in the lungs to become inflamed and to fill with fluid. White blood cells travel to the lungs to fight the infection, making it hard for the lungs to transfer oxygen into the bloodstream. Although not as contagious as flu, you can get it if infected people cough or sneeze near you, or you can develop secondary pneumonia following a respiratory infection.

- **Know the symptoms:** coughing, breathlessness and fever, accompanied by confusion and unsteadiness, especially in over-65s.
- **Beware complications:** including fluid build-up around the lungs, severe breathing difficulties or septicaemia if the infection spreads.
- **Cut your risk:** ask about a pneumococcal anti-influenza vaccination, treat chest infections promptly, don't smoke.

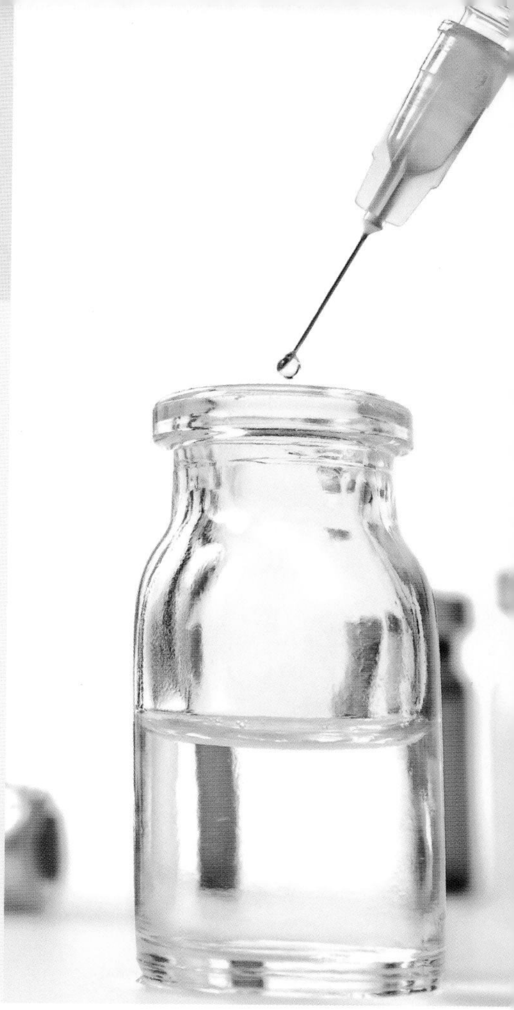

Whatever the diagnosis, as well as taking any prescribed medication and getting some rest, take these steps to get you back on your feet.

- **Drink for health** Take plenty of fluids to counteract dehydration, which occurs as the body combats the bugs. This will also help to loosen and thin any mucus in your lungs, so it's easier to cough up.
- **Increase the humidity** A humidifier in the room helps loosen mucus and aids breathing. Inhaling steam – run the hot taps in the bathroom then add drops of eucalyptus or menthol – also helps.
- **Try a traditional remedy** If you have a sore throat or a tickly cough, honey, lemon and ginger in warm water is a soothing remedy. Lemon is a good source of vitamin C, honey reduces the coughing and ginger helps to relieve congestion. Gargle before swallowing.
- **Take the salt** If you're left with blocked sinuses (sinusitis), try a natural seawater nasal spray, which cleans out the nostrils and can be used freely. A 2011 study by Polish researchers found that douching with saline solution can greatly reduce nasal swelling.

Ask about vaccination against pneumococcal pneumonia, the most common type.

An annual flu jab is essential if you have lung disease.

TAKING ACTION for lung problems

Breathing involves a constant interaction between your lungs and the world outside of your body. This makes your lungs vulnerable to attack by pollutants and a variety of diseases.

Older people are especially susceptible because of age-related changes to their lungs as well as a reduced coughing reflex and lowered immunity. But if you do experience breathing difficulties, there's much you can do to ease your problem. Of course, it can be frightening if you struggle to draw a breath. Your doctor will be able to help ensure that you get an accurate diagnosis and effective treatment, so do report any worrying symptoms as soon as you notice them. Left untreated, breathing problems can also have a knock-on effect, leading to anxiety and depression.

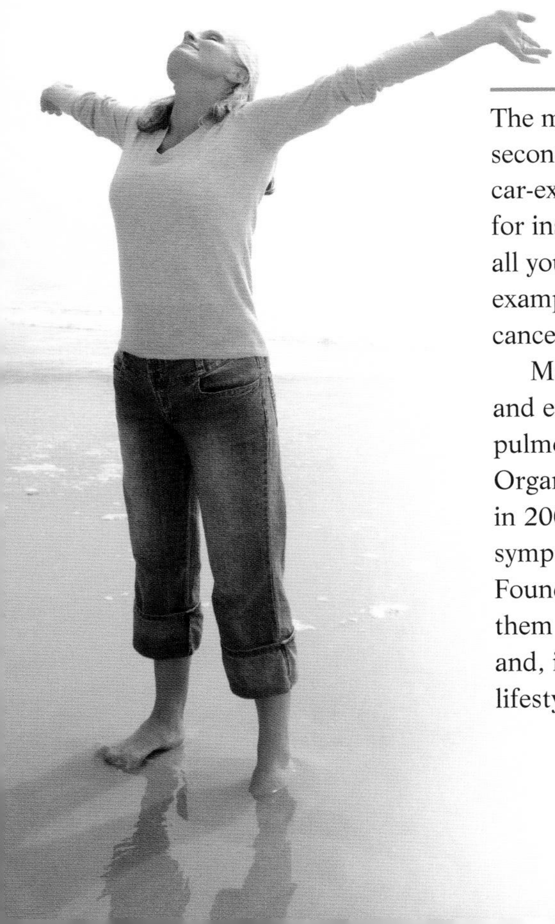

LONG-TERM CONDITIONS

The most common cause of lung problems is smoking, or breathing in secondhand smoke. But they may also be linked to air pollution from car-exhaust fumes and exposure to asbestos, which was once used for insulation and fireproofing. Sometimes the air you've breathed in all your working life can affect your lungs later on. Farmer's lung, for example, is an allergic reaction to a fungus in mouldy hay, while lung cancer can be caused by exposure to asbestos in the workplace.

Many long-term lung problems, including chronic bronchitis and emphysema, come under the umbrella term chronic obstructive pulmonary disease (COPD) – a condition that the World Health Organization estimates affected 64 million people worldwide in 2004. It often goes undiagnosed because people think their symptoms are just part of ageing. According to the Australian Lung Foundation, COPD affects one in seven people over 40 – and half of them don't even know it. Yet it's possible to manage the condition and, in some cases, significantly lessen symptoms by making simple lifestyle changes.

take CARE! PULMONARY EMBOLISM

Any condition that makes the blood sticky or slows down circulation in the veins in the legs can lead to pulmonary embolism.

If you get little exercise or have been bed-bound for any reason, you may be more at risk of pulmonary embolism. An embolus is a 'wandering' blood clot. If a clot (thrombus) develops in the deep veins of the leg, part of it may break off, travel round the body, and block part of one of the blood vessels in the lungs.

Small clots produce no symptoms; medium clots cause sudden breathlessness. A clot big enough to block lung circulation can cause collapse or even sudden death. Smaller wandering clots can break off from a larger clot in the legs and cause sharp pains when you breathe, as the lungs start to bleed temporarily. You may also cough up blood. Treatment is with anticoagulant medication (heparin injections followed by warfarin tablets), which must be continued for several months and stops clots forming so easily. It doesn't dissolve the clot, but prevents it from getting larger and new ones from forming. The body's own healing mechanisms can then get to work to break up the existing clot. Our bodies have a very efficient system for dissolving clots, so most people make a complete recovery, even from a large embolism.

- **Cut your risk** Eat a low-fat, high fruit-and-veg diet; exercise regularly, especially your legs; and watch your weight. Ask your doctor about compression stockings.

Managing COPD

In COPD conditions, the airways are damaged and narrow, making it increasingly hard to breathe in and out. The bronchi (large airways) also become inflamed. See your doctor if you experience symptoms such as a chronic cough, phlegm and breathlessness. You will probably be asked to do a spirometry test: this measures how much air you can expel from your lungs in the first second of breathing out (your FEV1 rate).

If you have COPD, you'll see your doctor regularly so that your condition can be monitored, and you will need to keep taking your medication even if you feel better. Make sure that you stay up to date with jabs, including your yearly flu jab and a one-off pneumococcal vaccination. Keep your inhaler with you always, and ask your nurse or pharmacist to check you're using it properly – many people don't.

But there's more to managing COPD than medical care – there's so much you can do to help yourself. The most important step is to stop smoking – and avoid places where others smoke so that

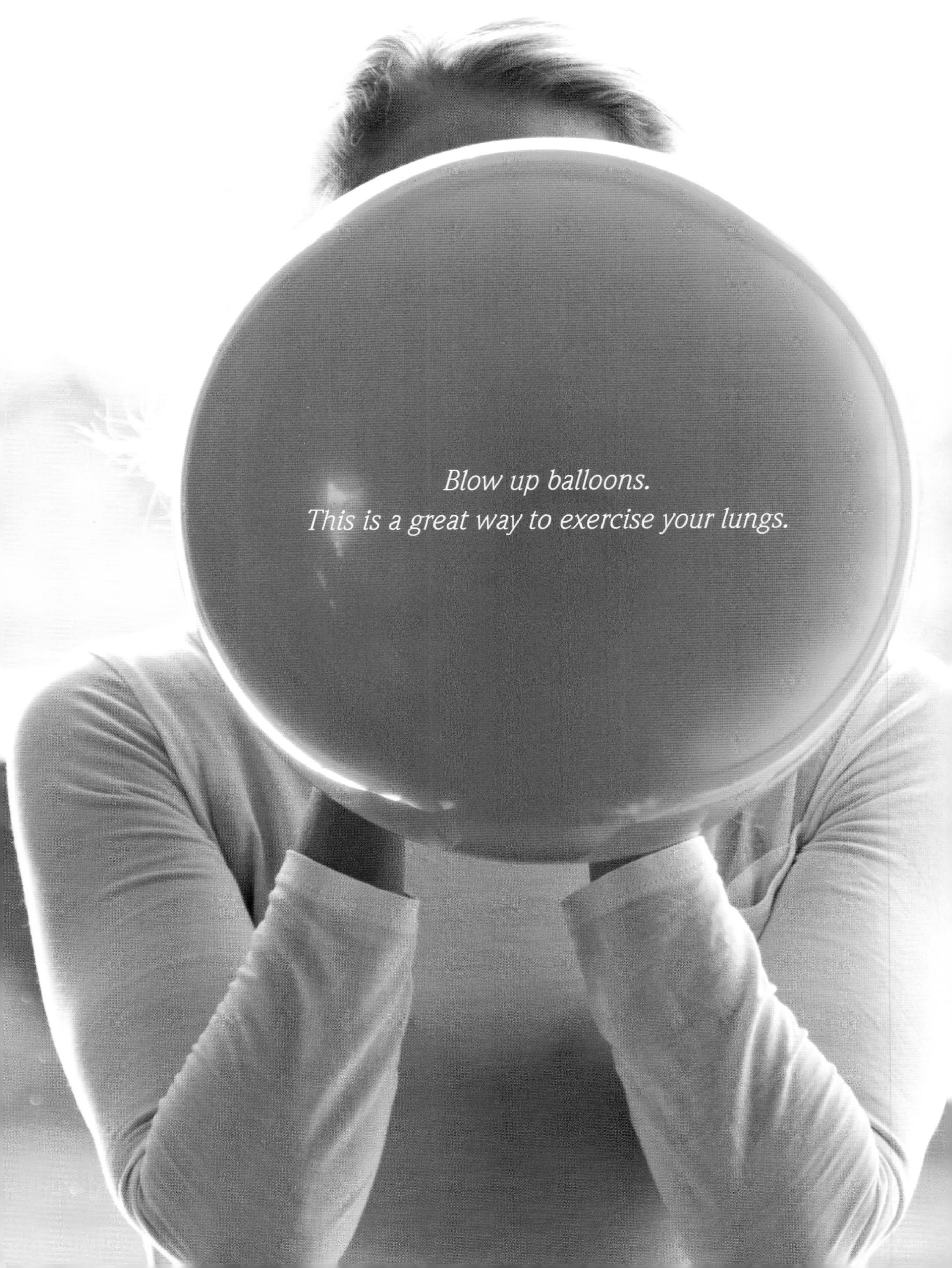

Blow up balloons.
This is a great way to exercise your lungs.

you don't breathe in secondhand fumes. Avoid stress as much as you can, and get plenty of rest – using an extra pillow or sleeping on your side might ease your breathing and help you sleep. Stay away from people with colds and flu since COPD makes you more vulnerable to chest infections. And try these ideas:

- **Do the whistle test** Exhale with your lips pursed – just as if you're whistling. This slows breathing and makes it more efficient. Blowing up balloons is an excellent way to exercise your lungs.
- **Check the forecast** Cold spells lasting for a week or more, and periods of hot weather and humidity, can aggravate breathing problems. Try to plan fewer outdoor activities for these times. Aim to maintain a constant temperature indoors.
- **Say no to scented products** Don't use air-freshener plug-ins or sprays, scented candles, hairspray and perfumes. Use cleaning products only if there's good ventilation in the room.
- **Keep on moving** Inactivity makes things worse. Try to walk, even if only around the house or garden. But pace yourself: keep it slow and steady if that's all you can manage.
- **Watch your weight** Carrying extra weight can exacerbate breathlessness; try to shed some of it. If you're underweight, make an effort to gain some weight: research has shown you'll have fewer symptoms as a result.
- **Eat well, breathe well** Aim to eat food that is high in protein and make sure you get sufficient (but not too many) kilojoules. Eat little and often to avoid getting breathless during meals and feeling bloated. Drink lots of water to keep your airways moist and your sputum thinner.

LUNG CANCER

Anyone can get lung cancer – worldwide, it's the most common cancer – but smokers are most at risk. It's more common in older people: most cases occur in people over 60. Lung cancer develops in the airways. It can grow within the lung and spread outside it. The two main types are small-cell cancer and non–small cell cancer. Symptoms include a cough that

what's NEW

LUNG CANCER SCREENING Spotting lung cancer early gives real hope for a cure. A Cornell University study found that 88 per cent of patients whose lung cancer was picked up by CT scans were still alive after ten years. Now, proposed pilot CT screening trials of 50 to 75-year-olds at high risk of the disease could, if successful, pave the way for screening programs to be introduced elsewhere. When such a screening program was trialled in the USA, it showed a 20 per cent reduction in lung cancer deaths. But it's not ready to go mainstream yet, as many 'false positive' diagnoses were made, exposing people without the disease to the risks of dangerous testing.

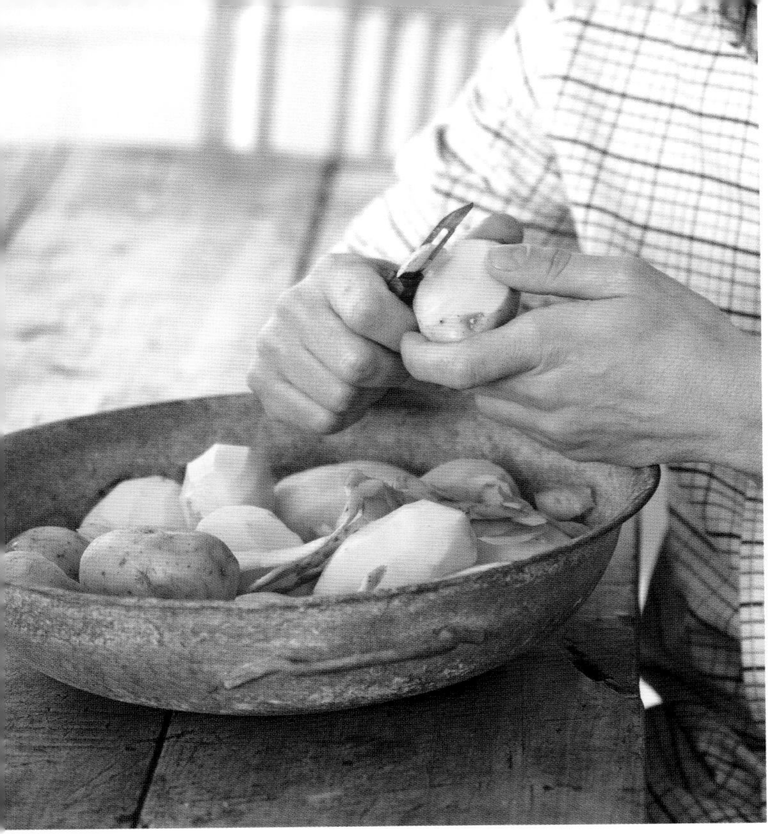

doesn't go away, coughing up blood, breathlessness, unexplained weight loss, excessive fatigue and chest pain.

There may be other reasons for these symptoms, but it's important to see your doctor as soon as you can to get a diagnosis. You may need tests such as a CT or MRI scan, a bronchoscopy (in which a thin, flexible tube is passed into the lungs through your nose or mouth so that photographs or samples may be taken) or a biopsy. If you do have lung cancer, you may need to have surgery, chemotherapy or radiotherapy – depending on where the cancer is, the type of tumour and how far it has spread.

Conserve energy by doing simple activities, such as peeling potatoes, sitting down.

What next?

A diagnosis of lung cancer can come as a huge shock, hitting you with conflicting emotions: fear, anger, resentment, disbelief, even guilt. But there is much you can do, and a great deal of support available – practical and emotional – to help you through. There are strategies to cope with breathlessness, fatigue and anxiety – by changing how you breathe (*see* right) – and practical actions to improve daily life.

Don't try to sort everything out at one go; it may take time to deal with each issue. You'll feel more in control if you're well informed about the implications of your lung cancer. You can write out a list of queries to ask your doctor, such as:

- Can I be cured?
- What treatment will be most effective for my type of lung cancer?
- Will there be side effects from my treatment?
- What practical support is available?
- How will this affect my daily life; will I be able to go shopping, see friends, carry on my hobbies, go on holiday?

Lung cancer organisations can help you find local support, and reputable web forums (such as those of official bodies or government sites) are a way to contact others in the same situation. Make sure any websites you use are approved by experts, unbiased and updated regularly. They should not try to sell you anything.

BE prepared ... Managing BREATHLESSNESS

There are many ways to make life easier if breathlessness has become an everyday problem. With the right support and strategies, your daily routine may be largely unchanged and you can continue to do the things that you enjoy.

People with long-term lung conditions may find their lungs can't provide enough oxygen for their muscles to perform even simple tasks. If you're permanently short of breath, it can make you feel very tired and eventually everything becomes a struggle. But there's no need for it to be like this. Here are some ways to take the strain off your lungs:

● **CONSERVE ENERGY** Do simple activities such as brushing your teeth, peeling potatoes or showering sitting down. And instead of drying yourself with a towel, put on a towelling bath robe.

● **THINK AHEAD** When you're going downstairs, carry everything you need in a bag or basket to reduce trips upstairs. Similarly, gather everything you need for household tasks before you start. And carry a cordless or mobile phone so you don't have to walk to take a call.

● **USE YOUR BREATH** When climbing stairs, pace your breathing. Breathe in time with the steps you take; use a rhythm that suits you, depending on how breathless you are. For example, breathe in for one stair and out for one stair, or in for two stairs and out for three. During the hardest part of any action – blow as you go.

● **FIND SUPPORT** When you need to stand up for prolonged periods, lean from the hips with your forearms resting on something of the right height – chairs, windowsills, kitchen work surfaces and supermarket trolleys are often ideal supports.

● **BEAT THE BLOAT** Limit your intake of gas-forming foods such as onions, raw apples and cucumber. A bloated stomach reduces lung space and might make breathing uncomfortable.

● **AND RELAX ...** Learn relaxation techniques, visualise a favourite walk or listen to music to reduce anxiety, which makes breathlessness worse.

Using oxygen

If low blood-oxygen levels are causing your breathlessness, you could benefit from using oxygen at home. This can be delivered to you in several different forms – for example, an oxygen concentrator, oxygen cylinders (portable and non-portable) and liquid oxygen.

● **SAFETY FIRST** Make sure no one smokes when you're using oxygen: it is highly combustible, plus the carbon monoxide in tobacco smoke makes the oxygen less effective.

Even if you need to use oxygen, you may still be able to travel by air if your doctor says you're fit enough to fly and provides written support. You can pre-arrange to buy on-board oxygen before you travel (planes carry emergency supplies only). Make sure your travel insurance covers medical costs arising from your lung condition.

● **REMEMBER** Keep your inhalers and medication in your hand luggage; move about every hour and exercise your legs; drink plenty of water.

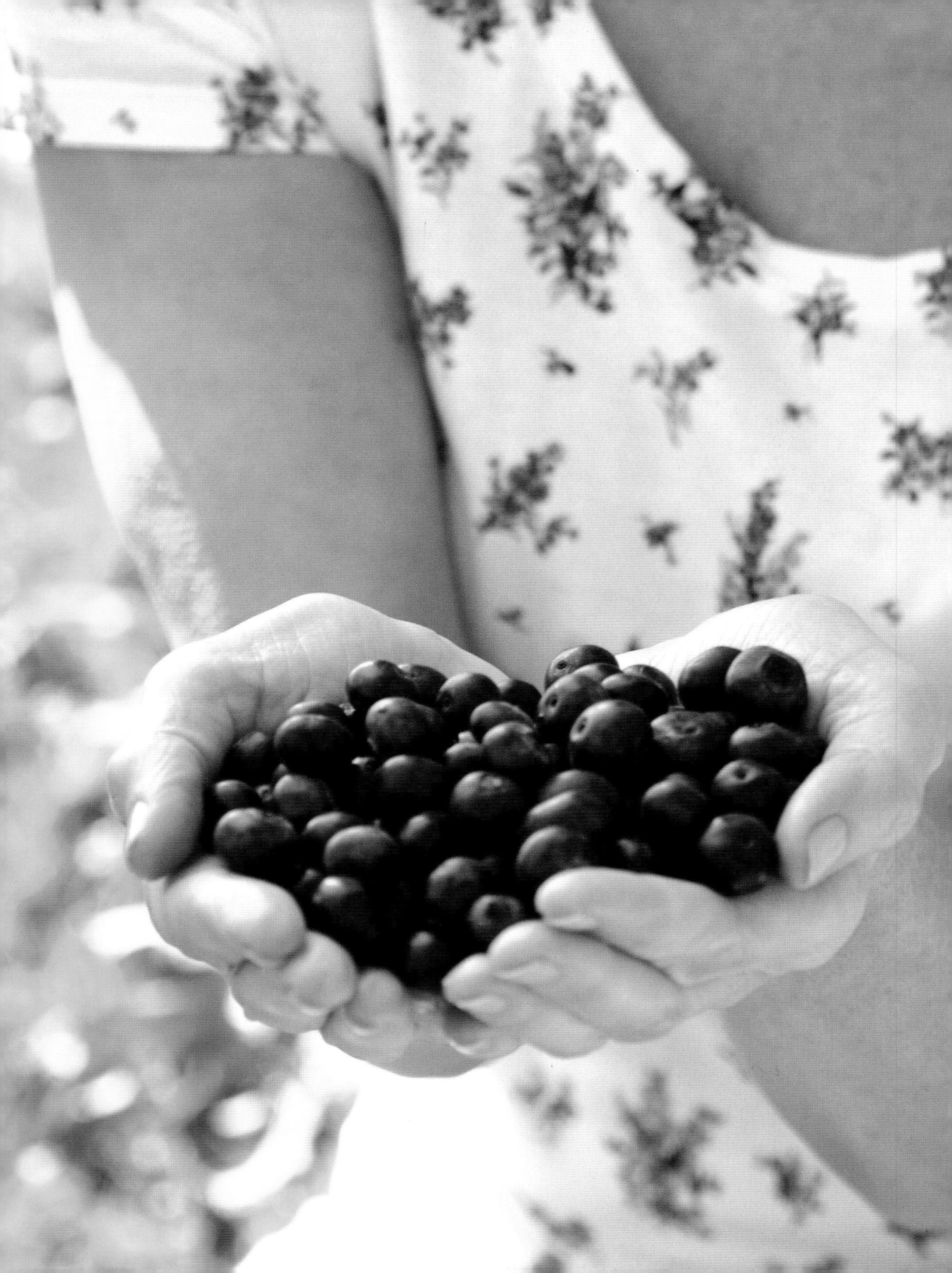

4

Eat, drink & LIVE WELL

You are what you eat. The health of your body reflects your diet. All the more so as you grow older: adopting sensible eating habits is probably the single best thing you can do to live longer – feeling fit and energetic, and free from chronic disease. The physical and lifestyle changes that generally occur after the age of 60 may mean you need to make a few dietary adjustments, but this isn't difficult and there's much pleasure to be had from discovering new ways to cook and eat.

Olive oil was a key element in the diet of Jeanne Calment, who lived to 122.

FOOD FOR LIFE
your diet, your body

Eating well doesn't mean following faddy diets. All the scientific evidence suggests that simply choosing to eat a wide range of delicious healthy foods can help keep you strong and fit well into old age.

As you grow older, a balanced diet becomes increasingly important. It improves your physical performance, as measured by your walking speed and leg strength; it boosts your bone health; it reduces your risk of some of the conditions associated with age, such as diabetes, high blood pressure, heart attack and various cancers; and lastly, for all these reasons, it increases life expectancy.

The basic principles of a healthy diet – as recommended by the World Health Organization (WHO) – can be summarised in three simple steps:

- **Eat more plants** That means more fruit and vegetables, legumes (such as beans, peas and lentils) as well as nuts and cereals (of the wholegrain variety).
- **Cut the white stuff** Reduce your consumption of salt and sugar.
- **Be fat-aware** Cut back on fat, and when you do eat fats, choose unsaturated rather than saturated or trans fats (*see* page 86).

Eat foods that are naturally rich in iodine, such as shellfish.

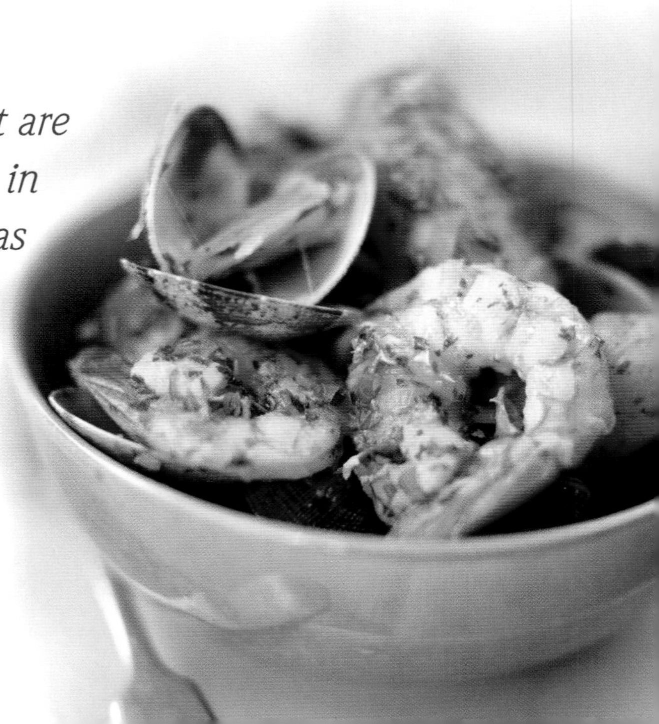

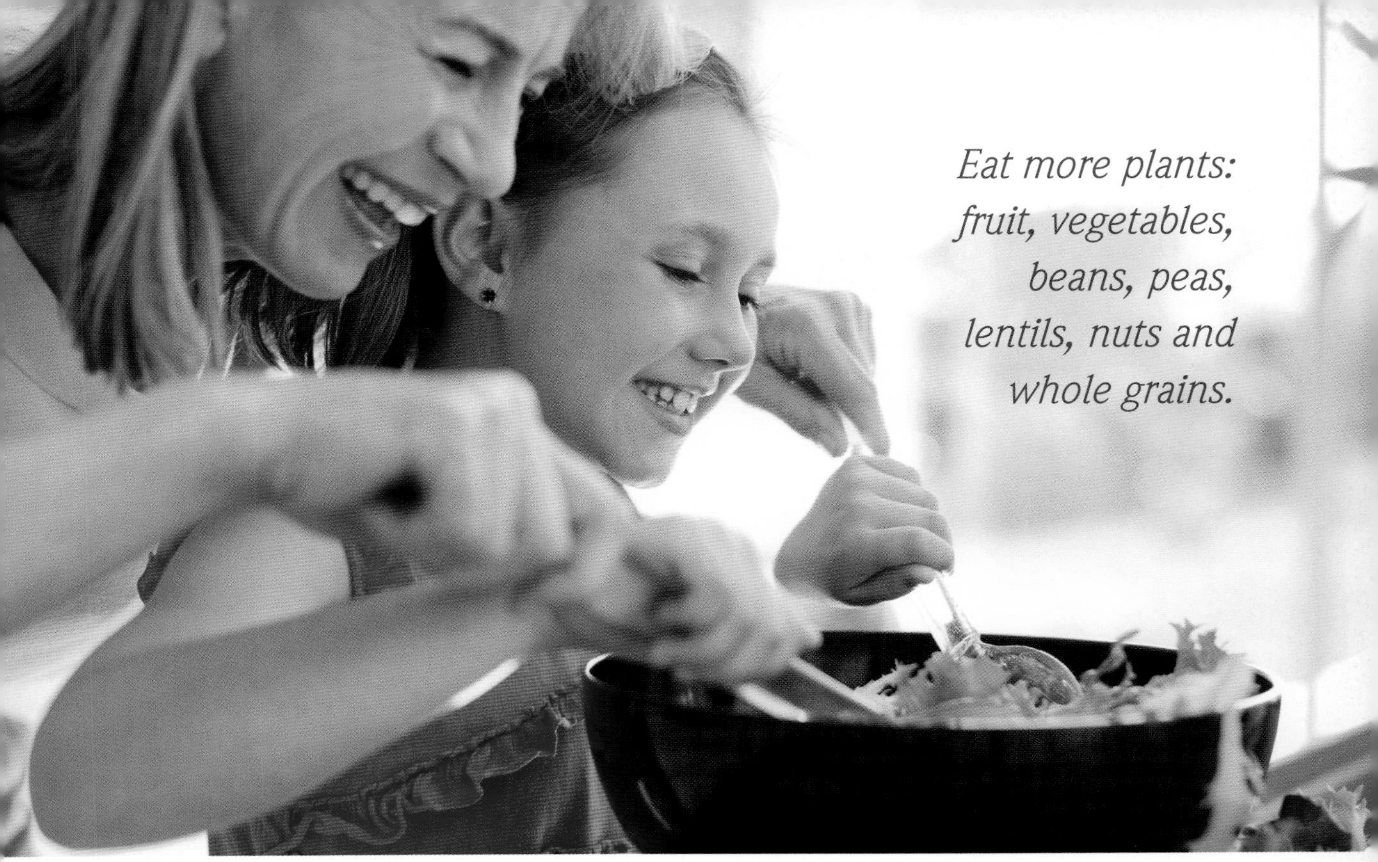

Everyone has individual energy needs, which vary according to our size, gender and lifestyle. WHO recommends maintaining a healthy weight, and 'energy balance'. In other words, you should make sure that your kilojoule intake from food and drink doesn't exceed what you use up in physical activity.

You should also ensure that you take in enough iodine: iodine deficiency is now common in our modern Western diets and can lead to thyroid problems in older people. One way to do this is to ensure that any salt you use is iodised (meaning it contains added iodine). It also helps to eat foods that are naturally rich in iodine, for example, fish, shellfish and seaweed, cows' milk, yogurt, eggs, strawberries, baked potatoes with the skin on and turkey breast.

FROM THE MED TO OKINAWA

There's lots of research showing that one particular diet appears to boost longevity. The traditional Mediterranean diet is rich in exactly the kind of foods that WHO recommends for everybody. It includes lots of fruit and vegetables, legumes, nuts and whole grains. It also has minimal meat but plenty of fish, moderate amounts of red wine and poultry, and olive oil, which is rich in healthy monounsaturated fats. In research conducted at the University of Cambridge, using data from a large US study, the diets of nearly 400,000 people who were all retired were scored on how closely they corresponded to a Mediterranean diet. Ten years later, those who had the highest scores were 20 per cent less likely to have died than those who had the lowest scores.

Or take the Okinawa islands in Japan, famed for having the highest percentage of people over 100 years old in the world. Okinawa's centenarians age slowly, and delay or escape many apparently age-related conditions such as dementia and cancer. When they become frail and die, they tend to do so rapidly rather than after suffering years of ill health.

'Happiness depends on a leisurely breakfast.'

John Gunther, US journalist

Okinawans may have genes that promote longevity and, like traditional Mediterranean peoples, they are generally active, have supportive communities and revere their elders, all of which are known to contribute to better ageing. But scientists believe that their diet is also crucial in maintaining health in later life. It is mainly vegetable-based, high in water and fibre, low in kilojoules but nutrient-rich in vitamins and minerals. Staples include sweet potatoes, rather than rice as in the rest of Japan, along with seaweed, health-promoting spices and green tea.

Lessons of Okinawa

When Okinawans abandon their traditional habits, the health benefits disappear. This has been seen in both the younger generation living in Okinawa and in migrants to Brazil and Hawaii, who suffer from increased obesity, high blood pressure, high cholesterol, diabetes and heart disease, and have a consequently shorter life expectancy. But take heart from the fact that this works the other way round, too: if your diet isn't ideal now, then you can effect a huge change to your health by altering the way you eat.

A study at the Medical University of South Carolina tracked 15,708 people aged 45 to 64. At the start, 8.5 per cent scored on four healthy habits including eating at least five serves of fruit and vegetables daily and doing regular exercise. After six years, a further 8.4 per cent had adopted healthy lifestyles. Four years after that, these 'late adopters' were 40 per cent less likely to have died, and 35 per cent less likely to have had a heart attack or a stroke, than those who didn't follow a healthy lifestyle.

8 SUPER FOODS for the third age

Why 'super foods'? Because these foods contain high levels of health-boosting 'phytochemicals': anti-oxidants, vitamins, minerals and compounds such as flavonoids that protect against heart disease, cancer and perhaps cognitive decline.

1 BERRIES contain polyphenols – anti-oxidants that help reduce the risk factors for cardiovascular disease. Blueberries and grape juice improve memory and cognitive function in older people, according to Jean Mayer at Boston's Human Nutrition Research Center on Aging.

2 CRUCIFEROUS VEGETABLES – broccoli, Brussels sprouts, cabbage – may boost longevity. A study of 135,000 people in Shanghai, China, found that the risk of death over five or ten years reduced the more fruit and vegetables the participants ate, particularly cruciferous vegetables.

3 HONEY promotes healing of wounds and burns, reduces coughing and may help lower cholesterol and ward off heart disease and cancer. When researchers at the University of Wales analysed the diets that 655 men had reported 25 years earlier, they found the subsequent death rate among the 41 men who had recorded eating honey to be less than half that of the remainder.

4 GREEN TEA helps reduce blood-cholesterol levels and protects against heart disease; it also seems to guard against tooth loss, aid weight management and protect against sun damage.

5 WALNUTS contain anti-oxidants and omega-3 fatty acids that may improve brain function. A Californian study of 87 people with high cholesterol found that eating walnuts for six months improved cholesterol levels.

6 RED WINE contains anti-oxidants that help mop up harmful free radicals – chemicals that promote 'furring up' of the artery walls. Having one or two drinks a day has been linked with a lower death rate from cardiovascular disease.

7 GARLIC helps fight infection and reduce high blood pressure, and may protect against cardiovascular disease and cancer. In one study of 65 patients with an average age of 60 and at risk of cardiovascular disease, those given a garlic extract showed evidence of healthier blood fats after a year.

8 TOMATOES are rich in anti-oxidants, especially the compound lycopene, which is linked to a lower risk of cancer and cardiovascular disease. Cook them with olive oil – the nutrients are better absorbed that way.

Boost longevity with brussels sprouts.

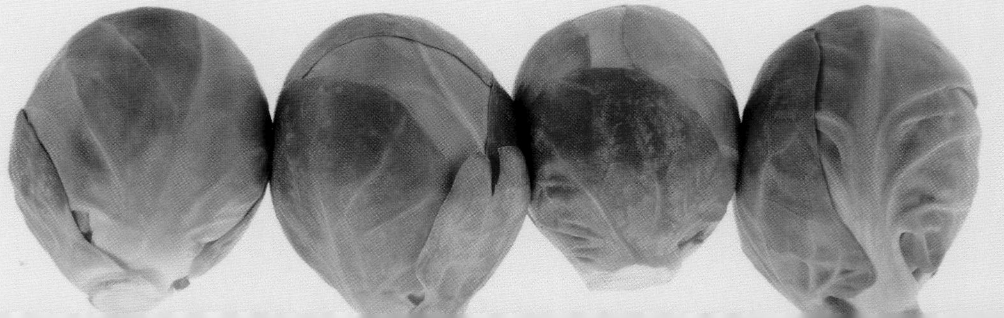

Quiz How does **your diet** fare?

Most of us think we eat more healthily than we actually do. This quiz will help you to check your diet rating. Pick the answer that's nearest to your experience.

1 Which is closest to your typical breakfast?

- ☐ **A** Nothing, or just coffee or tea
- ☐ **B** Porridge or wholegrain cereals/toast, fruit, yogurt
- ☐ **C** White toast and marmalade, sugar-coated cereals or a fry-up

2 How many wholegrain serves do you eat in a typical week? (A serve is 1 slice of wholegrain bread, half a wholemeal pita, 3 tbsp wholegrain breakfast cereal, 3 tbsp cooked brown pasta or 1 tbsp uncooked oats.)

- ☐ **A** None
- ☐ **B** More than 7
- ☐ **C** 1 to 7

3 How often do you eat takeaway or fast foods (such as burgers or kebabs)**?**

- ☐ **A** Three or more times a week
- ☐ **B** Less than once a week
- ☐ **C** Once or twice a week

4 If you fancy a snack, which of these would you be most likely to choose?

- ☐ **A** Chips, biscuits or cakes
- ☐ **B** Fruit, raisins, carrot sticks and hummus, unsalted nuts or yogurt
- ☐ **C** Cheese and crackers

5 Which of these do you use most for cooking?

- ☐ **A** Butter or lard
- ☐ **B** Olive oil or rapeseed oil
- ☐ **C** Polyunsaturated vegetable oils (such as corn oil or sunflower oil)

6 How often do you eat seven or more portions of fruit and vegetables a day?

- ☐ **A** Twice a week or less
- ☐ **B** Daily (or almost)
- ☐ **C** 3 or 4 times a week

7 How often do you eat processed meats? (Processed meats include sausages, meat pies, burgers, hot dogs, salami, bacon and ham.)

- ☐ **A** Three or more times per week
- ☐ **B** Less than once a week
- ☐ **C** Once or twice a week

8 If you're thirsty, which of these would you choose?

- ☐ **A** Fizzy, diet or sugared drinks (for instance, cola or squash)
- ☐ **B** Water (still or sparkling) or tea
- ☐ **C** Pure fruit juice, milk or coffee

9 In a typical week are you likely to eat?

- ☐ **A** Only fish in batter or breadcrumbs or occasionally fish fingers or fish cakes, if I eat any fish at all
- ☐ **B** One or two portions of oily fish: salmon, trout, mackerel or sardines
- ☐ **C** No oily fish, but at least one portion of frozen uncoated white fish/shellfish or canned tuna

What's your favourite snack?

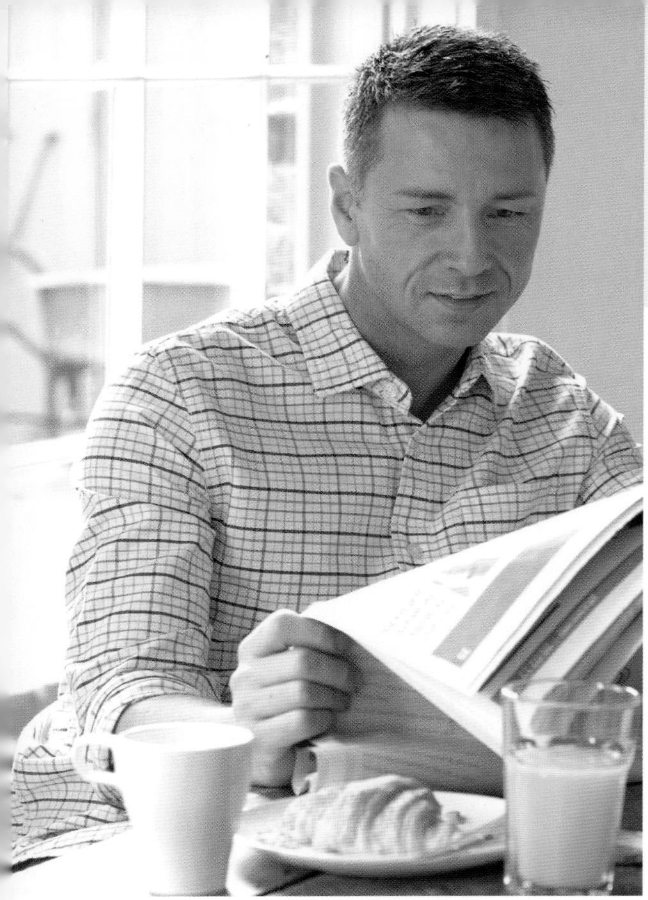

How healthy is your breakfast?

WHY IT MATTERS

1 People who eat breakfast are less likely to be overweight. Scientists across the world have found that skipping breakfast may increase the chance of becoming overweight or obese by 75 per cent.

2 Whole grains help to control body weight and reduce the risk of cardiovascular disease, diabetes and cancer; studies involving nearly 2 million people showed that three daily serves of whole grains reduced bowel cancer risk by around 17 per cent.

3 Fast foods increase weight gain, obesity, type 2 diabetes and heart disease. A University of North Carolina study found people who ate the most fast food gained on average 5.6 kg more in weight and 5.3 cm extra round the waist over ten years compared with those with the lowest intakes.

4 Snacks can actually help you maintain a healthy body weight and may add nutritional value – if, of course, they're healthy. Chips, biscuits and cakes tend to contain salt, trans fats and sugar.

5 Saturated fats raise blood cholesterol and heart disease risk, whereas olive oil is a major ingredient in the Mediterranean diet. Studies in Spain, Italy and Greece suggest that irrespective of the rest of their diet, people with a high olive oil consumption are less likely to have a heart attack.

6 WHO recommends eating at least 400 g of fruit and vegetables (excluding potatoes) every day to cut your risk of heart disease, cancer, diabetes and obesity.

7 Almost all processed meats contain cancer-promoting chemicals and are linked with an increased risk of cardiovascular disease. WHO recommends avoiding them altogether.

8 Sugary and diet drinks promote obesity. Tea is as thirst-quenching as water and is associated with a reduced risk of cardiovascular disease and diabetes; the effects of coffee on health are less clear.

9 Eating fish has been linked with better cognitive function (thinking power) in later life. The omega-3 fatty acids in oily fish reduce the risk of cardiovascular disease, but more than two portions a week may increase diabetes risk (limit oily fish to minimise your intake of mercury and other pollutants).

SCORE

MOSTLY A Your diet is lacking in many respects. Now's the time to start making some healthy food switches to boost your chances of a healthy old age.

MOSTLY B Your dietary habits are excellent, keep it up.

MOSTLY C Your diet's not bad, but introducing a few small changes would make it much healthier.

The art of eating

It's not just *what* you eat that affects your health, it's *how* you eat as well. In many Mediterranean countries, for example, dining tends to be a leisurely, social affair, often including children, extended family and friends. Meals are frequently taken outdoors, and ingredients are generally fresh, purchased with care, cooked lovingly and attractively presented. Portions are reasonably sized, and alcohol, most often red wine, is usually drunk with meals.

What could be a more delightful way to improve your health? Food taken seriously becomes one of life's pleasures, rather than a chore or a hasty refuel. There's another advantage to being older: if you don't have to rush to the office, you have more time to savour your food. You can eat less, but enjoy it more.

Even if you live alone, you can make mealtimes more enticing by taking care over how you present your food. Lay your table with care and eat slowly so you can savour every bite – and if you're trying to lose weight, there's a bonus to eating alone: you're less likely to over-eat than people who eat alongside family or friends, according to a small study at Glasgow Caledonian University.

DID **you** KNOW?

Older people generally need fewer kilojoules, so it makes sense to pack your diet with nutrient-rich foods. The Australian National Health and Medical Research Council recommends that women aged 51 to 70 eat about 6200 kJ of energy a day; for men, the figure is about 6500 kJ a day.

THE PERFECT BALANCE

Few of us are going to adopt a radically different diet, whatever the health benefits. It is mostly a question of altering the proportions of the elements in your diet while avoiding over-eating (which is unhealthy and uncomfortable).

● **RAMP UP THE VEGETABLES** Fruit and vegetables provide fibre ('roughage') and vital vitamins and minerals, as well as offering protection against virtually all the diseases of ageing. They should comprise about a third of your food intake. Not eating enough fruit and vegetables is a direct factor in 11 per cent of deaths from heart disease, according to WHO. A 2011 Cancer UK report blamed 6.1 per cent of all cancers in men and 3.4 per cent in women on a lack of fruit and vegetables. So:

- Eat at least seven portions a day – some experts say nine portions. A portion is a medium-sized vegetable or piece of fresh fruit or two small fruits, such as plums or peach halves, or six apricot halves (note that portion sizes are roughly the same for unsweetened stewed/canned fruit).

- If you have problems with chewing or your digestion, eating raw fruit and vegetables could be difficult. Experiment with homemade, vitamin-packed soups and smoothies.

- **CHOOSE CARBS WITH CARE** Starchy carbohydrate-laden foods such as potatoes, rice and bread provide most of the body's energy. Carbohydrates should comprise a third of your kilojoule intake. Choose whole grains (wholegrain bread, brown rice), which provide fibre and contain more vitamins and minerals than refined varieties.

- **PACK A PROTEIN PUNCH** The final third of a healthy diet comes from other foods, with protein-rich meat, fish, poultry, eggs, beans and lentils making up the largest proportion. Protein foods are vital as we age – older adults require about 25 per cent more protein per kilogram of body weight than younger people, more at times of illness or other stress. That's because muscle is made of protein, and muscle declines from around 45 per cent of total body weight in youth to about 27 per cent by age 70. Lack of protein contributes to muscle weakness, impaired wound/fracture healing, reduced immunity, longer recuperation from illness and loss of skin elasticity.

Eat outdoors. What could be a more delightful way to improve your health?

- **DAIRY MATTERS** You lose bone mass progressively with age, so a good intake of calcium and vitamin D is essential to maintain bone health. Dairy products such as milk, cheese and yogurt are rich in

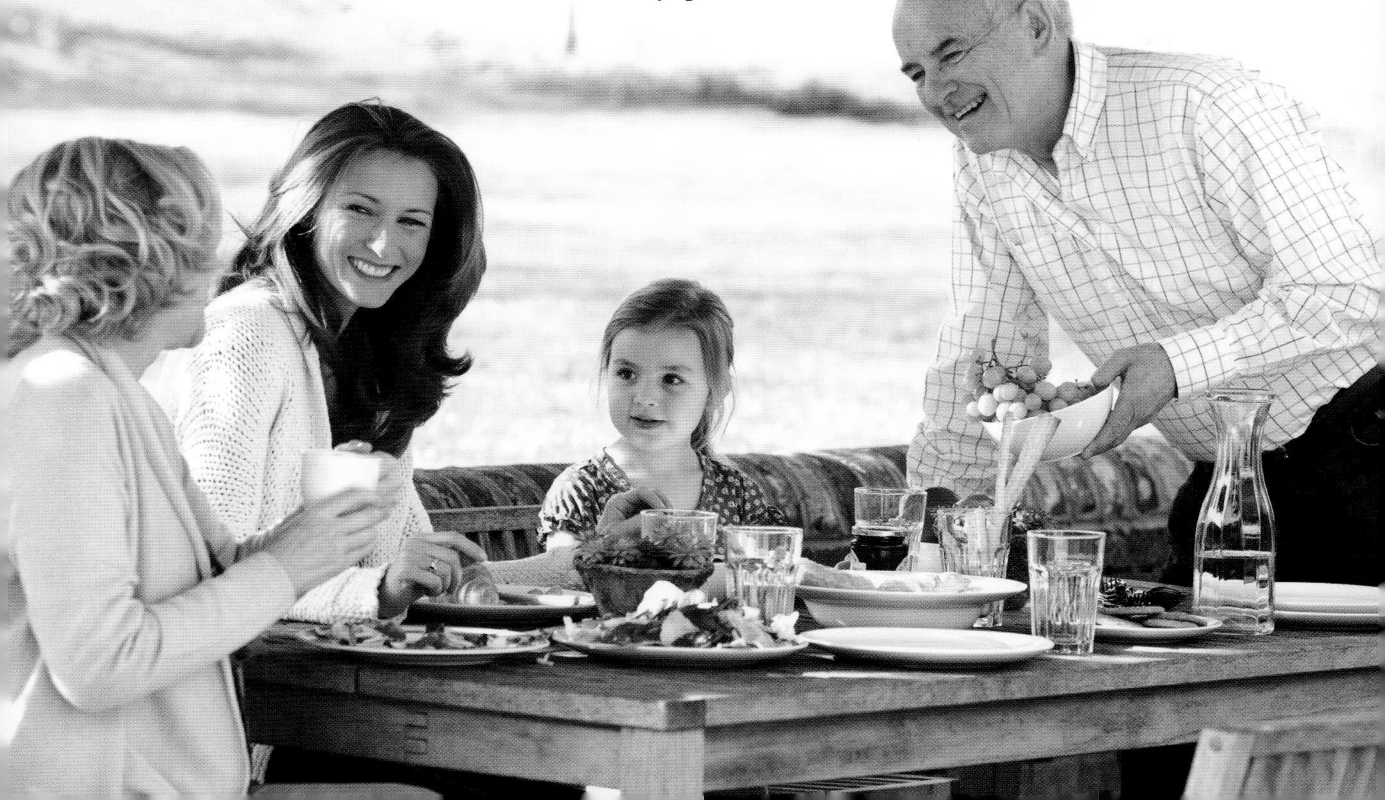

focus ON ... FAT

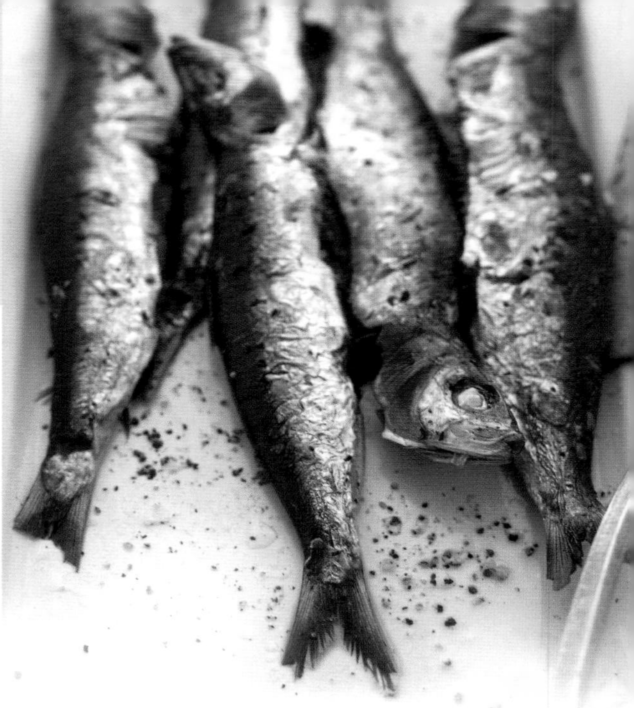

Fat makes food tasty, but moderation is key. Eating too much of certain types of fat is harmful, while other fats are vital, whatever your age. The healthiest choices come from plant and fish sources.

The good, the bad and the ugly

There are two main types of fat: saturated and unsaturated. Both contain the same number of kilojoules, but saturated fat is often classed as 'bad' fat. Here's what you need to know to be fat aware:

- **SATURATED FAT** – foods rich in saturated fat, such as cheese, cakes and pastry, lead to obesity, raise blood cholesterol and increase your risk of cardiovascular disease and type 2 diabetes. They should all be eaten sparingly. When you shop for food, compare the fat contents and choose lower-fat options (less than 1.5 g of saturated fat per 100 g).

- **UNSATURATED FATS** – largely found in plants and fish. These are healthier, but you still need to know what's what. There are two types: **monounsaturated** and **polyunsaturated**.

  Monounsaturated fat – in olive oil, avocados, salmon, walnuts – lowers blood cholesterol, cuts heart disease risk and helps with diabetes. A Harvard Medical School study of women aged 60-plus found those who ate more monounsaturated fat were protected against cognitive decline.

  Polyunsaturated fat – comes in various forms. We need good **omega-3 essential fatty acids** for health, and to help us fight against heart disease and diabetes. Omega-3 also boosts mental performance and memory, and protects against cognitive decline and depression. The best source is mackerel, closely followed by other oily fish (salmon, sardines and pilchards), as well as some plant foods such as flaxseeds (linseeds) and walnuts.

  Then there are **omega-6 fatty acids**, which are found in many vegetable oils such as palm, safflower and sunflower oil. While essential, we eat too many. The human diet once had a ratio of omega-6s to omega-3s of about 1:1 – in modern diets it's 15:1 or more. The result: a higher risk of all sorts of diseases, including cancer. Switch to olive oil – and avoid processed and takeaway foods, which often contain cheaper oils.

Oily fish is a rich source of brain-boosting omega-3.

- **Banish trans fats** Created by a process called hydrogenation, these are the biggest threat to health. Found in some spreads and baked goods, they act like a kind of toxic saturated fat, significantly increasing the risk of heart disease. Some manufacturers are phasing them out, but if you spot the words 'hydrogenated' or 'partially hydrogenated' on the packet, steer clear.

calcium and supply valuable protein, but they contain vitamin D only if they are fortified (and you should choose low-fat forms to avoid unhealthy saturated fats; for the same reason, keep your intake of butter and cream low). If you can't or don't like to eat dairy foods, alternative sources of calcium include canned fish that are eaten along with their bones (salmon or sardines – also good for vitamin D), leafy green vegetables, baked beans, sesame seeds, almonds, tofu and dried figs. Oily fish, eggs, and fortified cereals and spreads are good sources of vitamin D.

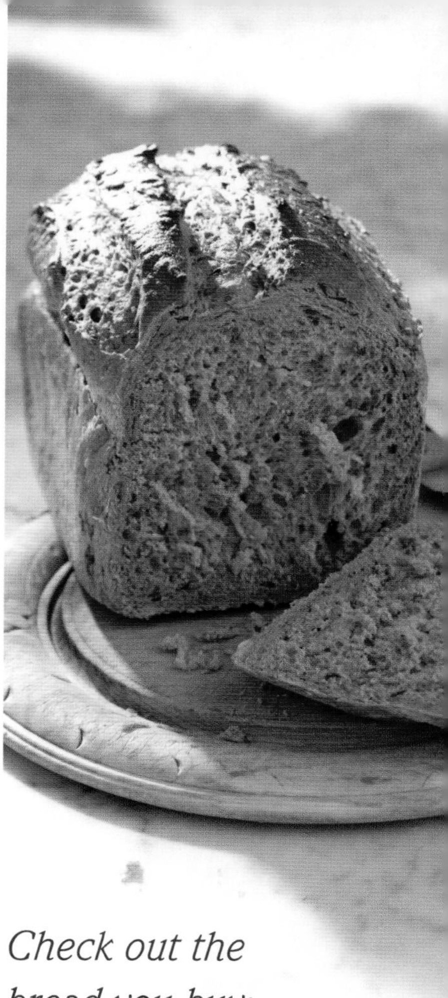

● **EAT THE RIGHT FAT** Fats should make up the smallest part of your diet. There's been much health advice about the importance of limiting saturated fats, the type found in animal products. But not all fats are bad for you, and some are essential. The monounsaturated fat found in olive oil, and the type of polyunsaturated fat called omega-3 fatty acids, for instance, are proven health-boosters that actively protect against various diseases (*see* left).

● **BE SALT-AWARE** Most of us eat far more salt than the daily 2.3 g maximum recommended. Excess salt is a known factor in raised blood pressure and heart disease. Most of the salt we eat comes not from what we add in cooking or at the table but from the hidden salt in processed foods, so the easiest way to cut down is to stop eating these foods or at least check the labels for salt content before you buy.

The chemical name for salt is sodium chloride, so it's sometimes listed as sodium. High-salt foods are those containing more than 1.5 g salt, or 0.6 g sodium, per 100 g. And check out the bread you buy: even apparently healthy loaves can contain a high level of salt. One advantage of retirement is that you may now have the time to make your own bread (a bread-maker cuts out the effort), and can control the amount of salt in it, as well as other ingredients. Give it a go! Many people, once they start, find baking bread to be an absorbing hobby and soothingly therapeutic.

Check out the bread you buy: even healthy loaves can contain a high level of salt ... try baking your own.

● **CUT BACK ON SUGAR** Finally, there is the small matter of sugar – most of us eat far too much of the wrong kind. The natural kind present in fruit and milk is generally healthy, but the refined sugar in processed foods such as cakes, biscuits, sweets, chocolate, ice cream, fizzy drinks and pastries is high in kilojoules but has little nutritional value. Watch out, too, for hidden sugar –

take CARE! THE PERILS of BACON

A bacon sandwich is a thing of pleasure, there's no denying it. But it's doing your health no favours – nor are most other processed meat products.

According to scientists advising the World Cancer Research Fund, bacon and hot dogs should be avoided as much as possible. The same applies to ham, salami, most sausages and some minced meats preserved with salt or chemicals.

Processed meats often contain added chemicals, usually sodium nitrite, to help preserve them. In the body these are converted to carcinogens called nitrosamines. Researchers at the Harvard School of Public Health found that each additional daily 50 g serve of processed meat raised the risk of heart disease by 42 per cent and diabetes by 19 per cent. And an article in the *British Journal of Cancer* reported that Swedish researchers have found that just two rashers of bacon a day can up your risk of pancreatic cancer by 19 per cent.

● **Natural remedy** If you can't give up the occasional bacon sandwich, try having a grapefruit or an orange at the same time – the natural vitamin C helps block nitrosamines.

in foods that don't taste sweet – bread, frozen meals, tomato sauce and canned soup and vegetables. Too much sugar contributes to tooth decay, so learn to look on sweet foods as very occasional treats, and aim to keep your sugar intake as low as possible.

SUPPLEMENTARY BENEFITS

It's usually possible (and preferable) to get all the nutrients that you need from a balanced diet. But this can sometimes be difficult, especially as you get older and your body becomes less efficient at absorbing some vitamins and minerals. For one thing, you may need fewer kilojoules (which is why it's important to ensure that those you get are packed full of nutrients) – and illness, medications or surgery may deplete stores or impair absorption just as your needs increase. Here are four supplements worth considering in later life:

● **CALCIUM** Many older people are advised by doctors to take a calcium supplement (usually combined with vitamin D, which helps with absorption) if they don't get enough calcium, to prevent the bone-weakening condition osteoporosis. It is usually best to take a supplement that contains magnesium because you need a balance between the two minerals for optimum bone health.

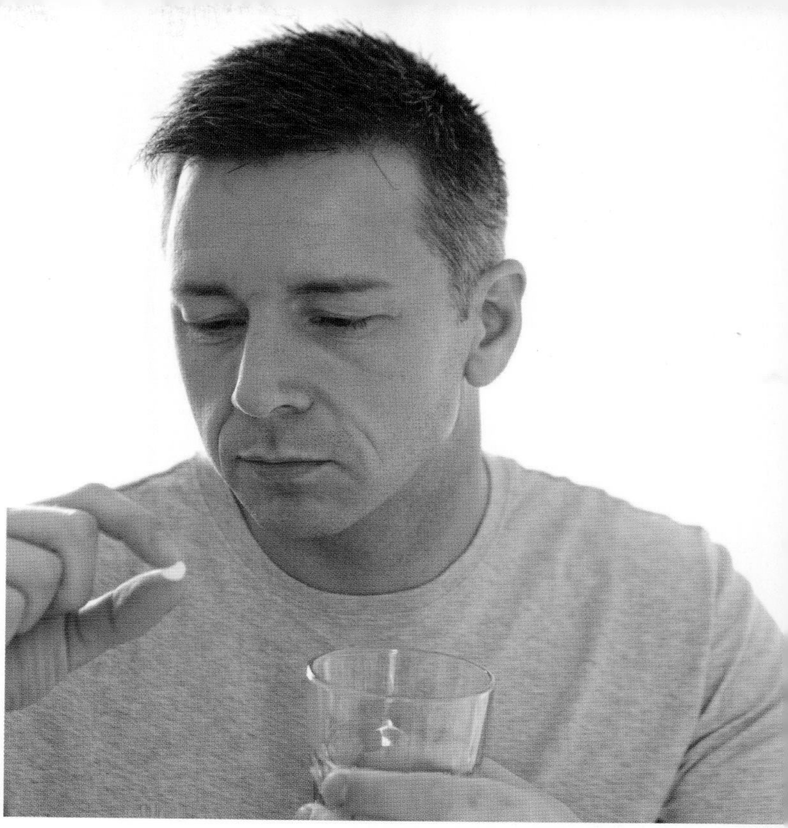

● **VITAMIN D** This nutrient has many health benefits including increased muscle strength, function and balance (according to a Swiss study, taking vitamin D supplements reduces falls among older people by about a fifth). Other studies suggest it may also offer protection against various cancers, multiple sclerosis and Parkinson's disease. Vitamin D can be made in the body by the action of sunlight on the skin – as we get older, our skin synthesises vitamin D less well, which is why it's a good idea to eat foods rich in vitamin D (such as oily fish) or take a supplement. Vitamin D absorption may be aided by a diet rich in monounsaturated fatty acids, such as olive oil, rather than polyunsaturates.

According to a Swiss study, taking vitamin D supplements reduces falls among older people by about a fifth.

● **OMEGA-3** If you don't like oily fish, consider supplements of fish oils or omega-3 fatty acids. They are essential for the health of the heart and the brain. Cod-liver oil supplements are a good source of omega-3s, but also contain vitamin A, so you shouldn't take them with other supplements that contain vitamin A.

● **PROBIOTIC** A probiotic supplement can boost gastro-intestinal health by maintaining a good level of 'friendly' bacteria in the gut – this helps keep conditions such as thrush in check. Probiotics are particularly useful after taking antibiotics, which deplete the number of friendly bacteria in your intestines.

It's important to realise that not all supplements are beneficial (and it's certainly not the case that more is better). In one study of nearly 39,000 older women followed for nearly 20 years, overall mortality was reduced among those taking calcium supplements but increased among women taking iron.

Eat at least two serves of protein a day to help your body heal.

EAT WELL
to get well

To speed recovery from illness or surgery, your body needs good food. At first you may have little appetite, but you must try to eat enough to help the healing process and raise your energy levels. You'll get better more quickly if you do.

When you're ill, it can be hard to make the effort to eat healthily. You won't want large meals, so have small portions and wholesome snacks at frequent intervals. Try to keep your fridge and pantry well stocked – good stand-bys are dried milk, canned fish, canned fruit, vegetables and pulses, oatcakes and long-life juice. If you can't get to the shops, ask a friend or neighbour to help, and make use of internet shopping options to have your groceries delivered.

Make sure everything you do eat packs a hefty nutritional punch: at times of recuperation, it's especially important to ensure your diet contains adequate supplies of all the food groups. If you've had surgery, your body may need more kilojoules, protein, vitamins A and C, and possibly zinc – these all aid wound healing. And:

- Eat at least two serves of protein a day (grilled chicken or fish, cold meats, eggs, nuts or cheese are all good options).
- Fill up on wholegrain bread and peanut butter or cottage cheese, cereal with yogurt and fruit, porridge with dried fruit and honey.
- Make a pot of nutrient-rich chicken or meat soup – it's easy to swallow and will last a few meals (reheat only what you need).
- Have vitamin C-rich fruit (citrus, strawberries, tomatoes) and vitamin A-rich vegetables (dark green leaves, carrots) every day.
- If you feel nauseous or have a disturbed sense of taste, cold food – chicken sandwiches, cottage cheese or tuna – may be more appealing.
- Avoid coffee, fizzy drinks and sweets and biscuits, which can dull the appetite.

'Tell me what you eat, and I will tell you what you are.'

Jean Anthelme Brillat-Savarin, French gastronome

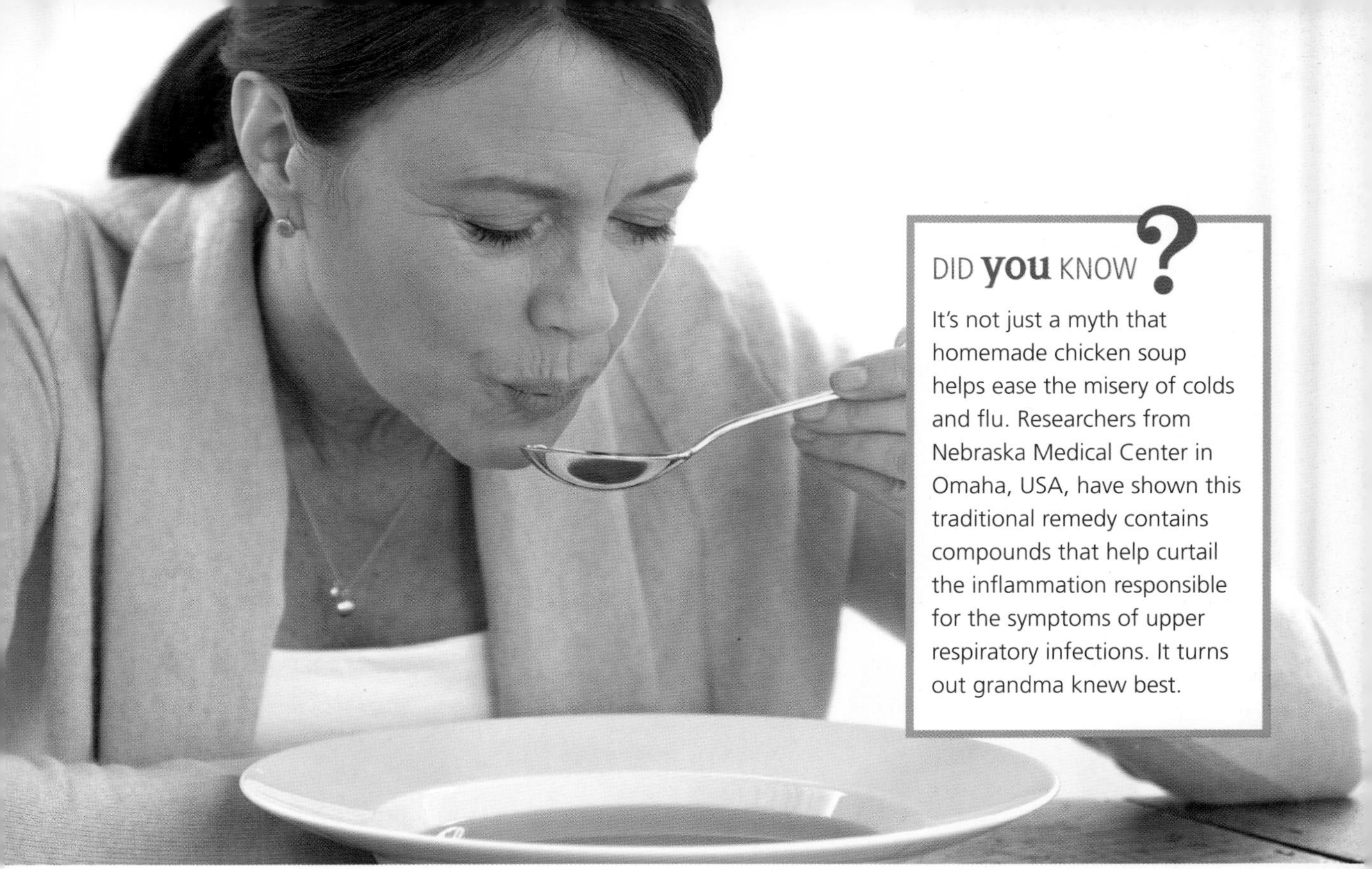

DID **you** KNOW?

It's not just a myth that homemade chicken soup helps ease the misery of colds and flu. Researchers from Nebraska Medical Center in Omaha, USA, have shown this traditional remedy contains compounds that help curtail the inflammation responsible for the symptoms of upper respiratory infections. It turns out grandma knew best.

Chicken soup – good for the body as well as the soul.

FOOD SAFETY AND YOU

At any age, food poisoning is a hazard but older people in particular are more at risk. One survey in the UK found that people over the age of 60 were more likely than younger people to use food after the safe date – a vestige of the days of 'waste not, want not' – which increases your chances of getting ill. And older people are also more likely to suffer complications from eating food that is beyond the safe date, because their immune systems are less robust. The Australian Food Safety Information Council warns against leaving perishable foods, such as cold meats, out for a later snack and advises older people to ensure food is cooked until it's steaming hot.

The foods that are most likely to be contaminated are raw or undercooked poultry and meat, shellfish, soft cheeses, pâtés, delicatessen meats, smoked fish, ready meals, prepacked sandwiches, bags of salad, and dairy products such as eggs and milk. Vulnerable

take CARE! DIET and MEDICATIONS

Many medications, both prescribed and over-the-counter remedies, interfere with your digestive system, exacerbating existing conditions or causing side effects.

Whenever you are prescribed a new medicine, read the enclosed leaflet carefully. You may already know that aspirin and other non-steroidal anti-inflammatory drugs (NSAIDS), often prescribed to treat arthritis, can irritate the stomach lining and cause pain, bleeding or ulcers. This is one reason why you take some medicines with food. These are not the only medications that can affect the digestive system: for example, alendronate, often prescribed for osteoporosis, may cause oesophageal ulcers (you are advised to remain upright for half an hour after taking it).

Many medications, including opiates, iron tablets and diuretics, are linked to constipation. Opiates and numerous others can also cause nausea, and some medicines produce loose stools or diarrhoea, which can then interfere with absorption of other medications.

- **Talk to your doctor** Be sure to report any unusual symptoms as he or she can usually suggest a solution, whether it's adjusting your dosage, changing the medication or finding other ways to alleviate or minimise the problem.

A two-way process

Different foods interact with as many as 200 medications, altering their action or increasing their toxicity.

- **Warfarin and vitamin K** The anticoagulant warfarin, for example, is rendered less effective by foods that contain large amounts of vitamin K, especially liver, Brussels sprouts, broccoli and green, leafy vegetables such as spinach and cabbage. You don't need to avoid these foods altogether – though it's advisable not to start eating large amounts suddenly – but your warfarin doses need to be monitored and adjusted regularly.
- **Alcohol and sedatives** Drinking alcohol with a sedative may increase the sedative effect.
- **The juice effect** Avoid grapefruit juice if you're taking some medications, including amiodarone (often prescribed to stabilise heart rhythms) and some statin cholesterol-lowering and blood pressure-lowering medications. The juice contains substances that interfere with enzymes, reducing the speed at which medications are metabolised and increasing their concentration in the blood. Pomegranate and cranberry juice can also interfere with some medicines.

Natural remedies

Herbal remedies can affect medications, too, including warfarin, as can some supplements. So it's wise to tell your doctor about everything you're taking if you're prescribed a new medication. St John's wort, often used to relieve depression, is a particular culprit.

Avoid drinking grapefruit juice as it can increase the concentration of some medications in the blood.

people, including anyone with immune problems, are advised to avoid completely foods with a high risk of listeria contamination, such as soft cheeses and pâté.

Spot the symptoms, reduce the risk

Symptoms of food poisoning tend to start one to three days after eating contaminated food, but can occur as soon as an hour or as long as 70 days later. They include diarrhoea, nausea, vomiting and stomach cramps. Rest and increased fluids is the basic treatment but if you can't keep fluids down for more than a day, you're still vomiting after two days or still have diarrhoea after three days, and if you pass blood or develop a high temperature, call your doctor.

The first step in preventing food poisoning is to wash your hands often, particularly after using the bathroom, before preparing food and after handling raw meat. Here are more ways to help you cut the risk:

Make sure meats are cooked properly to avoid giving your guests food poisoning.

- **BE FRIDGE SAVVY** Forty per cent of food poisoning cases involve food eaten at home. Keep your fridge at a maximum temperature of 4°C (check it at least every six months with a fridge thermometer). Keep raw meat and poultry separate on the bottom shelf. Defrost food thoroughly unless the packaging states it can be cooked from frozen.

- **RAW DATA** Check use-by dates, and throw foods away if they have expired (even if they look and smell fine). Use a separate chopping board for raw foods to avoid contaminating anything else. Take extra care with raw chicken: more than 50 per cent of it is contaminated with campylobacter, so don't let the juice splash around, and if you rinse chicken before cooking, stop – it's unnecessary and risks spreading germs.

- **COOK WELL** Make sure all foods are cooked properly, especially poultry, pork, burgers and kebabs. Anything you reheat should be piping hot all the way through. Never reheat food more than once, including takeaway meals and any dishes cooked by friends, neighbours or from outside sources.

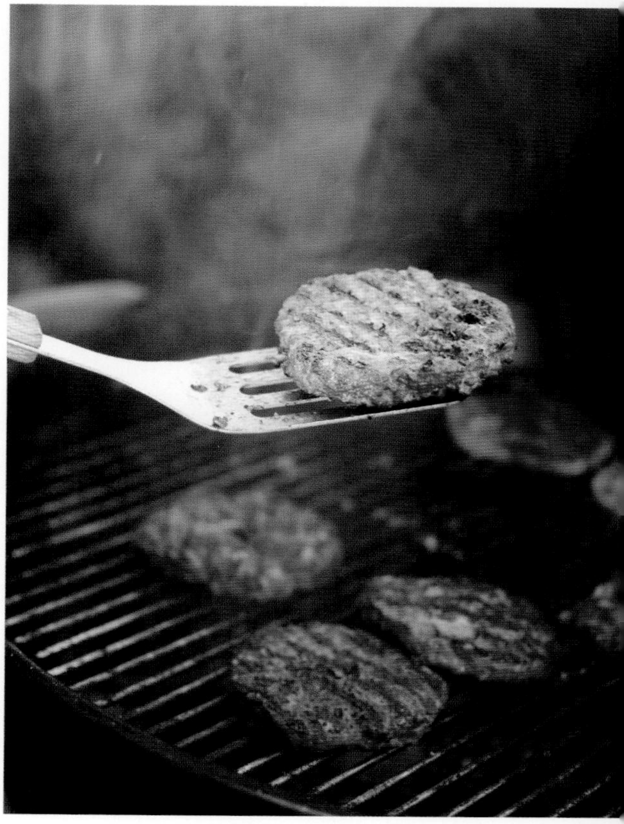

Build up your muscle strength to burn extra kilojoules.

YOUR WEIGHT
your life

Most of us put on weight as we get older, and fat is more likely to settle in the abdominal area and around the internal organs. But tweaking your diet and becoming a little more active will make a healthy difference to your shape and your life.

Few people are as slim at 60 as they were at 20. But your waistline is still something over which you can exert control. Researchers at Imperial College London looked at the food intake of nearly 50,000 people and checked their waist measurements over five years. Irrespective of weight, waist circumferences increased least in those who ate the most fruit and dairy products, and grew most among those who consumed the most white bread, processed meat, margarine and soft drinks.

A NEW METABOLISM

We tend to put on weight as we grow older because we don't adjust our habits to meet the body's changing needs. Our basic metabolic rate – the energy we expend just to sustain essential bodily functions such as heartbeat and respiration – slows down as we get older. (Once you reach your 80s, though, you tend to lose weight, because you shed body fat – a process that's accelerated by reduced appetite.)

This recalibration of your body's engine means that you need fewer kilojoules to maintain a constant weight than you did when you were younger, especially if your activity level reduces, which often happens after you retire, or if you develop any condition such as arthritis that affects mobility. If you continue to eat at the levels you did when you were younger and needed more fuel, then the excess will be stored as fat. And because we naturally lose muscle mass with age, this can also lead to fat gain – because muscle uses more kilojoules than other tissue. Strength training – for example, lifting free weights or using weight machines at the gym – can counteract this tendency by maintaining your muscle at a higher level for longer.

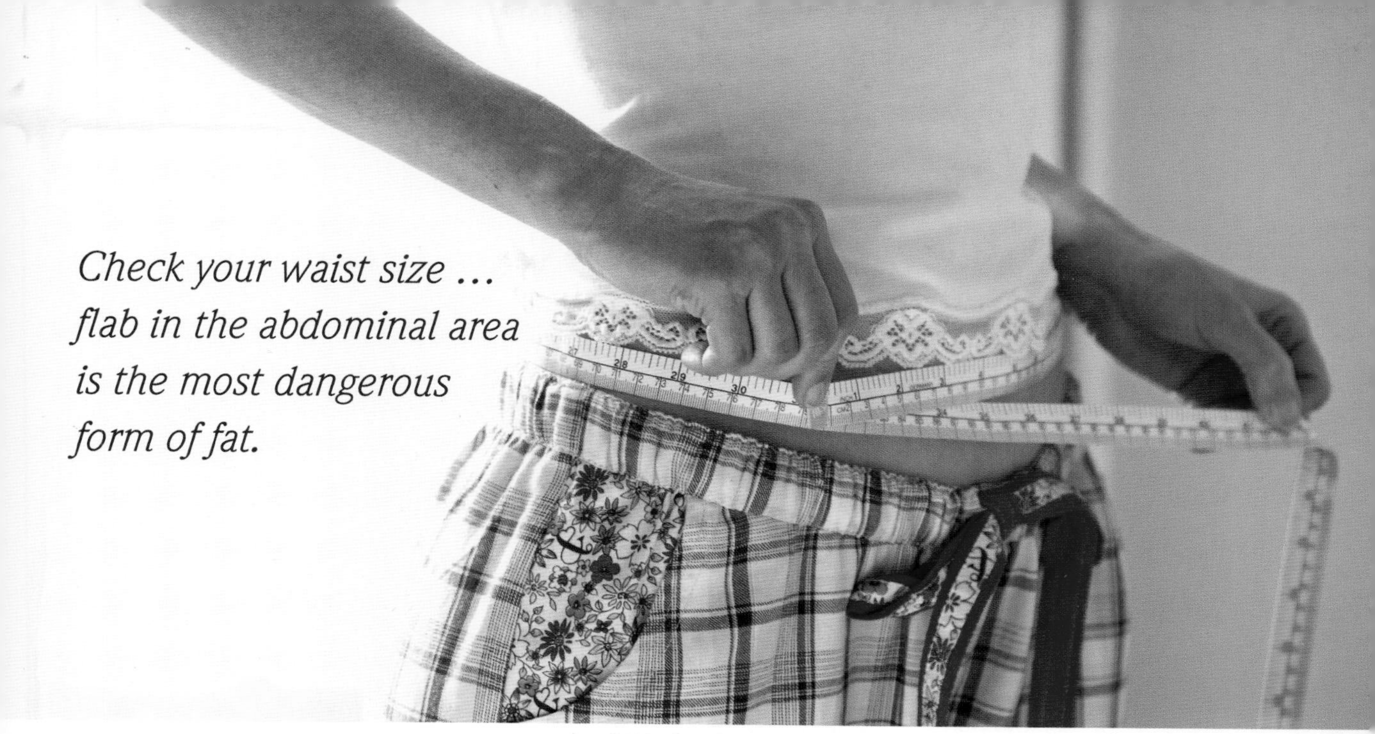

Check your waist size ... flab in the abdominal area is the most dangerous form of fat.

After middle age, fat is more likely to concentrate around your internal organs and in the abdomen, increasing your risk of cardiovascular disease, high blood pressure and diabetes. Other effects of age related to your metabolism include:

- Reduced liver and kidney function.
- Less effective immune responses.
- Decreased ability to metabolise medications, leading to higher blood concentrations and an increased risk of toxicity.
- Poorer ability to metabolise alcohol.
- Slight decrease in body temperature, which makes you less tolerant of extremes of heat and cold, and increases the risk of hypothermia.

Check your numbers

So you might have put on a few kilograms over the past few years. But is your health at risk? A few measurements and a couple of sums will give you a good indication:

● **MEASURE YOUR WAIST** Flab in the abdominal area is the most dangerous form of fat, and the best indicator of whether you may be at risk of diabetes and other diseases. The best way to check if you're in the danger zone is to take a tape measure and measure your waist. Ideally it should be less than 94 cm for men (90 cm for Asian men) and 80 cm for all women.

DID **you** KNOW?

Eating more slowly can help weight loss. In a study of 529 men followed for eight years at Fukuoka University in Japan, the faster eaters gained an average 1.9 kg compared with only 0.7 kg for medium and slow eaters. It takes about 20 minutes for your brain to recognise that your stomach is full. Many overweight people eat too quickly, so they may have already consumed too many kilojoules before they realise they're full.

CHECK YOUR BMI Body mass index (BMI) is the measure doctors use to calculate whether people are a healthy weight for their height. But it's not entirely foolproof; the BMI of a rugby player could be in the overweight range because of his heavy muscle. Conversely, older people who've lost a lot of muscle might figure in the 'normal' range but still be carrying too much fat around their waists, so check your waist size, too. However, BMI is a good general gauge and if yours is in the overweight or obese range, try to shed excess kilograms to reduce your risk of heart disease, diabetes and other conditions.

BMI FORMULA

Divide your weight in kilos by your height in metres squared (so if you weigh 60 kg and are 1.65 m tall, your BMI is 60 ÷ [1.65 x 1.65] = 22)

CHECK YOUR RESULTS AGAINST THIS CHART:

Underweight	=	<18.5
Normal weight	=	18.5–24.9
Overweight	=	25–29.9
Obese	=	30 or greater

DID **you** KNOW?

Eating soup can help you lose weight. Adding water to food reduces its energy density (the number of kilojoules by weight) and increases its overall volume, meaning you feel fuller on the same kilojoules. Scientists at Pennsylvania State University gave 24 women a chicken and rice casserole as a starter before lunch, the same dish with a glass of water, or a liquidised soup of the casserole plus the water. The average number of kilojoules consumed at lunch was 25 per cent lower following the soup than after the casserole (with or without water); and the women didn't go on to eat more at dinner.

LOSING THE KILOS

If you're trying to lose weight, get more exercise. Exercise doesn't just burn up the kilojoules while you're actually doing it, it also boosts your muscle metabolism, since muscle burns more kilojoules kilogram-for-kilogram than fat, even when you're at rest. Plus, you're most likely to stick with it if you opt for a form of exercise – such as walking – that you enjoy and find easy to manage (the same goes for diets, too). A study in the *Journal of Applied Physiology* found that a group of overweight or obese people aged 60 to 75 who dieted without exercising lost more lean muscle – something to be avoided if you're older – than those who dieted and exercised as well.

- It takes 14,650 extra kilojoules to put on each 0.5 kg of fat, so you'll need to knock that much off to lose it again. For each 2100 kJ you knock off your daily intake, expect to lose 0.5 kg a week.
- To lose the weight for good, slow and steady is best; if you're overweight, aim to lose no more than 0.5 to 1 kg a week.

focus ON ... GALLSTONES

Gallstones can cause intense pain in the upper-right abdomen, sometimes with vomiting, fever or jaundice. They're more common after 60, especially in women.

Gallstones are hard deposits that accumulate in the gallbladder. Your gallbladder's function is to aid the digestion of fats in the intestines by storing and concentrating bile, a green fluid produced in the liver that breaks down blood fats. Stones – particles mainly formed of cholesterol or bile pigments – are common (risk factors include lack of physical activity, obesity, crash diets and diabetes) and often cause no symptoms, so are noticed only on a routine X-ray or ultrasound, or during surgery. But sometimes they cause infection or inflammation of the gallbladder, or move and block a duct leading from the gallbladder, causing intense pain. This may resolve itself if the stone passes into the intestine. Unless that happens fairly quickly, you may need medication to dissolve the stones, shock-wave therapy or surgery.

There's always a new diet claiming to be the last word in weight loss, but how do you know what's best for you? When it comes to dieting, joining a group rather than going it alone may provide the impetus to succeed. A study published in *The Lancet* of 772 overweight and obese participants found that those who enrolled in a WeightWatchers program lost 5.1 kg after 12 months – more than double that lost by those following standard healthcare advice.

And researchers at Ben-Gurion University in Israel who assigned different diets to three groups of moderately obese participants found that the average weight loss was 3.3 kg on a low-fat diet, 4.6 kg on a Mediterranean diet and 5.5 kg on a low-carb diet (the only one that wasn't kilojoule-restricted). The low-carb diet yielded the best improvements in blood cholesterol, whereas among the 36 individuals with diabetes, the Mediterranean diet improved blood-glucose and insulin levels most.

REDUCING THE RISK OF DIABETES

You're much more likely to develop type 2 diabetes if you have an unhealthy diet and are overweight. The risk of diabetes also increases with age – and not just because we put on weight. Average blood-glucose levels start to go up after about the age of 50 because our

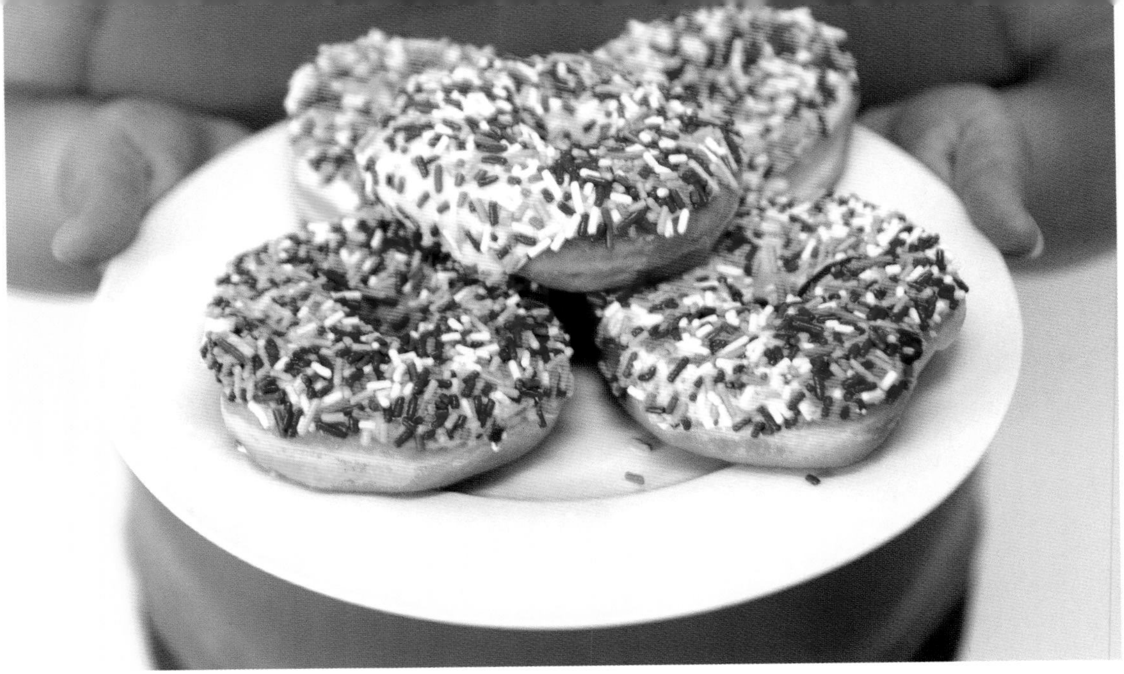

An unhealthy diet and being overweight are major risk factors for the development of type 2 diabetes.

cells become less sensitive to insulin, the hormone that regulates glucose levels. This means that glucose tolerance (the measure of how well we handle carbohydrates in food) decreases as we get older.

A vicious cycle of high blood glucose and increased insulin production along with insulin resistance can lead to diabetes. The risk is increased if you have abdominal fat (the 'apple shape'), high cholesterol and triglycerides in the blood, and high blood pressure; together these are called 'metabolic syndrome' and they place you at high risk of diabetes and cardiovascular disease. Making small lifestyle changes, such as becoming more active and losing a little weight, can reduce your risk of type 2 diabetes significantly.

What you eat is also crucial. Yet again the Mediterranean diet comes to the rescue – olive oil, wine and omega-3 fatty acids in fish all have proven benefits. Limiting your intake of saturated fat helps, too. Researchers in a study at Harvard School of Public Health estimate you could cut your diabetes risk by 16 to 35 per cent by replacing one daily serve of red meat with nuts, low-fat dairy products or whole grains.

what's NEW

THE DIABETES FAST Obesity-related diabetes may be reversible in its early stages. How? By the shock of an extremely low-kilojoule diet to remove excess fat in the insulin-producing cells of the pancreas. Scientists at Newcastle University put 11 people with type 2 diabetes and an average age of 50 on 2500 kJ a day for eight weeks. Their blood-glucose values became normal, as did their measures of pancreatic function. However, this type of diet could be dangerous and shouldn't be followed without medical supervision.

7 steps to the RIGHT WEIGHT

Achieving and maintaining a healthy weight depend on your energy balance – the kilojoules you take in must equal your kilojoules you use up. Here are some easy tricks to help you nudge yourself towards the right balance.

1 EAT WELL In a study at Harvard Medical School of over 120,000 people from 1986 to 2006, increased daily serves of vegetables, whole grains, fruit, nuts or yogurt tended to result in weight loss, whereas chips, potatoes, sugary drinks and red meat led to weight gain in each four-year period.

2 SHRINK THE PLATE Using a smaller plate tricks your brain into thinking you're getting more food. Studies show that the bigger the plate or bowl, the more food people serve – and when offered bigger portions, people tend to eat them.

3 UP THE PROTEIN In an Australian study 22 volunteers were first fed meals with a 10 per cent protein content, then 15 per cent. On the low-protein days, they were hungrier and consumed more kilojoules in total (the extra kilojoules came mostly from unhealthy snacks). Researchers conclude that people compensate for reduced protein with more fat and carbohydrate, which could increase the risk of gaining weight.

Put your knife and fork down between each mouthful.

4 GO SLOW Chew your food carefully, and put your knife and fork down between mouthfuls. Researchers in Athens tested levels of appetite-regulating hormones in 17 volunteers eating ice cream over 5 or 30 minutes. They found that eating quickly stopped the release of gut hormones that make people feel full.

5 SAY NO TO TV DINNERS Research shows that the more time you spend watching television, the higher your risk of obesity, regardless of total activity levels. In a University of Birmingham study, women ate more biscuits in the afternoon on days when they watched TV while they ate lunch.

6 THINK BACK Recalling your last meal dampens your appetite. Psychologists at the University of Birmingham have shown that volunteers reminded of what they ate for lunch ate less at their next meal; people who recalled what they had for lunch had fewer snacks later.

7 FOLLOW THE 80 PER CENT RULE Take a tip from traditional Okinawans, who practise *hara hachi bu* – eating until you are 80 per cent full. It's enough to stop you feeling hungry but averts over-eating.

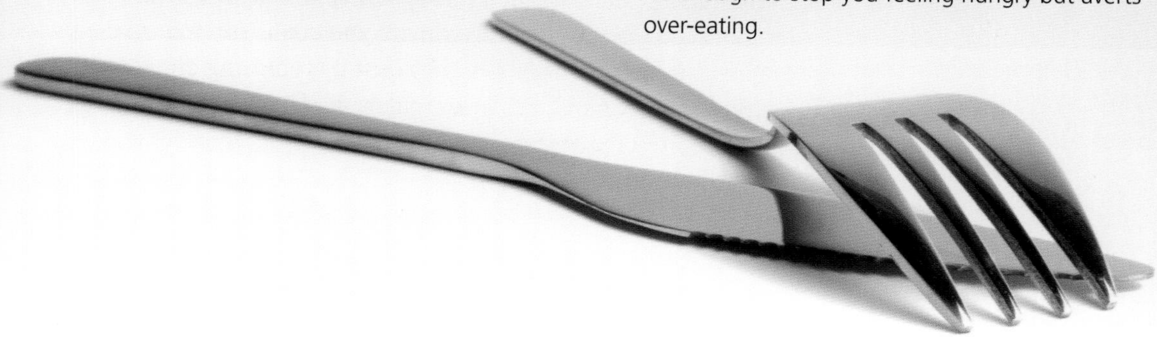

Try a probiotic yogurt or supplement to help combat bloating.

INSIDE TRACK
a healthy digestion

You may have already noticed that you are beginning to develop more digestive problems, such as constipation and indigestion. Although age has an impact on the way your body handles food, there is much you can do to keep the process smooth.

Food is moved through your body by a series of muscle contractions – rather like a Mexican wave. As you get older, these muscle contractions become weaker, which can hamper digestion. To keep your digestion on top form, follow three golden rules:

- Eat a healthy diet with plenty of high-fibre foods.
- Drink plenty of water.
- Keep active.

You may also find it helpful to:

- Take a probiotic – found in live yogurts and as a supplement. Some people find that probiotics, which contain 'friendly bacteria' to keep harmful bugs in your intestines under control, help with bloating or abdominal pain.
- Avoid stress, which is known to contribute to disturbed digestion and exacerbate symptoms of bowel disorders. Yoga or other relaxation techniques may help – a Canadian study showed that yoga reduced gastrointestinal symptoms in people with irritable bowel syndrome.

DEALING WITH CONSTIPATION

When the contents of your intestines remain in your colon too long, too much water may be reabsorbed, leading to constipation (infrequent bowel movements with hard, dry stools that are difficult to pass). If you have a tendency towards constipation, look to your diet – not having enough dietary fibre is often a major factor.

In about four out of ten cases, constipation is a side effect of some medications (*see* page 92). The problem may also be linked to conditions such as diabetes. Paradoxically, laxatives may also lead to constipation as the bowel comes to need them in increasing doses

Continued on page 102

focus ON ... INDIGESTION

As the muscle in the walls of the gastrointestinal tract weakens, 'heartburn' or indigestion (dyspepsia) becomes more common, making it harder for the body to process food. This can cause pain, nausea, belching or bloating. You may be able to minimise or even solve any problems by adjusting your diet or medication.

Eating too much or too fast, smoking, eating certain foods or alcohol can all lead to indigestion. Symptoms vary from pain in the upper abdomen to nausea, bloating or burping. Indigestion is not usually serious, but see your doctor if:

- The pain persists.
- You experience recurrent bouts, increasingly severe pain or weight loss.
- You vomit blood or have black tarry stools.

Three common causes of indigestion are:

- Gastro-oesophageal reflux, which occurs when the ring of muscle at the junction of your oesophagus and stomach weakens, allowing the acidic contents of your stomach to flow back up the oesophagus.
- Hiatus hernia – affecting a third of people over 50 – where part of the stomach protrudes upwards through a weakening in the diaphragm.
- Medication: anti-inflammatory medications may irritate the lining of the stomach or small intestines, in severe cases leading to an ulcer. Nitrates, taken to dilate the blood vessels, also relax the oesophageal sphincter, increasing your chance of reflux, too.

To determine the root of your pain, your doctor may refer you for tests such as an endoscopy, where a tube is passed into the stomach to examine the interior, or an ultrasound, X-ray or CT scan. Often, though, simple steps are enough to deal with it:

- **Avoid trigger foods** (spicy, fried or fatty foods, chocolate, garlic, onions, alcohol and caffeine).
- **Don't eat late at night,** or too quickly.
- **Eat smaller,** more frequent meals.
- **Lose weight** if you need to.
- **Raise the head of your bed** to prevent acid reflux at night.

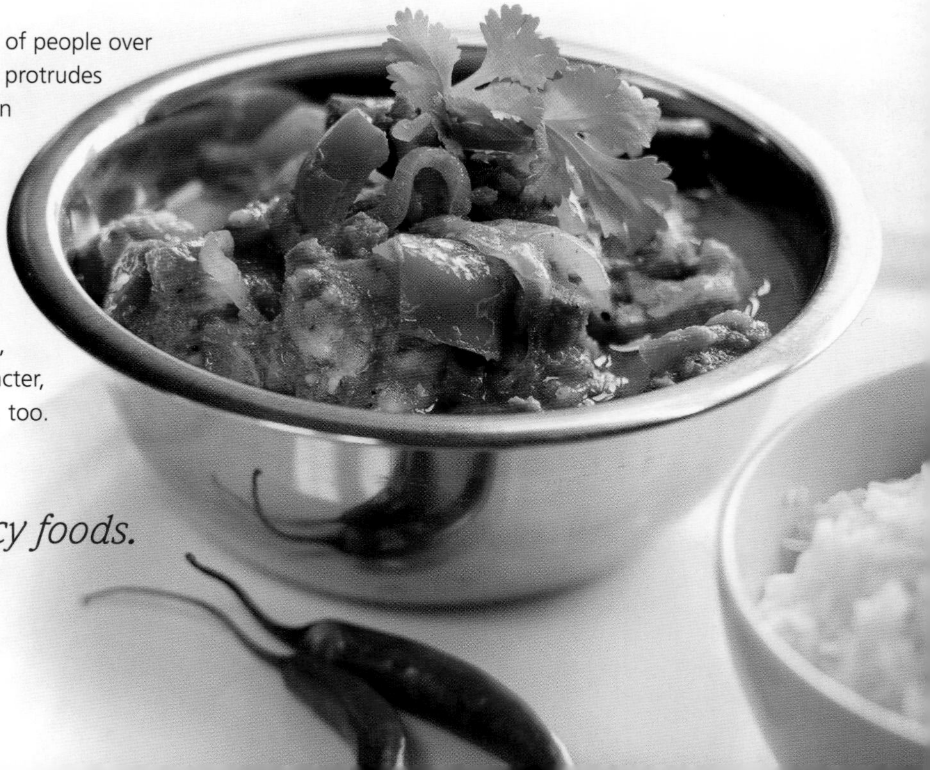

Try to avoid hot, spicy foods.

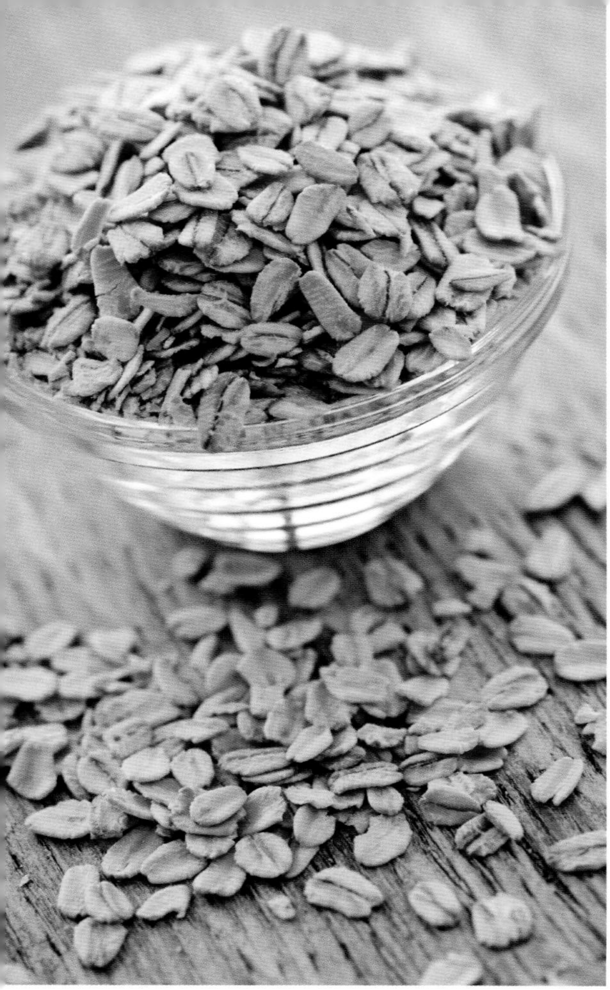

to achieve a result. Laxatives can also interfere with your digestion and absorption of nutrients, so should only be used in the short term. Here are some good ways to prevent chronic constipation:

- **Up the fibre** Pack in as much fruit and vegetables as you can, and try to eat three portions of whole grains daily (a portion is 3 tbsp of cereal or a slice of bread).
- **Choose unrefined** Pick brown rice rather than white and have wholemeal pasta.
- **Stay active** Move more in general – avoid sitting for long periods. Aim for 30 minutes' activity a day – it helps improve the regularity of your bowels.
- **Drink water** Your intestines need enough water to keep things moving, so carry on drinking.
- **Re-train your bowel** Make sure you have some undisturbed time and privacy at a set time each day, say, after breakfast. Never ignore the urge to have a bowel movement.

Fissures and haemorrhoids

If you're straining to pass hard stools, the effort can cause small tears or fissures in the anus. These may lead to bleeding and make it painful to pass a stool. Or you may develop haemorrhoids (piles) around the anus – small, painful or itchy swellings (actually varicose veins). Both usually clear up once the constipation is resolved. See your doctor if they are very painful; a steroid cream, painkillers or laxatives may help. Treatment for persistent haemorrhoids includes:

Up the fibre – try to eat three portions of whole grains daily.

- **Banding** Small rubber bands are placed around the base of the haemorrhoid, which cuts off the blood supply and causes it to drop off. One or two are treated at a time (treating many is painful).
- **Other options** These include sclerotherapy (injections), infrared coagulation and, occasionally, surgery.

DIGESTIVE CONDITIONS

Often as a result of straining due to constipation, small pouches (diverticula) develop in weakened areas of the wall of the large intestine (colon) – a condition known as diverticular disease. By the age of 50, around 50 per cent of people in the Western world

take CARE! Spot the signs of BOWEL CANCER

More than 85 per cent of cases of bowel cancer occur in people aged 60 and over. Risk factors include a high intake of red and processed meat, insufficient dietary fibre, obesity, inactivity, smoking, alcohol, some other bowel disorders and family history.

Ninety per cent of cases of bowel cancer can be treated if caught early, so never ignore changes in bowel habits and do go for regular screening (*see* page 127). See your doctor if any of the following last for more than three weeks:

- Diarrhoea, constipation or passing mucus.
- Bleeding from the rectum, blood in the stool, or dark, tarry motions.
- Abdominal pain or cramping.
- A lump in your abdomen, especially on the right side, or in your back passage.
- Unexplained weight loss, tiredness, weakness, fatigue, dizziness or breathlessness.

Some of these symptoms can occur with haemorrhoids, infection or polyps (raised growths) on the colon wall. Most polyps are non-cancerous (benign) but some can lead to bowel cancer.

Getting a diagnosis

You will usually need an endoscopy, in which a thin tube is passed through the anus into the rectum and colon to examine the inside of the bowel and, if necessary, take a biopsy. A CT or MRI scan may also be performed. Treatment usually involves surgery to remove the tumour, followed by chemotherapy to reduce the risk of the cancer coming back.

will have developed diverticula, and 70 per cent have them at the age of 80. The condition seems to be a direct consequence of diets that contain insufficient fibre – it's common in Europe and North America, but rare in Africa and Asia. It can be both prevented and treated simply by increasing the amount of fibre in your diet.

Usually there are no symptoms but one in four people experience intermittent lower abdominal pain and cramping, usually on the left side, along with bloating, diarrhoea or constipation, and wind; people can also experience bleeding from the rectum. If the diverticula become inflamed – diverticulitis – you may have severe, constant pain, a high temperature, nausea and sometimes bleeding. This needs treatment with antibiotics or sometimes surgery.

Irritable bowel syndrome (IBS) produces very similar symptoms, but this disorder tends to get less common as you get older. The cause is uncertain, and although it's uncomfortable, it's not dangerous. Symptoms can usually be eased by changing your diet, taking more exercise and reducing stress.

DID **you** KNOW?

Many people think they're constipated because they don't open their bowels daily, but in fact this is not unusual. Normal frequency varies from three times a day to once every three days.

A cup of coffee a day lowers stroke risk by up to 25 per cent, a Swedish study found.

LIQUID ASSETS
drinks and your health

Good nutrition is about what you drink, as well as what you eat. We don't always pay much attention to what's in our glass or our cup, but drinks of all sorts have an effect on our health.

One strange scientific fact known to most of us is that the human body is mostly water. Often the exact proportion is exaggerated – you may have heard at some time that people are 97 per cent water. In fact, the amount of water in your body varies throughout your life. A baby is about 90 per cent water, but this drops to between 50 and 70 per cent in adults. A man who weighs 70 kg, is carrying around 40 litres of water – so it's no surprise that your liquid intake is a vital element of your health.

WHAT TO DRINK

Water itself is the perfect drink: thirst-quenching, health-giving, kilojoule-free. There is no need to buy bottled water: it is not necessarily healthier than tap water and may even contain higher-than-average levels of micro-organisms. If you don't like the taste of tap water, try adding a slice of lemon or orange, or a little fruit juice.

Pure juice is the healthiest option if you want a sweet drink. But it contains fruit sugar (fructose) and is quite high in kilojoules, so drinking more than a glass or two a day could cause weight gain. Its sugar and acids can also be bad for your teeth. One large American study of women aged between 30 and 55 found that increasing the consumption of whole fruit and vegetables reduced the risk of diabetes, while drinking fruit juice actually slightly increased it.

Your daily cuppa

Coffee, especially if it's unfiltered (such as Greek or Turkish coffee, which is put in the pot and boiled), raises cholesterol levels, but most studies have found no associated increased risk of cardiovascular disease. And now it seems that coffee may actually protect against type 2 diabetes, Parkinson's disease and liver disease, according to scientists at Oregon State University. Tea also has benefits: in 2011 UK researchers who reviewed published studies concluded that three or four cups of tea a day reduces heart attack risk. Green tea is renowned for its health-boosting properties (*see* page 83), and even black tea contains some anti-oxidants. Herbal teas contain a wide range of phytochemicals with protective health effects.

There's little evidence that the caffeine content of tea, coffee and cocoa is harmful either – in fact, recent research suggests that caffeine itself is an anti-oxidant and may protect against heart disease and Alzheimer's disease. A study at the French National Institute for Health and Medical Research found that women aged 65 and over who drank more than three cups of coffee daily, or the equivalent as tea, showed less memory decline over four years than women who drank one cup or less. The benefits were not seen in men, but increased with age in women: 65-year-old women were 30 per cent less likely to have a decline in memory if they drank coffee; by the age of 80, that level of protection increased to a staggering 70 per cent.

Fizzy drinks – sugar-free or no?

Fizzy drinks are often linked to obesity, and diet or sugar-free versions are not necessarily healthier. Researchers at the University of Texas followed 474 people aged 65 to 74 for ten years, and found that those who opted for diet drinks put on more weight, and their waistlines expanded at a faster rate than those who didn't. People who drank more than two diet drinks per day had a six times bigger

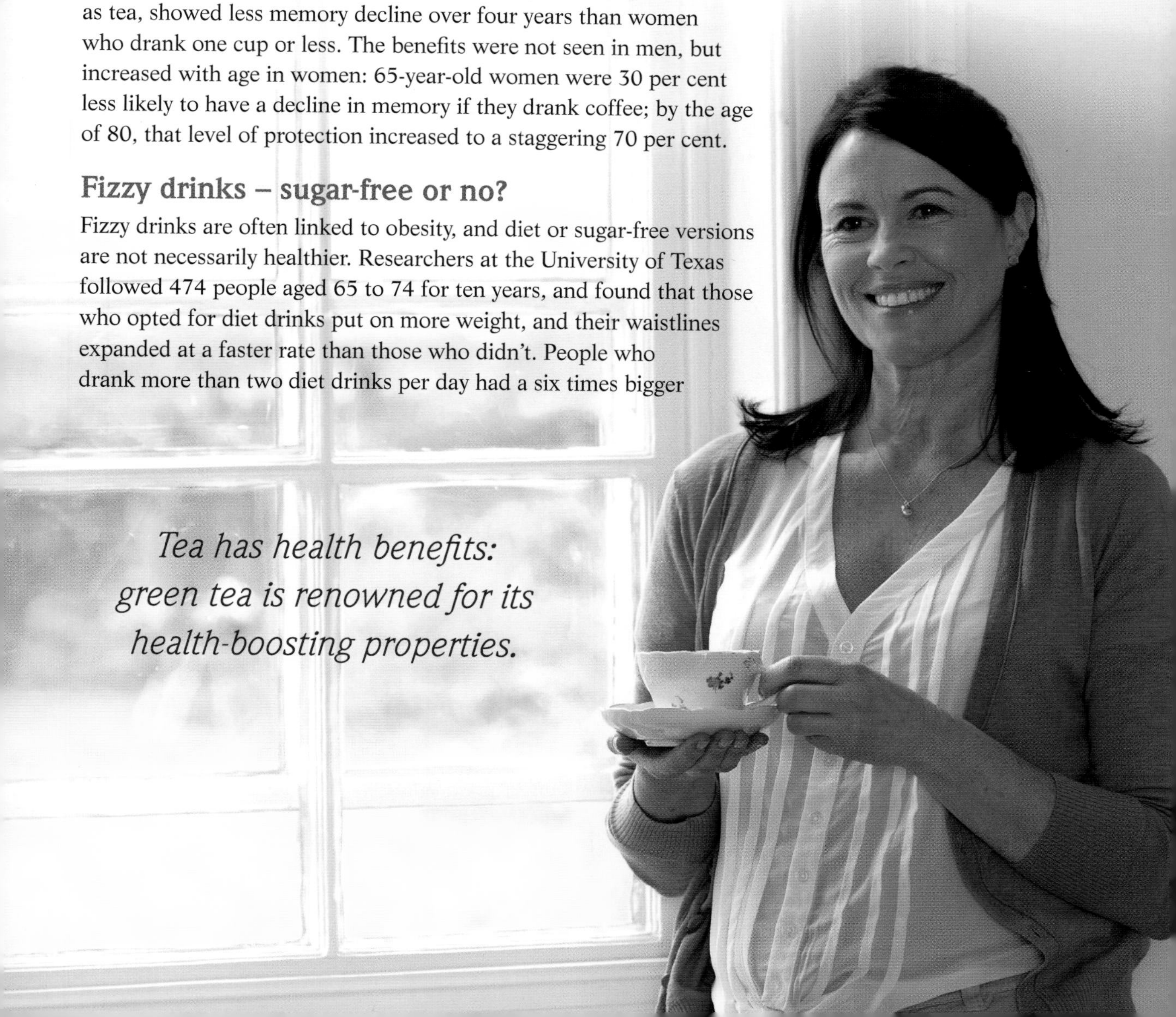

Tea has health benefits: green tea is renowned for its health-boosting properties.

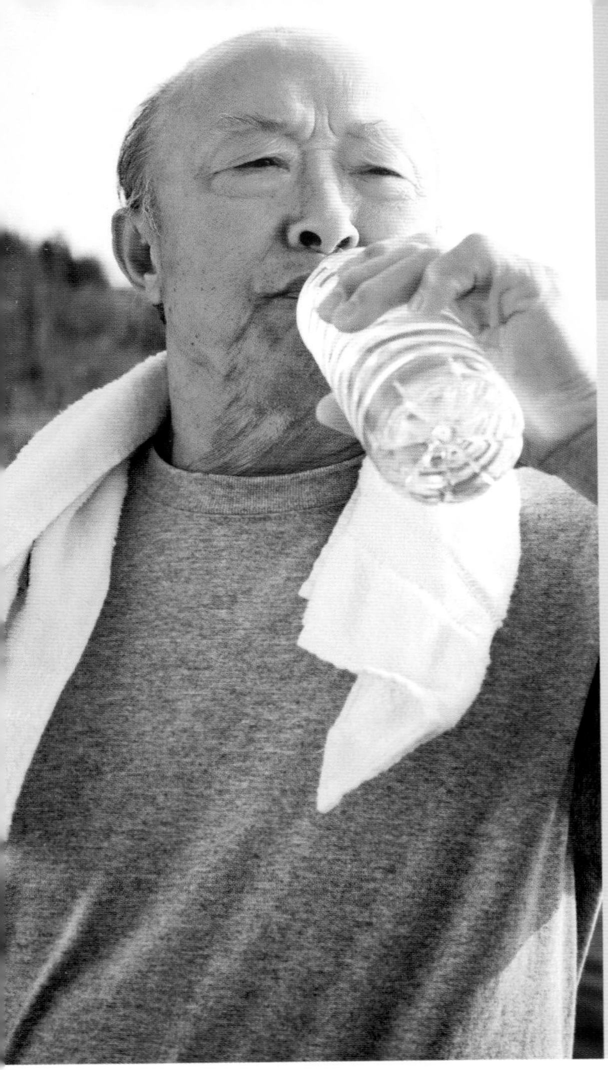

take CARE ! DEHYDRATION

Because much of your body's water is held in muscle tissue, reduced muscle mass with age also depletes the amount of water in your body.

Changes in your hormone levels and reduced kidney function mean that more water is lost in your urine, too, but this is largely balanced by reduced sweating capacity with age, so your water requirements do not generally change. However, your thirst sensation dulls with age, and it takes longer to restore the body's fluid balance, so you need to take extra care to drink enough to ensure you stay hydrated. Older people are more susceptible to dehydration from reduced water intake, illness, higher temperatures, exercise or the effect of medications, especially diuretics. To avoid dehydration:

- **Don't use thirst** as a guide to when to drink.
- **Check your urine** It's your best indicator of dehydration – if it's pale straw-coloured, you're getting enough, any darker and you need to increase the amount you drink.

increase in waist circumference by the end of the study than those who drank none. One explanation for these findings is suggested by a US study in which mice were fed food laced with aspartame, a common sweetener in diet drinks. After three months, the mice had increased blood glucose but reduced insulin levels – suggesting the early changes of diabetes.

Alcohol and you

As you get older, your body metabolises alcohol less well than when you were young. This is due to changes in the way your body distributes fluid and to a reduction in your liver enzymes. So when you drink, the levels of alcohol in your blood may be higher than they would be in younger people consuming the same amount, and the alcohol may stay in the system for longer. In addition, the liver and brain become more sensitive to toxic effects as you age and alcohol–medication interactions become more common.

But that's not to say you shouldn't enjoy a drink. Various studies have found moderate drinking is beneficial. One US survey involving 1824 people aged 55 to 65 at the outset showed that moderate drinkers had a lower death rate after 20 years than heavy drinkers or teetotallers. To keep your drinking moderate:

- Alternate alcoholic drinks with soft drinks.
- Stay away from salty nuts and chips.
- Keep one or two days a week alcohol-free.
- Stick to recommended daily limits: 1 to 2 standard drinks. One standard drink is one mid-strength can of beer or one 100 ml glass of wine.

it's a **MYTH ...**

... that you need **EIGHT GLASSES OF WATER A DAY**

The classic piece of advice is that we should all drink eight 240 ml glasses (more than 2 litres) of water daily. But there's actually no evidence to back up this widely held belief, according to kidney specialists Dan Negoianu and Stanley Goldfarb of the University of Pennsylvania. While it's important to stay hydrated, fluid in foods contributes, too, especially water-rich fruit and vegetables. What's more, the notion that only pure water counts has been debunked – in a British study of healthy volunteers, black tea was found to be just as hydrating as water.

URINARY INFECTIONS

Getting older increases your risk of a urinary tract infection (UTI), which usually occurs when bacteria from your bowel enters your urethra (the tube leading out of the bladder). UTIs are more common in women – who have a shorter urethra, in closer proximity to the anus, than men – and become more frequent after the menopause because loss of oestrogen thins the lining of the urinary tract. Other factors that increase the risk include diabetes, kidney stones, an enlarged prostate gland in men, incontinence and immobility. Infection may affect the urethra (urethritis) or move up the urinary tract to the bladder (cystitis), the ureters (the tubes running from the bladder to the kidneys – ureteritis) or the kidneys (pyelonephritis). Symptoms include:

- A burning pain on urinating.
- Cloudy, blood-stained or foul-smelling urine.
- A need to urinate more frequently and urgently.
- Sometimes, a raised body temperature.

Your doctor can confirm that you have an infection by a urine test, and prescribe antibiotics to treat it. The best thing you can do is to drink plenty of water to flush out germs. Staying well hydrated may help to prevent UTIs from taking hold in the first place.

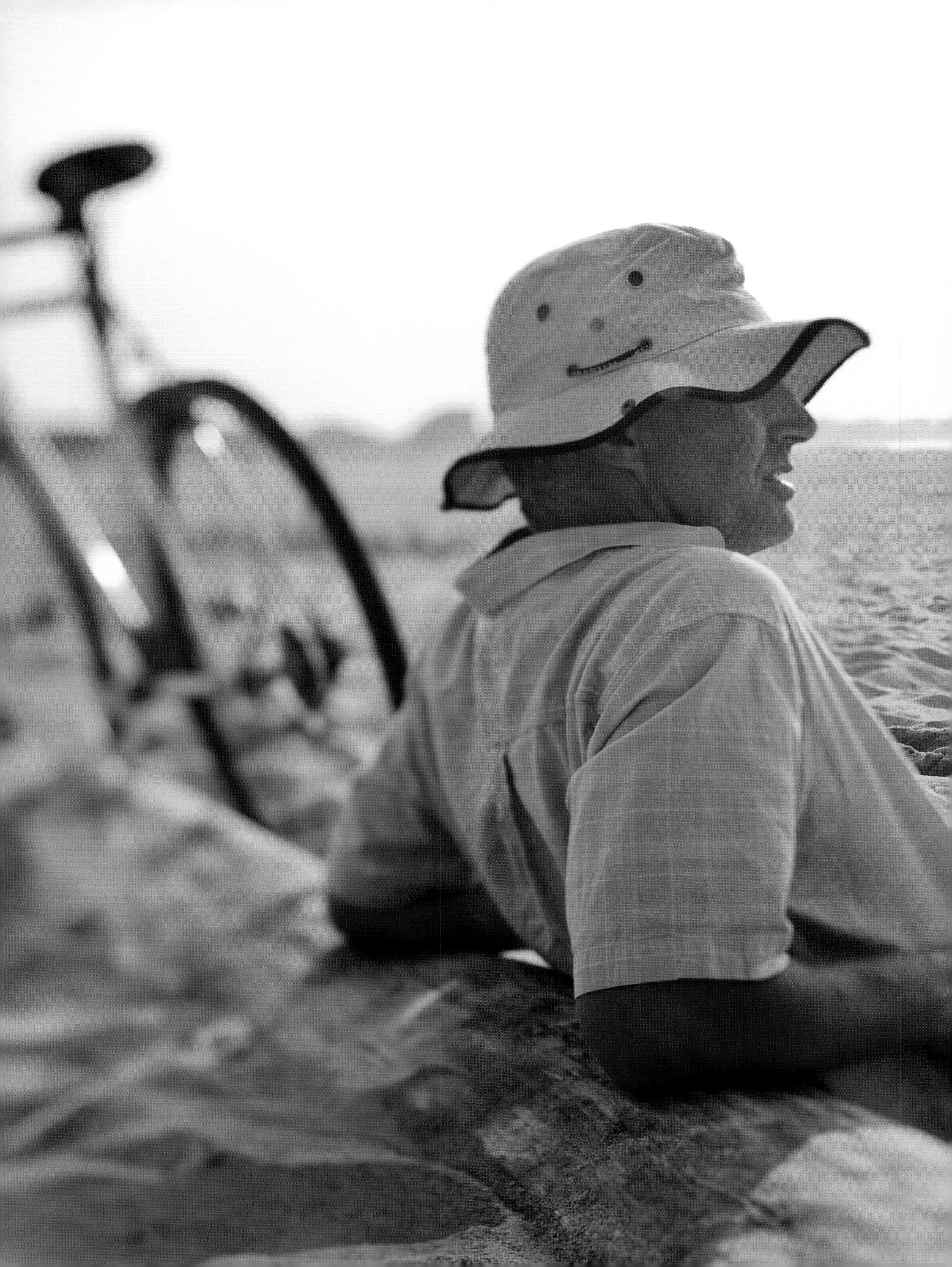

5

Boost your IMMUNITY

A strong immune system is your fortress against attack, helping you to build up resistance to all the bugs you encounter throughout life. But it needs careful maintenance, and even the healthiest immune system changes naturally with age. As you get older, there are important steps you can take to ensure that your very own bodyguard continues to defend your organs and tissues against external attack.

Get laughing to increase your production of infection-fighting T cells.

YOUR BODY'S frontline defence

Without your body's amazing ability to repel invaders, you would be prey to every marauding germ. The immune system's defence mechanisms are naturally formidable, but they need maintenance and support to function at their best – especially as you get older.

The role of your immune system is to guard your body against incursions of viruses, bacteria and parasites. Its instant reaction to such dangers is called the 'immune response'. The immune system does its work inside your body: the inner linings of your gut and lungs, for example, trap invading bacteria, while the helpful bacteria found in your bowel prevent takeover by harmful organisms. The fight carries on in your urine, which flushes germs out from your bladder, while in your blood vessels, white blood cells called neutrophils are highly efficient at seeking out and killing infectious intruders.

You have built-in immune protection from birth – mechanisms that are always ready to fight invaders on your behalf. But your immune system can also learn: it has the ability to identify and defeat new and different enemies. This 'acquired' or 'adaptive' immunity means that your body is forearmed once it has encountered a particular form of attack on its systems. Next time, it will be better equipped to fight it off. This is a positive advantage as you get older and have encountered most common infections.

Germ warfare

The work of the immune system is described here in military terms. This is no idle metaphor: the body really is subject to invasion by organisms that intend – albeit blindly – to destroy or take over the corporeal territory that belongs to you. And it is a biological fact that you have forces at your disposal whose function it is to resist: white blood cells, or lymphocytes. The two main types of lymphocyte – T cells and B cells – are made in the bone marrow; B cells mature there, while T cells are deployed to the thymus gland (located above

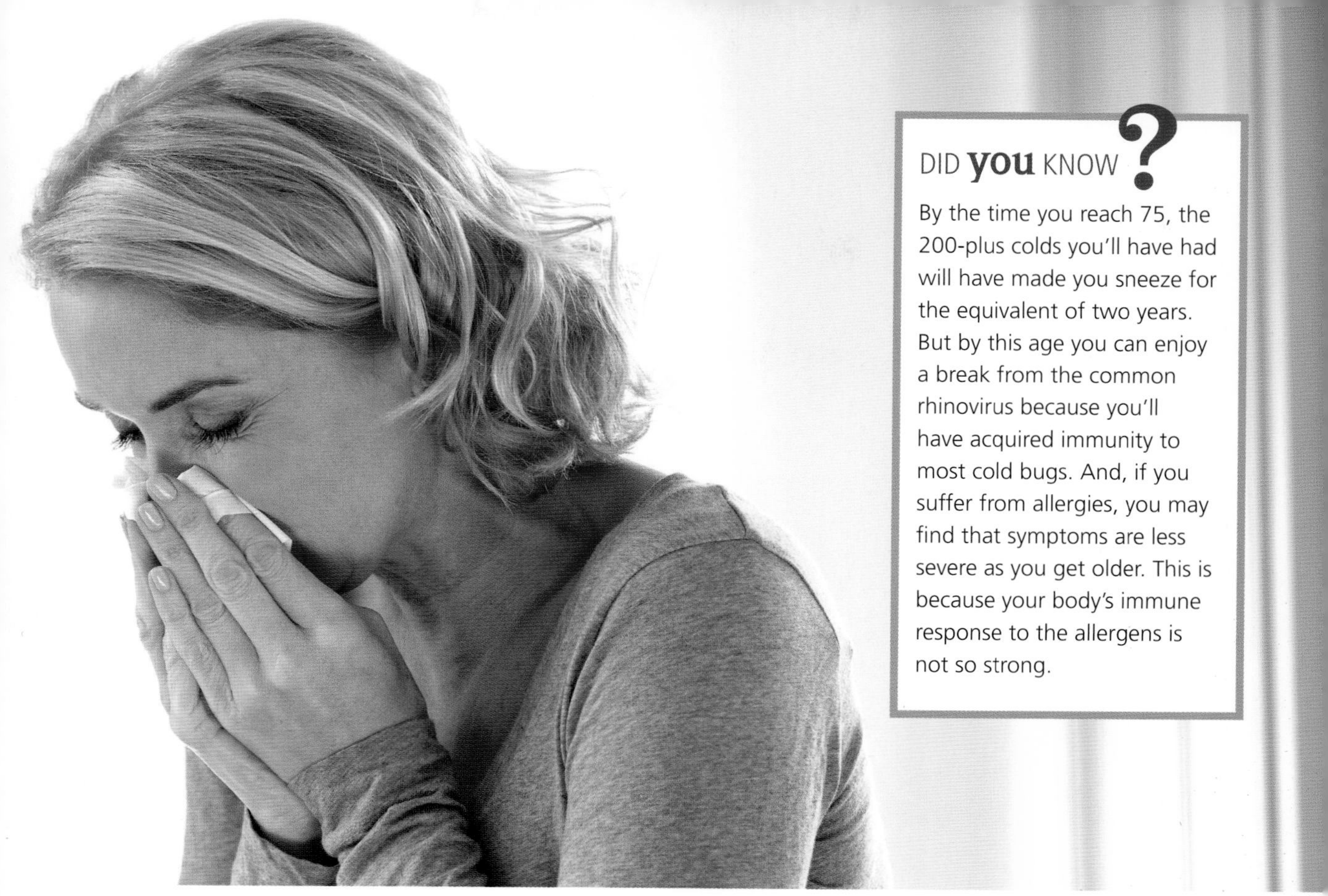

DID **you** KNOW?

By the time you reach 75, the 200-plus colds you'll have had will have made you sneeze for the equivalent of two years. But by this age you can enjoy a break from the common rhinovirus because you'll have acquired immunity to most cold bugs. And, if you suffer from allergies, you may find that symptoms are less severe as you get older. This is because your body's immune response to the allergens is not so strong.

Good news ... colds may be common in younger people, but by the age of 75 you'll have built up immunity to most cold bugs.

the heart), where they mature fully then move to the spleen and lymph nodes, ready to battle against infection. Before the T cells can get to work, they need to learn how to detect specific foreign invaders; this crucial 'education' process occurs in the thymus.

The disappearing thymus

As your body ages, your thymus gland shrinks – by the time you reach 60 only a few wispy remnants remain – and your body makes far fewer T cells. It is not fully understood why this happens, but there may be an underlying evolutionary reason. It may be that the thymus needs to be active in youth before the body has had time to build up resistance to foreign substances (antigens); once the immune system is developed, it shrivels away – allowing the body to apportion its energy elsewhere. But at some point in the future, it may be

take CARE! Keep tabs on your **IMMUNE SYSTEM**

Do you usually feel well? Or do you easily fall prey to all sorts of niggling health problems? Use the quick checklist below to get a picture of how your immune system is functioning. If you answer yes to one or more, take steps to boost your immunity. See your doctor if the problem persists.

- ☐ You succumb easily to the coughs and sneezes of those around you, and when you get a cold, you can't shake it off for ages.
- ☐ You're constantly tired and lacking in energy, and have no interest in taking up anything new.
- ☐ When you look in the mirror, your tongue is coated rather than an even pink.
- ☐ Getting off to sleep is a problem; when you do sleep, you don't often feel rested on waking.
- ☐ Your skin is dry, blotchy and uneven rather than being clear.
- ☐ You have no appetite; nothing seems to make your mouth water.

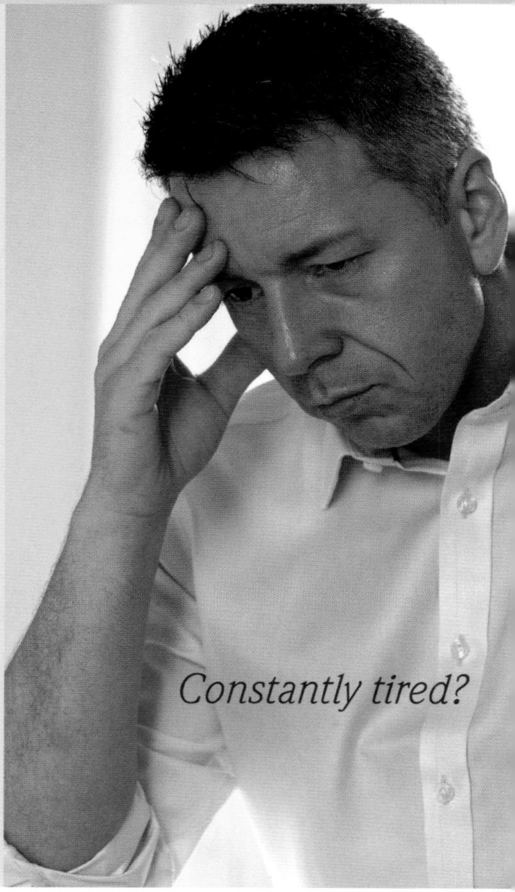

Constantly tired?

possible to restore and rejuvenate the components of the immune system, renewing your body's supply of T cells. Scientists around the world are looking closely at immune regeneration and some are investigating ways in which the thymus can be functionally restored.

What T and B cells do

Our bodies produce different types of immunity cells. Killer T cells attack and kill other cells if they've been infected by viruses or bacteria, stopping the invader from reproducing and spreading the infection. Helper T cells stimulate the B cells to make antibodies (proteins that lock onto the invaders, marking them so the body knows to kill them off). Another group, known as 'naïve T cells', are fresh cells developed in response to a newly encountered bug; they become specialised 'memory T cells' after a first encounter, and proliferate in order to respond quickly to further similar attack. In newborn babies, the ratio of naïve to memory T cells is high, but by adulthood most naïve T cells have already 'met' antigens (foreign substances) and have converted to memory cells. Older people have almost no naïve T cells at all: it is as if the body assumes it has seen every kind of attack that is likely to come its way. But this also means it can be caught off guard by, say, a new strain of flu.

it's a **MYTH ...**

... that a **FEVER WEAKENS** your **IMMUNE SYSTEM**

A fever can actually help your immune system fight infection in two ways. First, a higher body temperature speeds up the functioning of certain cells, including the ones that fight illness, so they respond faster to invading bugs. New research published in the *Journal of Leukocyte Biology* in 2011 confirms that mild fever actually plays a vital part in the immune system's response in times of attack. The higher temperature also makes it harder for the foreign pathogens to reproduce and multiply. To allow your immune system to get on with its job unhindered, rest is essential – because the body uses a large amount of energy to overcome the infection.

AN OLDER IMMUNE SYSTEM

As your immune system changes with age, it also cannot respond quite as quickly or as efficiently as before – a process called immunosenescence. You may notice, for example, that it sometimes takes you longer to throw off an illness, or that any wounds may be slower to heal than they were when you were younger.

There are many possible explanations for this, including age-related chemical modifications within your cells, differences in the proteins on the cell surfaces, even alterations in entire organs. Taken separately, each may be quite trivial, but added together they can have a radical affect on your overall health.

Are immune problems a cause of ageing, or one of its effects? Scientists don't yet know, but what is certain is that illness and disease are not an inevitable part of ageing. The science of the ageing process – immunogerontology – poses exciting but perplexing questions about why our immune system changes over time.

Evidence from those who live the longest lives suggests that individuals can make a real difference to their health and longevity. By monitoring your immune responses as you get older, and making some sensible lifestyle changes to keep them strong, you can become your immune system's biggest ally in the battle to defend your health.

DID **you** KNOW?

The herb echinacea – which can be taken as a supplement – has been shown to enhance immune function by increasing immunoglobulin production, while black elderberry liquid appears to inhibit two different strains of influenza virus. However, echinacea should not be taken by anyone with an auto-immune condition, such as rheumatoid arthritis, lupus or multiple sclerosis.

BUILD YOUR STRENGTH

You can support your immune system by working on the many aspects of your lifestyle that affect it. Here are the best ways to keep the immune system healthy:

- **Stay smoke-free** Active and passive smoking both make you more prone to infections, which are also likely to be more severe than in those not exposed to smoke. This was clearly illustrated by a 2010 study in Cincinnati, Ohio, which found that both smoking and exposure to secondhand smoke in nurses had negative effects on the immune system's ability to function.
- **Be active** Ask yourself whether you get enough exercise. If you're generally fit and mobile, aim to include a combination of aerobic and muscle-strengthening activities. Good choices for over-65s include 30 minutes of brisk walking, yoga, dancing or even pushing a lawnmower most days – or digging the garden on a couple of days a week. For anyone less mobile, doing any activity, however light, is beneficial. This may also help you keep to a healthy weight – carrying excess kilos raises your risk of diseases such as diabetes, cancer and heart disease. And part of the reason for that may lie in the way excess fat cells affect the immune system, causing dangerous inflammation, which in turn damages your tissues.
- **Prioritise sleep** A good night's sleep is essential if your body's defence system is to work to the best of its ability; conversely, prolonged sleep deprivation can wear down your immune responses – and you'll produce fewer antibodies to combat infections, as one recent Brazilian study has shown. (*See* pages 241–245 for ways to improve your sleep.)
- **Eat for immunity** A well-balanced diet that answers all your body's nutritional needs helps to protect you against infection – choose lots of fruit, vegetables, fibre and whole grains, and foods that are low in saturated fats and sugars (*see* pages 118–122).

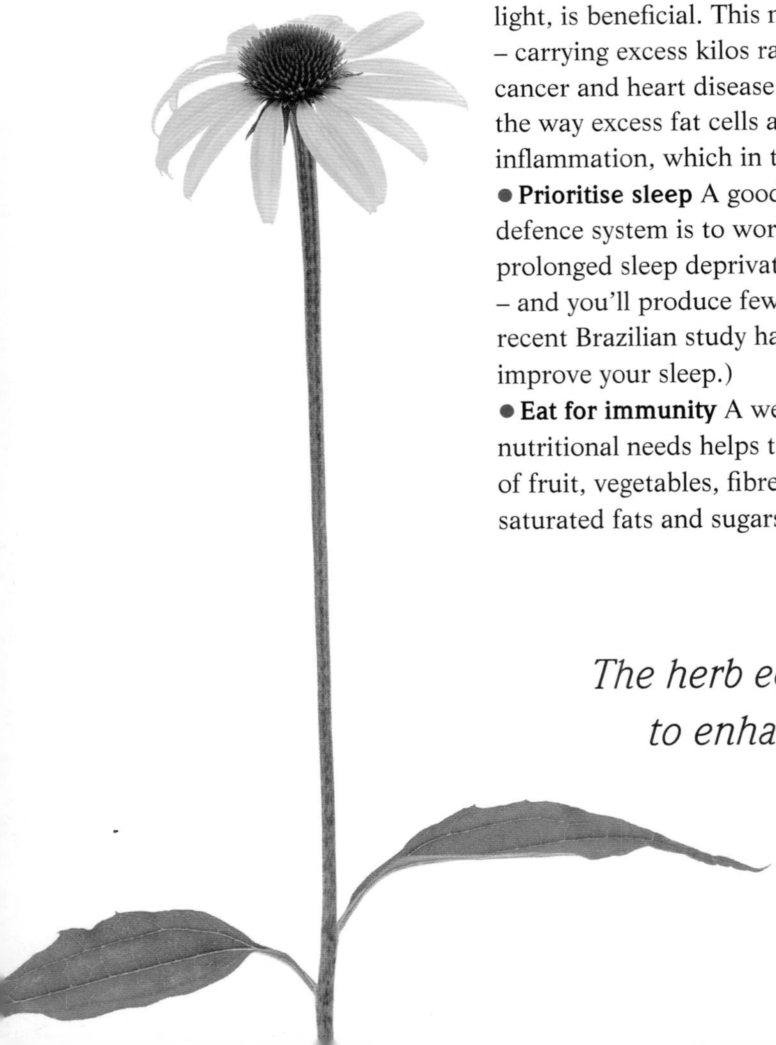

The herb echinacea has been shown to enhance immune function.

5 ways to PEP UP your IMMUNE SYSTEM

There are many ways to keep your immune system in the best possible working order. Here are five immunity boosters that may surprise you:

1 CHERISH YOUR FRIENDS A ten-year study of 1500 people over 70, conducted by Flinders University in Australia, found that those with stronger friendship networks lived longer than those with fewer friends, suggesting that friends have a positive influence on lifestyle choices, such as smoking or exercise, as well as offering emotional support. All of these are good news for your immune system.

2 KNOW YOUR LIMITS Persistently taking on more than you can easily manage causes stress, which has a negative impact on health, as studies worldwide from the 1960s to the present day have shown. The stress hormones cortisol and adrenaline suppress the immune system. Stress affects the body's ability to respond to infection, and can lead to a loss of appetite, changes in sleep patterns and depression. Learn to say no when you feel overloaded. And if you can't avoid the stresses in your life, practise relaxation techniques or learn meditation.

3 PUT ON A CD Listening to your favourite music can help your immune system. A study at Wilkes University in Pennsylvania found that when the music stopped after 30 minutes of listening, levels of IgA – an antibody that helps fight infections – increased, remaining elevated, while stress levels were reduced proportionately.

4 ENJOY SEX There seems to be a link between sexual activity and a sense of wellbeing. A study by the University of Chicago Pritzker School of Medicine of 3000 Americans aged 57 to 85 showed that those who were having sex rated their general health higher than those who weren't. The reason: having sex provides a healthy boost of IgA protein. Those who were in a close relationship or married were more likely to say they felt in very good health, the same study found.

5 BE AN ANIMAL LOVER Stroking a pet not only fulfils the basic human need to touch, but has also been found to benefit the immune system by boosting protective IgA levels, another study by Wilkes University found.

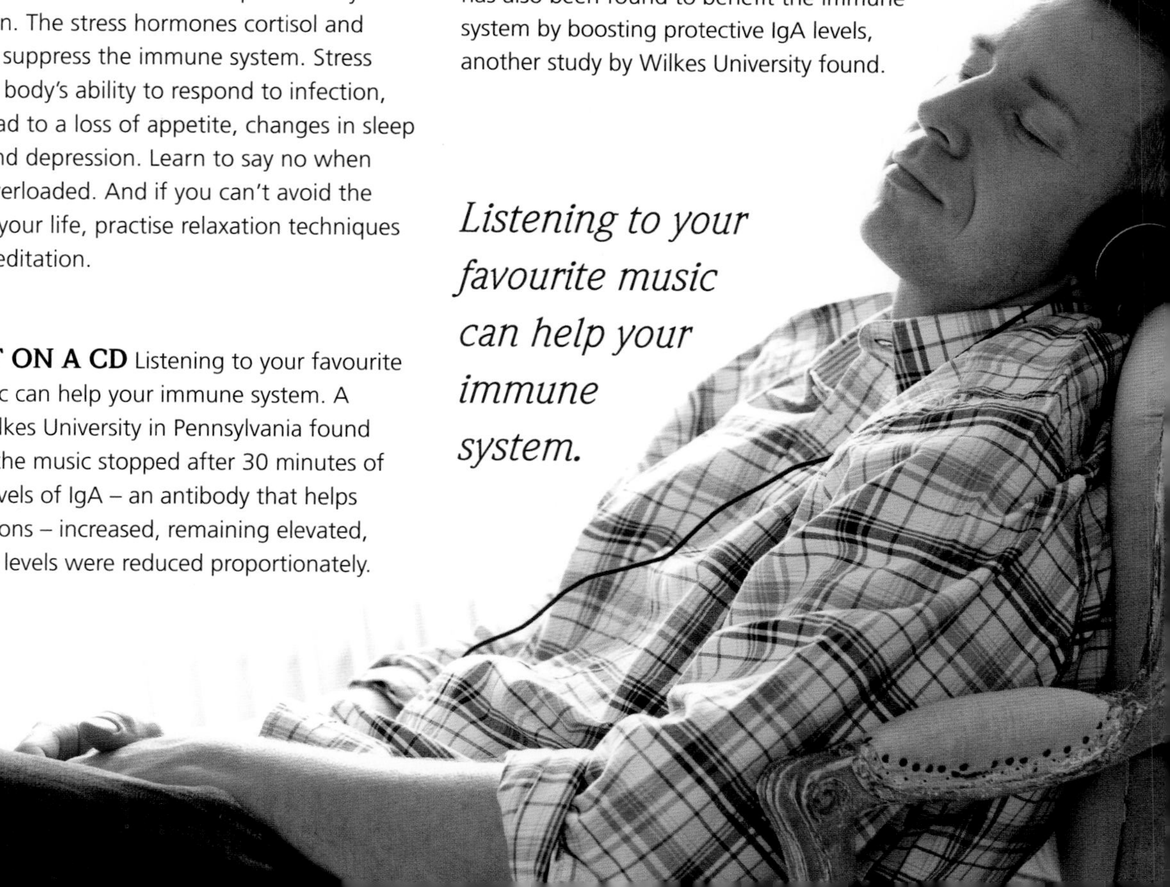

Listening to your favourite music can help your immune system.

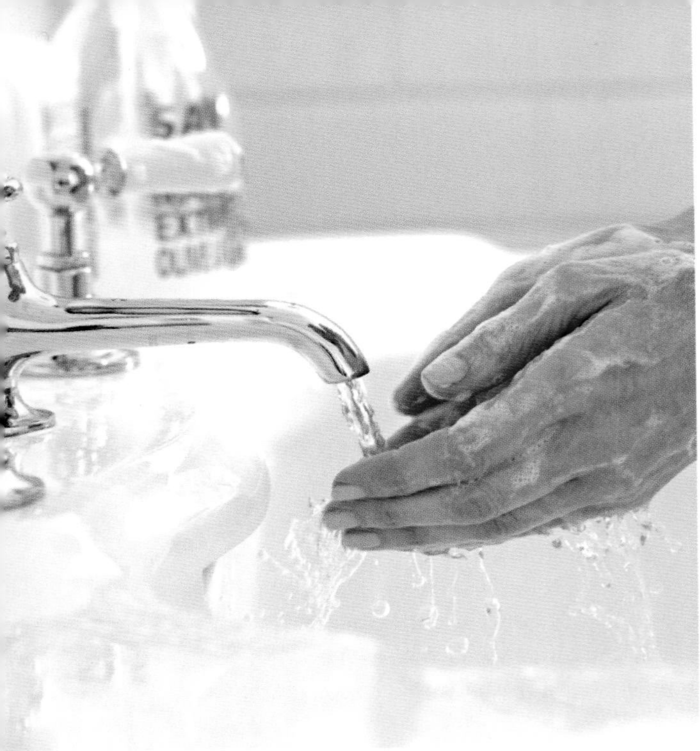

- **Keep clean** Be scrupulous about hygiene when you prepare, cook and store food. Thoroughly clean the inside of your fridge regularly and check the temperature is sufficiently low (0°C to 5°C). When you're preparing food, take care over kitchen cleanliness and wash your hands frequently. This will reduce the number of pathogens able to get into your body.
- **Reduce toxins** Keep tabs on the amount of toxic chemical products such as detergents and bleach that you use around the house – if you don't need it, don't use it. Avoid mixing different chemicals such as bleach and limescale remover, as this can give off noxious gases.
- **Get protection** Another crucial precautionary measure: take advantage of vaccinations for older people – an annual flu jab, and a one-off pneumonia jab. Take up screening too, such as eye tests, breast screening and the faecal occult blood test (*see* page 127).

Wash your hands thoroughly after using public transport and when you come home from an outing.

DODGE THE GERMS

Older people tend to mix less in groups – you're now much less likely to be going out to work in an office or spending the day in a classroom, for example. This means that you come up against fewer bugs for your immune system to fight off on a day-to-day basis. But there is still plenty of potential for encountering 'new' pathogens – through close contact with your grandchildren, mingling with crowds of people in shopping centres or using public transport or facilities such as libraries and swimming pools. A disease you missed in childhood – such as rubella (German measles) or chickenpox, or a cold bug that your memory T cells have not encountered before – can cause problems for your immune system, which, because of depleted numbers of naïve T cells (*see* page 113), can lead to more serious complications than in younger people.

It makes sense, therefore, to do all you can to avoid such infections:

- Wash your hands thoroughly after using public transport, and when you come home from an outing.

focus ON ... SHINGLES

Anyone who has had chickenpox in the past can develop shingles, but it's more likely to strike when you're older. Inactive particles of the original virus lie dormant in a 'junction box' in the nerves beside your spine over a lifetime – kept in check by the immune system – until they are reactivated, sometimes for no apparent reason.

The result of this reactivation? Shingles (due to the herpes zoster virus) – the infection of a nerve and the area of skin supplied by that nerve, on one side of the body, commonly the chest, abdomen and upper face (including the eye). Usual symptoms are a localised band of pain and a rash of red blotches that quickly turn into blisters.

There's often confusion over how shingles develops. Here are two facts it's worth knowing:

- You cannot catch shingles from someone who has shingles.
- You can catch chickenpox from someone with shingles if you haven't had chickenpox before; the virus is passed on by direct contact with the blisters.

As many as one in four people over 60 who gets shingles develops post-herpetic neuralgia (PHN), where the nerve pain persists after the rash has gone. The likelihood of PHN increases with age.

● **HELP YOURSELF** If you have shingles, taking painkillers, using calamine lotion and wearing loose clothing may all help reduce pain. In addition, ask your doctor to prescribe an antiviral medicine to prevent PHN. This is usually given within 72 hours (ideally, within 14) of the rash appearing, or later if you are older and have severe shingles, or if it affects your eye. It doesn't kill the virus, but stops it from multiplying and reduces the length of the illnesss and the risk of PHN.

● **NEW HOPE** A US study of 75,000 over-60s who had been vaccinated against herpes zoster (the shingles virus) found their risk of the disease was halved, confirming previous studies. The vaccine is available in Australia on a private prescription from your doctor and costs about $200.

- Go shopping and use public transport outside peak hours.
- Open windows to get fresh air circulating when the room is full of people.
- Keep away from your grandchildren when they have infections, if you possibly can.
- If you can't stay away, go for minimal physical contact – avoid hugging and kissing family and friends when they are infectious. And take extra care with hygiene.
- Pay particular attention to the tips on pages 114–116 if you have been around anyone with an infectious illness.

Losing **excess** weight can strengthen your immune system by 50 per cent, say US scientists.

WAYS TO PEP UP
the immune system

A number of nutritious ingredients can make a real difference to how well your immune system functions, as well as helping it to counteract any of the detrimental changes that come with age. Take extra care now to ensure that your diet is packed full of them.

After the age of 60, your eating habits, likes and dislikes may change. There are many reasons for this: your sense of taste may alter, you may eat your meals at different times because you don't have to fit into a work routine, you may have less of an appetite and feel full quicker. And if you take medicines, they may hinder the absorption of some nutrients, leading to a lack of some vitamins and minerals. None of these changes needs to be a problem. But it is increasingly important to select the foods you eat with a view to boosting your immune system. And do make sure your food is as fresh as possible – it can lose vital nutrients if it's left around for too long, whether on the shelf or in the fridge.

● **BEAT FREE RADICALS** These are normal by-products of your metabolism, but can upset healthy cell functioning and suppress your immune system if left unchecked. The way to combat them is to take in more anti-oxidants such as vitamins A, C and E, as well as compounds called flavonoids. Citrus fruits supply vitamin C, which boosts your system's ability to kill viruses and bacteria. Other orange and dark green fruits and vegetables provide beta-carotene, which the body converts into vitamin A, the main anti-oxidant needed to keep the skin and mucous membranes that line your gut in good health. Avocados, nuts, wheatgerm, seeds and seed oils, and egg yolks all contain vitamin E, which boosts the body's response to invading bugs.

● **GO FOR ZINC** Even a mild deficiency in zinc – which is quite common as you get older – can impair your immune function and make you more open to infections. Shellfish, pumpkin seeds and wholemeal bread are all zinc-rich foods, as are pine nuts.

5 SUPER FOODS for inner strength

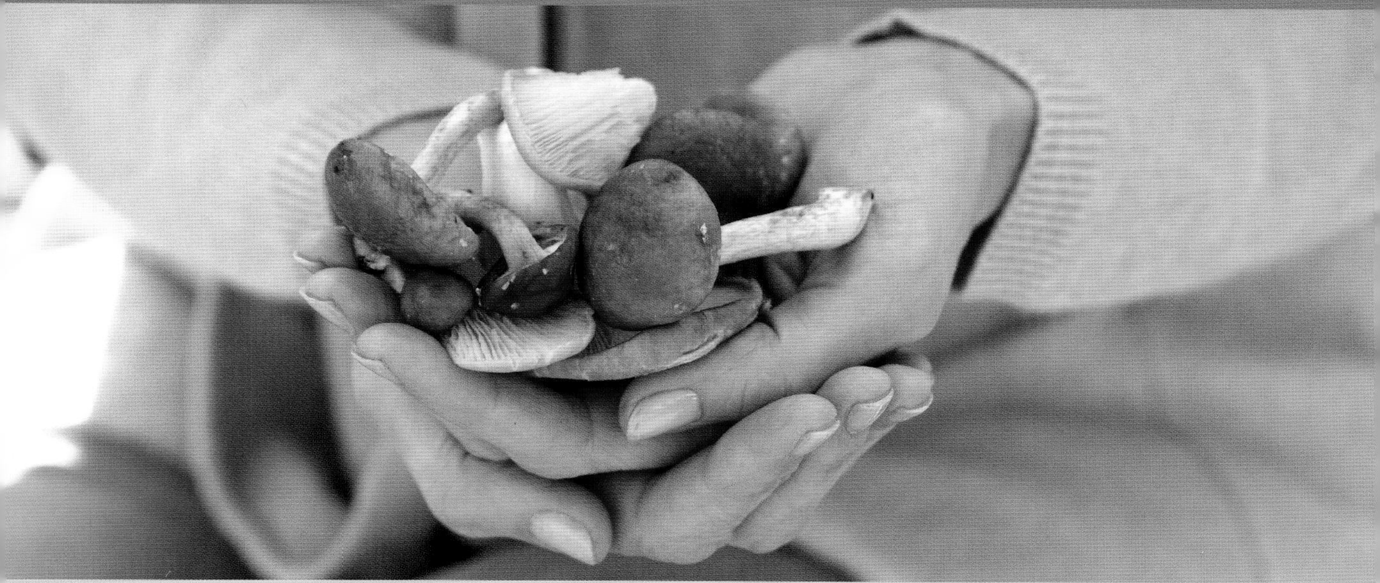

Mushrooms can stimulate your immune system ...

1 PROBIOTIC CHEESE A 2010 study at the University of Turku in Finland showed that eating probiotic cheese can help improve the immune response – an innovative way to thwart deterioration of the immune system. Aged cheese is a first-rate source of probiotics as, during the ripening process, bacteria spontaneously grow. Aged and vintage Gouda are excellent sources. You can also buy cheese to which probiotic bacteria have been added.

2 APPLES The old saying 'an apple a day keeps the doctor away' is true, according to a 2010 study by the University of Illinois. It found that pectin, the soluble fibre found in apples, caused immune cells to become anti-inflammatory, speeding healing from infection. Apples also contain flavonoids, which work as anti-oxidants in the body.

3 GOLDEN KIWI FRUIT Research by the Norwegian Institute of Public Health found that this type of kiwi fruit is packed with ingredients that protect you against damage from free radicals.

4 MUSHROOMS A study at Pennsylvania State University showed that five different types of edible mushroom stimulate the immune system: white button, crimini, maitake, oyster and shiitake – confirming previous research.

5 OLIVE OIL A 2011 study at Alagappa University, India, clearly illustrated that olive oil – an excellent source of vitamin E and mono-unsaturated fats – is good for both the heart and the immune system, guarding against oxidative stress (which produces free radicals) as well as DNA damage.

DID you KNOW?

Cutting kilojoules may be the key to boosting immunity. Scientists at Tufts University, USA, studied 46 overweight, but not obese, men and women aged 20 to 42 who spent six months on a kilojoule-restricted diet. Not only did the participants shed weight, but their immune response was boosted by 30 to 50 per cent (indicated by a skin test that measured how well their T cells reacted to antigens before and after the study).

When Indian scientists conducted an analysis in 2011 of 15 trials, they confirmed what many people already swear by – that zinc supplements reduce the duration and severity of the common cold when taken within 24 hours of the onset of symptoms.

● **DON'T FORGET THE IRON** Being low in iron adversely affects your immune system by reducing the activity of white cells. Red meat, liver, egg yolks, pulses and dark green leafy vegetables are all good sources.

● **RAISE YOUR GLASS** To wash down all this immunity-enhancing food you can enjoy a glass of wine. Moderate intake has been found to raise IgA levels (the antibody that has a critical effect on immunity).

● **WATCH THE FAT** A diet that is high in saturated fats can suppress your immune system. Opt for healthier fats – the type found in oily fish such as salmon or tuna. And try flaxseed (linseed) or walnut oils for cooking.

● **EAT FIBRE-RICH FOODS** Fibre speeds up the rate at which waste passes through your body, cutting the time any potentially cancer-causing substances are in contact with your intestine. Aim for 25 g a day for women and 30 g for men A review of 25 studies by Imperial College London confirmed that a high intake of fibre, particularly cereal fibre and whole grains, was associated with a reduced risk of colorectal cancer.

THE SUNSHINE VITAMIN

Vitamin D was for a long time known only for its role in bone health. But now scientists are finding out much more about the crucial part it plays in preventing illnesses from flu to cancer. Vitamin D is what is termed a 'fat-soluble' vitamin. This is important because it means it can be stored in your body for future use. There are only a few foods that contain vitamin D naturally. In fact, 90 per cent of vitamin D is made in our skin with the help of sunlight – and that is where the problem arises: insufficient sunlight leads to low levels of vitamin D. That might not seem like a common problem in sunny Australia, but with so many people being careful about sun exposure, some are missing out.

Quiz How **toxic** is your lifestyle?

Many everyday things we do pose no significant problem to our immune system by themselves (though some certainly do). But added together they can have a harmful impact. Take the test to see the impact of your lifestyle on your immune system.

	Every day/Always	Sometimes	Occasionally/Never
1 Do you often feel stressed or anxious?	☐	☐	☐
2 Do you smoke?	☐	☐	☐
3 Do you feel unusually thirsty?	☐	☐	☐
4 Do you have more than one glass of alcohol in an evening?	☐	☐	☐
5 Do you drink coffee, tea and other caffeinated drinks?	☐	☐	☐
6 Do you often use household products such as chemical sprays, detergents and bleach?	☐	☐	☐
7 Do you keep your windows tightly closed?	☐	☐	☐
8 Do you ever forget to wash your hands after touching your pet?	☐	☐	☐
9 Do you walk or cycle along busy roads?	☐	☐	☐
10 Do you eat red meat?	☐	☐	☐

Score 2 for each 'Every day/Always', 1 for 'Sometimes', and 0 for 'Occasionally/Never'

11 or more: Your immune system is taking quite a battering. Act now to protect your health by quitting smoking and reducing the amount you drink, if necessary. Other changes are less demanding – staying well hydrated, cutting down on salt and red meat, getting plenty of fresh air and checking your cleaning products for toxicity.

6–10: You could be kinder to your immune system. Making a few changes to your lifestyle could make a big difference. Why put unnecessary pressure on your body?

Under 5: You obviously have a good understanding of immunity health hazards; your immune system will thank you for it.

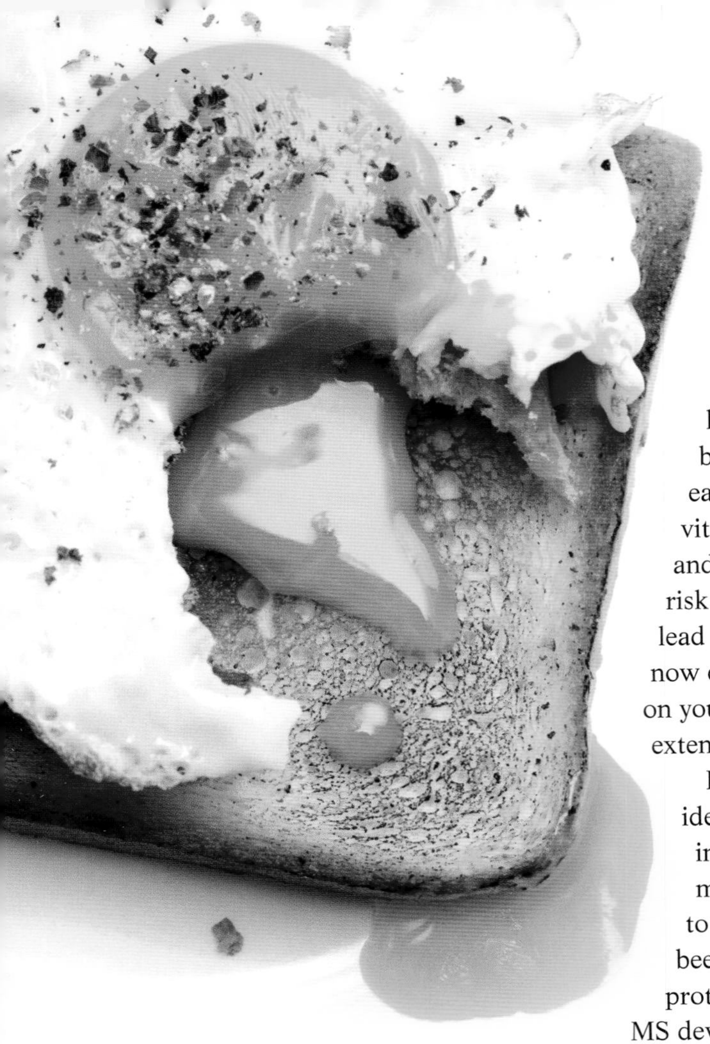

Why you need D

It's easy to become deficient in vitamin D, especially when you're older. You might stay indoors more than you used to; you may be taking medications that interfere with its production (such as some steroids, cholesterol-lowering medications and calcium channel blockers); you may have thinner skin that burns easily so you cover up more. But without enough vitamin D to help with the absorption of calcium and phosphorus in your diet, you're at increased risk of bone and muscle weakness, which can in turn lead to falls and fractures. What's more, science has now established that vitamin D has significant effects on your whole immune system: in fact, its influence extends to almost every cell in your body.

Researchers in the USA and elsewhere have identified certain cancers that are more common in those with low vitamin D levels, and there's mounting evidence to link multiple sclerosis (MS) to a lack of sunshine. Taking D supplements has been shown to lower levels of C-reactive protein (a protein linked to inflammation in the body), arrest MS development, turn off proliferating cancer cells, prevent respiratory infections … The list goes on. So it pays to adopt the following strategies:

Eat egg yolks to boost levels of essential vitamin D.

- **Snatch sunshine** How long you need to be in the sun to get enough vitamin D varies from person to person depending on their skin type, location, the time of day/year and so on. Ask your doctor for a specific recommendation.
- **Eat oily fish** Top choices are salmon, sardines, pilchards, herring, trout, tuna and mackerel (especially important in winter months).
- **Enjoy eggs** The yolk of an egg is rich in vitamin D.
- **Try fortified foods** Some cereals and juices come with added vitamin D.
- **Supplement** You can supplement with vitamin D all year round; the National Health and Medical Research Council recommends 10 mcg (400 IU) a day for people aged 51 to 70 and 15 mcg (600 IU) for people over 70 years of age. (*See also* page 89.)

SHOULD I GET VACCINATED?

When you are given a jab, a non-infectious substance, which contains the same antigens as a foreign invader, is introduced into your body. Your immune system is then 'taught' to recognise the bug by creating an army of memory T cells and antibody-producing B cells to protect against future infection (*see* pages 112–113).

Early vaccination is something that will carry you through to your later years. That's because your body remembers the instructions to combat an unchanging invader. But the flu vaccine needs to be given on an annual basis because there are many different strains of flu virus and the dominant strain changes each year. Here are the three most important things to know about vaccination as you get older:

- **ARM YOURSELF AGAINST FLU** It's important to get your annual flu jab once you're 65 or if you have asthma, COPD or some other lung problem. Flu can be more severe as you get older and you are more likely to develop complications. The best time to get your jab? In the autumn before the flu season starts.

- **GET THE 'PNEUMO' JAB** Anyone over 65 is advised to have a pneumococcal conjugate vaccine (PCV), to protect against pneumococcal bacterium, which can cause several dangerous infections, including pneumonia. This is a one-off jab that provides lifelong protection.

- **PREPARE BEFORE YOU TRAVEL** When you holiday abroad, be sure to have the required vaccinations and booster shots. Check with your doctor that they will continue to protect you for the duration of your stay, bearing in mind that your immune system may not be as well equipped as it used to be to respond to new bugs. This is especially important if you're heading for exotic places likely to be populated by bugs you have previously not met.

what's NEW

TARGETED JABS Austrian researchers have found that older people do not react as well as younger people to vaccinations because their antibody responses are slower and less strong. Consequently, new types of vaccines – and novel methods of vaccine delivery – are being explored. Trials in the USA of a new, high-dose flu vaccination designed specifically for people aged 65 and above have indicated that it produces a stronger immune response (higher antibody levels) than the standard flu vaccine. This suggests that there could soon be more effective vaccinations routinely available and tailored to the ageing population.

2.8 million cancers could be prevented worldwide if people lived healthier lives.

CANCER
a better outlook

More people are living longer, so it's not surprising that cancer is much more common – it's a disease more likely to occur in later life when cells have had time to mutate. But improved scientific understanding of the way cancer works is producing real benefits in prevention, treatment and survival, taking away much of the fear a diagnosis used to bring.

Cancer occurs when your cells grow, divide and proliferate uncontrollably. This is usually triggered by damage to your DNA – the molecular blueprint that 'instructs' your cells how to behave. Only a small proportion of cancers are caused by inherited genes.

This is good news because it means that you can substantially reduce your risk of cancer simply by avoiding exposure to the things that cause DNA damage – such as the toxic substances in cigarette smoke. In fact, more than 40 per cent of cancers are caused by lifestyle factors, which are things you can change, according to Cancer Research UK. And adopting a healthy lifestyle also helps to boost your immune response, cutting the risk of other illnesses.

If you change just six things ...

There is plenty of advice about making healthy choices in this book, but according to the Australian Cancer Council, the following are the most important changes you can make to cut your risk of cancer.

- Give up smoking.
- Include more fruit and vegetables in your diet.
- Drink alcohol only in moderation.
- Exercise regularly.
- Make sure you maintain a healthy weight.
- Limit exposure to intense sunlight and don't use sunbeds.

SPOT IT EARLY

Early diagnosis of any cancer usually means easier treatment and a more successful outcome. You know your body well, so are in the best position to notice any unusual symptoms. Look out, in particular, for specific cancer 'red flags' – such as suspicious lumps as indicators of breast cancer, dark red blood in stools that may suggest bowel cancer, or altered moles or itchy spots which can indicate skin cancer. Knowing what is normal for you will ensure that you notice anything unusual promptly. Tell your family doctor if you spot an unexplained or persistent change – don't simply put it down to age and the expectation that your body will behave differently as you get older.

'Attitude is a little thing that makes a big difference.'

Winston Churchill,
British prime minister

NEW TREATMENTS

Advances in the way cancer is diagnosed and treated have led to huge improvements: more than 40 per cent of people with cancer today will still be alive in ten years. Treatments aim to cure the cancer, control it or relieve symptoms. Surgery is used to remove the tumour; chemotherapy drugs kill cancer cells; radiotherapy uses high-energy rays to destroy cancer cells; biological therapies use natural body substances to the same end; while hormonal therapies alter the way hormones in the body affect cancer cells.

Continued on page 128

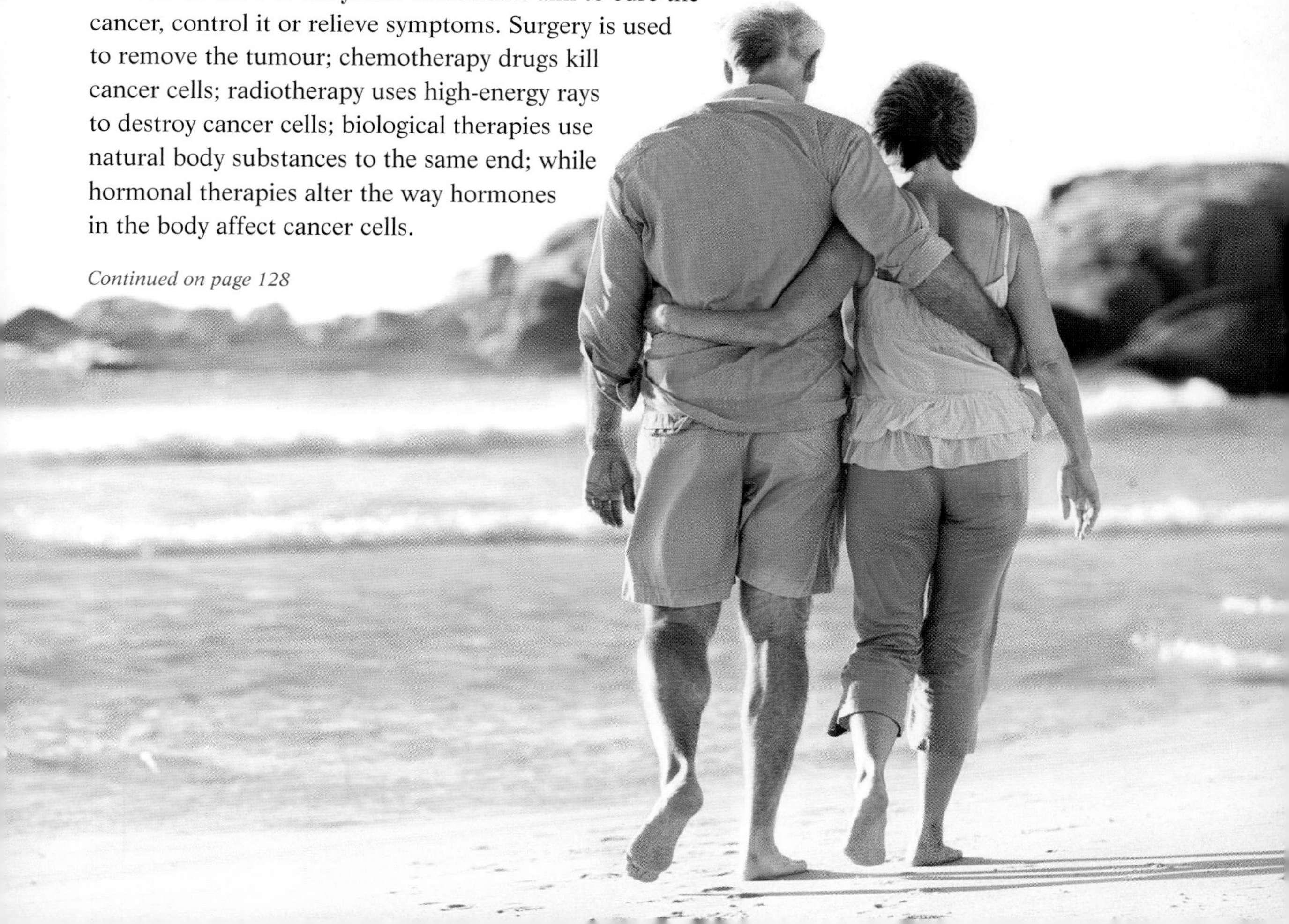

SCREEN for common cancers

In Australia, the most common types of cancer are prostate, bowel, breast and lung cancer and melanoma. There are screening programs for bowel, cervical and breast cancer, and a controversial test for prostate cancer, while people at risk of melanoma can have regular skin checks with their doctor.

Prostate

According to the Australian Cancer Council, the risk of being diagnosed with prostate cancer by the age of 85 is one in four. Age is the most significant risk factor but your risk also goes up if you have a family history of prostate or breast cancer, or are of black African ancestry.

See your doctor urgently if you experience any of these symptoms: having to rush to the toilet to pass urine, difficulty or pain in passing urine, passing urine more often than usual, especially at night-time, or blood in your urine. The good news is that prostate cancer has a high survival rate of 77 per cent after the milestone marker of five years.

Checking the blood

The current screening (available on request) is a blood test for prostate specific antigen (PSA). A raised PSA level may mean you have prostate cancer, but some experts believe the test is unhelpful because:

- Two out of three men with raised PSA levels do not have prostate cancer – the cause may also be enlarged prostate, prostatitis or urinary infection.
- The PSA test can miss cancer.
- Further tests are needed to confirm cancer.
- There's no evidence that testing reduces mortality.

Your doctor can help you decide whether or not to take the screening test. Research into ways of improving screening has come up with promising results – Surrey University discovered that a urine test for eN2 protein (found only in men with cancer) was 66 per cent accurate in predicting prostate cancer.

Breast

In Australia, more than 10,000 cases of breast cancer are diagnosed each year; it is the most common cancer in women. It can affect women of all ages but those over 70 are most at risk. Men can get it too (though this is rare). Yet there is much cause for optimism. Better understanding and treatment mean that more people are now recovering and living long and full lives. If caught early, 85 to 90 per cent of people survive at least five years – the point at which the chance of the cancer returning is much lower.

Look for symptoms

- Be breast aware – look out for any lumps or bumps, or changes in appearance or feel. This goes for men as well as women. Report anything unusual to your doctor straight away.
- Australian women aged 50 to 70 are invited to screening by the screening program every two years. (Between 40 and 50 and after 70, you can still have screening, but need to ask for it.) The test is by mammogram – the breast is pressed between two plates so that an X-ray can be taken. It can be uncomfortable but only for the short time the X-ray is being taken. Further tests such as an ultrasound or a biopsy may be needed to confirm the cancer.

Breast cancer screening is somewhat controversial because of the number of women falsely diagnosed and put through unnecessary treatment. But screening can pick up the disease at an early stage, so the advice is still to take up

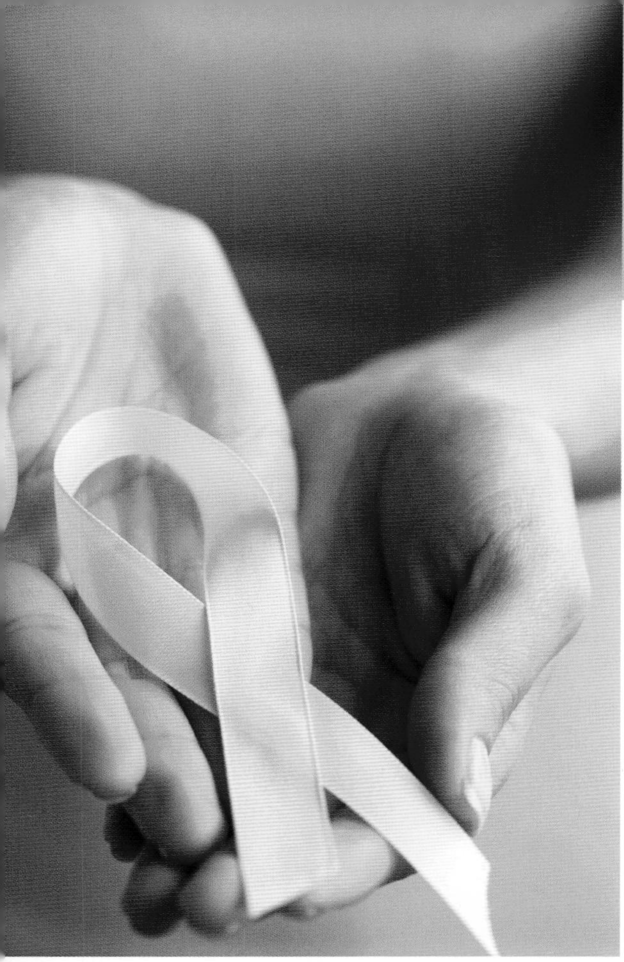

screening: survival rates for all people with screen-detected cancers are high: 85 per cent live at least 15 years. In the future the introduction of new digital equipment with improved image quality and reduced radiation dose will inevitably lead to more advanced techniques and more accurate diagnoses. Your doctor can help you to make an informed decision on screening, and understand fully the benefits and limitations.

Genetic tests are available to women with a strong family history of breast cancer; you usually need to have a living relative with breast cancer who can be tested first. Ask your family doctor for details and be aware that the test can have a big impact on you and other family members.

Bowel

Colorectal or bowel cancer becomes much more common with age: 86 per cent of bowel cancers occur in people over 60. Ask your doctor about the best screening test for you and whether it is available for free.

Take the test

- The faecal occult blood test (FOBT) is effective and safe – and it is done in the privacy of your own home via a testing kit. It detects traces of blood that you can't normally see, and is a valuable opportunity to identify cancer at an early stage and treat benign polyps before they become malignant (*see* page 103). The Australian Cancer Council recommends an FOBT every two years once you turn fifty.
- A new one-off flexible sigmoidoscopy (the flexi-sig) test can reduce the chances of 55 to 64-year-olds developing cancer by a third and cut death rates by 43 per cent, according to a study of more than 170,000 men and women in 14 UK centres, conducted by Imperial College London. Experts hope a screening program will one day become available in Australia.

Cervical

Cervical cancer is one of the few preventable cancers because pre-cancerous cell changes can be picked up before they have a chance to develop into cancer. Screening – in the form of the 'smear test' in which a sample of cells is taken from the cervix – is offered in Australia every two years until you turn seventy.

Targeted screening

If you are over 70, and your last two tests were normal, you won't be asked to come for more in Australia. If recent tests are normal, your doctor will advise you about what further screening you need. If you've never had a test, have one regardless of age. Ask your doctor to arrange this.

And better understanding of how normal cells escape their control mechanisms to become cancerous has opened the door to selective treatments. These block the growth and spread of cancer by interfering with specific molecules involved in tumour growth, leaving normal cells untouched. Some block the growth of blood vessels to tumours (angiogenesis); some induce cell death; some help the immune system to destroy cancer cells; some deliver toxic medications directly to cancer cells. We are moving towards a new era of 'personalised' medicine that will enable doctors to predict how a patient will respond to targeted treatment, and the dosage needed.

CANCER AND THE IMMUNE SYSTEM

There are more than 200 different types of cancer, affecting every part of the body. The immune system can be weakened by some, such as leukaemia or lymphoma, if it spreads into the bone marrow where the white blood cells that help fight infection are produced. Equally, treatments such as chemotherapy and radiotherapy can weaken immunity by causing a drop in the number of these white cells. Medical experts are now trying to turns things around and use our own immune systems to fight off cancer.

The immune system quite naturally detects some cancer cells because they are different from normal cells. But once cancer has taken hold, it does not identify a sufficient number of cells to be able to destroy it. Outside assistance is needed. The answer may lie in immunotherapy – an exciting approach that aims to harness the power of the body's own immune system to target cancer cells. Scientists are working on ways to boost the immune system's anti-tumour responses to a number of different cancer types; these novel approaches range from monoclonal antibodies (laboratory-made antibodies that recognise cancer cells) to cancer vaccines. A prototype breast cancer vaccine has shown promising results, giving hope of effective breast cancer protection in the future.

what's NEW

GREAT LEAPS FORWARD New research conducted in Britain has thrown light on the workings of the immune response to rogue tissues such as cancers. Using a super-resolution microscope, scientists were able to study the workings of natural killer (NK) cells, and hope to use the information to develop effective new cancer treatments.

Another study, at the University of Texas MD Anderson Cancer Center in the USA, has discovered that specific helper T cells – Th17 cells – can alert the body to the presence of cancer cells and initiate an attack on these cells by custom-made T cells. The findings raise the future possibility of taking a patient's own Th17 cells, expanding them in the laboratory, then re-infusing them to boost the immune response to the cancer.

Finding out that you have cancer can affect you in many different ways: you may be frightened, confused or in denial. You will adjust, though, and get on top of your conflicting emotions, and may even be relieved finally to know what is wrong.

What is certain is that you will deal with every experience in your own way. It's bound to be an up-and-down ride: one day you may feel positive – the next, deeply down. Will I ever feel happy again? Do other people with cancer feel this way? What can I do to help myself? Being patient with yourself – and getting other people to understand your situation – can enable you to cope well. Here are some ways to help yourself get through it:

- **BE GENTLE WITH YOURSELF** Don't expect to get back to normal as soon as your treatment is completed: this may be the time when the emotional impact of it all hits you, and you need more support than ever. And don't try to achieve too much. Have a go at small tasks – you'll find you can do a little more each day, and that some days you can do more than others.

- **FIND THE SUPPORT YOU NEED** People may not always react in a way that suits you, and you may find some personal relationships become strained. Being clear about the support you need makes it easier for people to help. Bear in mind that you may need to talk to others outside your close family. Join a support group or chat online.

- **WORK WITH YOUR TEAM** You may experience cancer fatigue. It's very common – and can be the most troublesome symptom – affecting you mentally, physically and emotionally. Always report it to your medical team to find out how to manage your specific feelings of exhaustion. Discuss any nausea, too – there are effective ways to control sickness, but the team needs to ascertain the cause.

- **DON'T ASSUME THE WORST** You may have pain, which can be frightening. But the amount of pain doesn't necessarily relate to how advanced the cancer is: a very small tumour might be pressing on a nerve, for instance, or the pain might not be related to the cancer at all. Do report any pain to your doctor, who will be able to help.

- **KEEP EXERCISING** Check with your doctor, of course – but physical exercise is generally beneficial for cancer patients. In a 2011 study of prostate patients in Boston, Massachusetts, USA, those who walked at normal to very brisk rates substantially improved their chances of survival.

- **PAMPER YOUR IMMUNE SYSTEM** This is more important than ever. In particular, after your treatment, take steps to ensure you don't get run down. Take special care to avoid infections. Reduce stress, in every way possible. Eat fresh food (but don't go for raw foods and macrobiotic diets, which can actually cause nutritional deficiencies and weaken your defences). Get plenty of rest, even if you can't sleep.

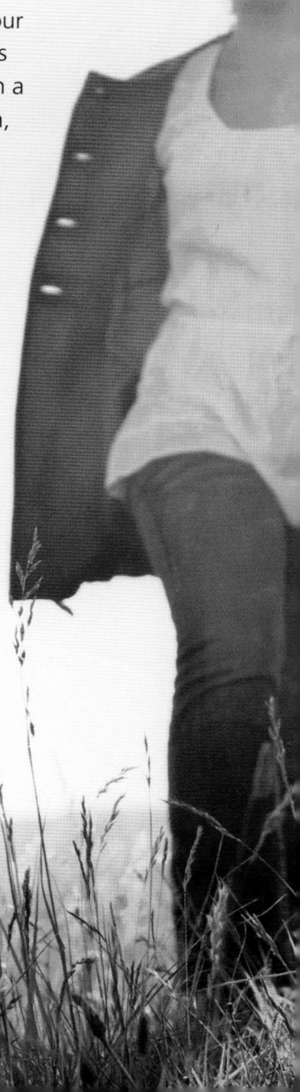

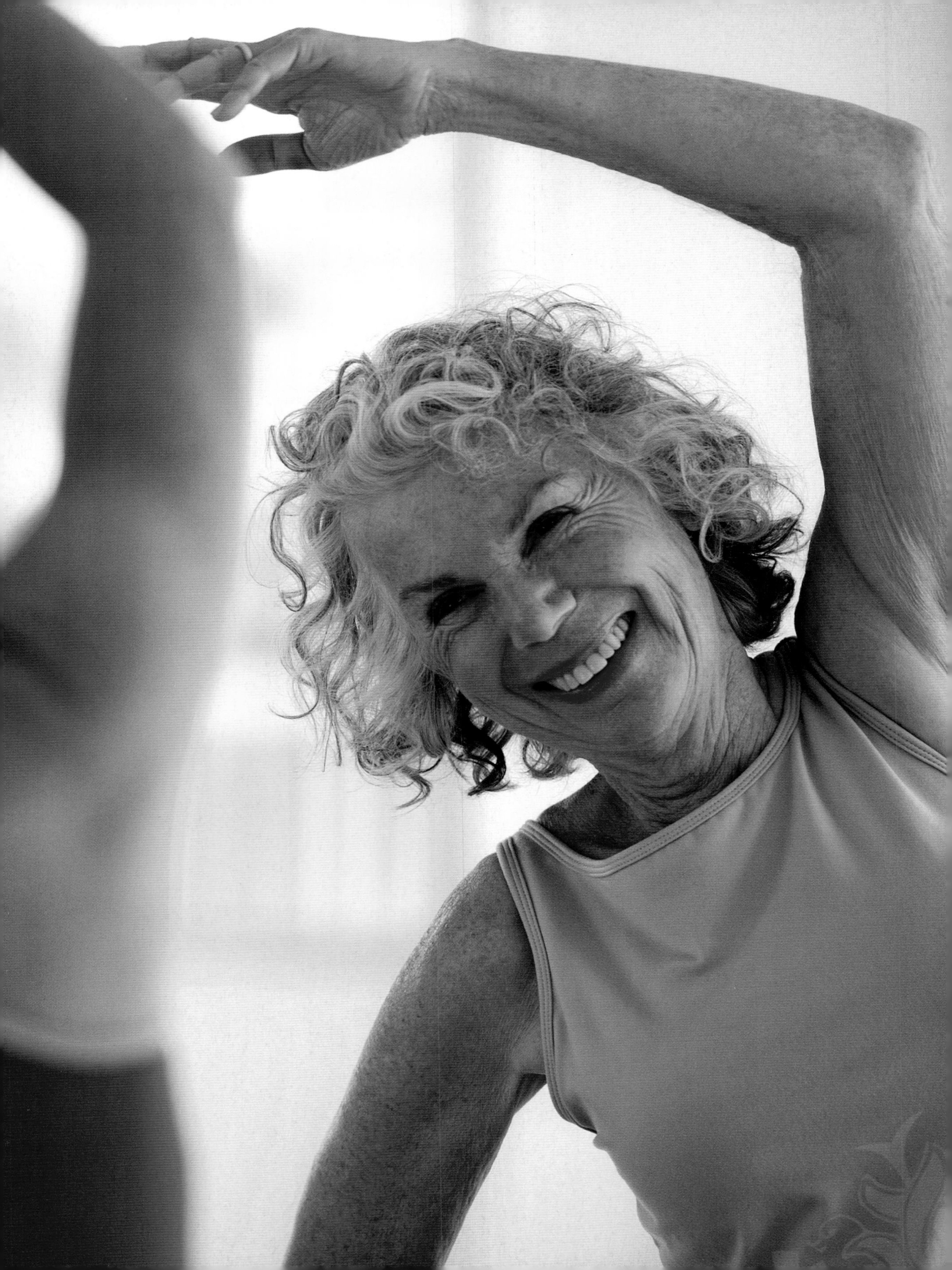

6

Keep on MOVING

Studies now confirm what Hippocrates, the father of medicine, wrote 2500 years ago: keeping active boosts your health and can prolong your life. What's more, scientists today know why the right type and amount of exercise is so beneficial. It helps to combat many age-related diseases and other physical changes that occur as you get older. Staying mobile also enables you to enjoy life's pleasures, such as travel or country walks, and these are the things that help to keep you feeling young. So what are you waiting for? It's time to get started.

30 minutes of exercise a day may cut the risk of Parkinson's disease by 40 per cent.

THE MAGIC of movement

It's a simple, proven fact: staying active keeps you well. It helps you counter the physical and mental changes of ageing, enabling you to look younger, feel more energetic and fend off illness. If there were a magic youth pill, its name would be 'physical activity'.

Why is it so important to keep moving? As you grow older your metabolism (the rate at which you burn energy) starts to slow down. That's because your vital organs, such as the brain and heart, and your tissues – for instance, bone and, crucially, muscle – tend to shrink as you age. If you are also now less active, you will have a lower energy requirement, so if you consume the same number of kilojoules as you always have, the kilograms will start to pile on. And that's a no-no because they become ever harder to shift. When it comes to burning energy, fat is more sluggish than muscle tissue, which is energy hungry – even when you're at rest. Excess fat is also more dangerous, putting you at risk of both disease and muscle and joint disorders.

How exercise helps

Weight control is just one of the benefits of keeping active. You'll also find that your breathing improves. That's because being on the move increases your body's demand for oxygen, and this challenges your heart and lungs to work harder, increasing their efficiency.

Your disease risk could fall dramatically, too. A ten-year study of 143,000 people with an average age of 63 by Harvard School of Public Health found that half an hour a day of moderate activity – jogging, swimming, tennis or cycling, say – was linked to a 40 per cent lower risk of Parkinson's disease. And Texan researchers who studied 12 sedentary individuals and 12 elite older athletes with an average age of 70 found, not surprisingly, that the older athletes had more youthful, less rigid hearts and better heart function. But encouragingly they also found that just a year of progressive and vigorous exercise training significantly improved heart function in the sedentary group – even though it didn't actually reduce cardiac stiffening.

Quiz Take the **fitness test**

Your answers to the questions below give a good indication of your general fitness. If you answer no to more than five, it's time to find ways to become more active, which will boost your strength and stamina, and help with balance.

1 Can you stand on one leg (with your arms folded across your chest, your eyes closed and your other knee bent) for longer than 20 seconds? (Stand close to a chair back or worktop that you can grab if you start to wobble.)

2 When you're out and about, do you take the stairs rather than the lift or escalator?

3 Can you walk for 30 minutes without feeling tired?

4 Are you able to carry large cartons of milk or jugs of water in each hand without feeling the strain?

5 Do you find it easy to stand up and sit down seven times in quick succession?

6 Is it easy to twist round and look behind you without moving your feet?

7 Without bending your knees, can you touch your toes?

8 Can you dance to fast music for 5 minutes and not feel winded?

9 Did you spend less than 4 hours yesterday sitting down watching TV, using a computer or just passing time?

10 Would friends and family be more likely to describe you as an energetic optimist or a worn-out pessimist?

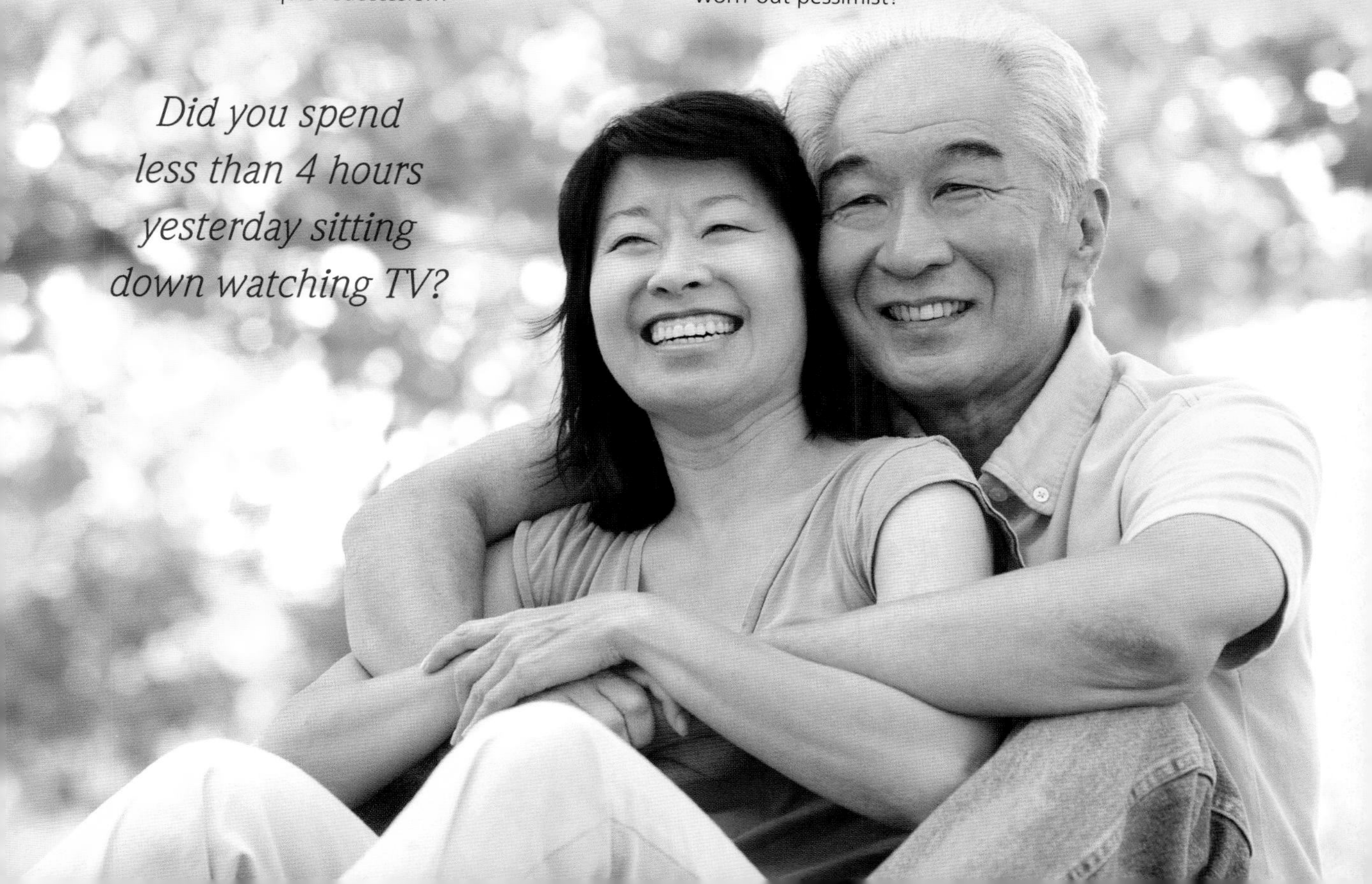

Did you spend less than 4 hours yesterday sitting down watching TV?

'To get back my youth I would do anything in the world except take exercise, get up early or be respectable.'

Oscar Wilde,
English playwright

THE FOUR PILLARS OF EXERCISE

There are four main types of activity you need to incorporate into any exercise plan, each of which has specific benefits.

● **FOR HEART AND LUNGS: cardiovascular exercise** Any activity that involves your whole body or uses your large muscle groups, and which increases your heart and breathing rate while getting you slightly breathless, is good exercise. Why? Because it increases your stamina by improving your heart's ability to pump blood around your body and supply oxygen to your organs. This also helps counteract furring and stiffening of the arteries. Try walking, running, cycling, swimming, aerobic classes, dancing or using gym equipment such as a treadmill or elliptical trainer.

● **FOR STRONG MUSCLES: resistance exercise** Exercise that forces your muscles to resist movement, either through the use of gravity-resistance aids, such as weights or bands, or by using your own body weight, will help keep your muscles strong and reduce the risk of wasting (good muscle tone also makes you look younger). Options include lifting free weights, working with stretchy 'resistance' bands or using weight machines in the gym. Yoga and Pilates both use your own body weight to help build muscle, and many gyms hold aerobic classes such as BodyPump that incorporate work with weights.

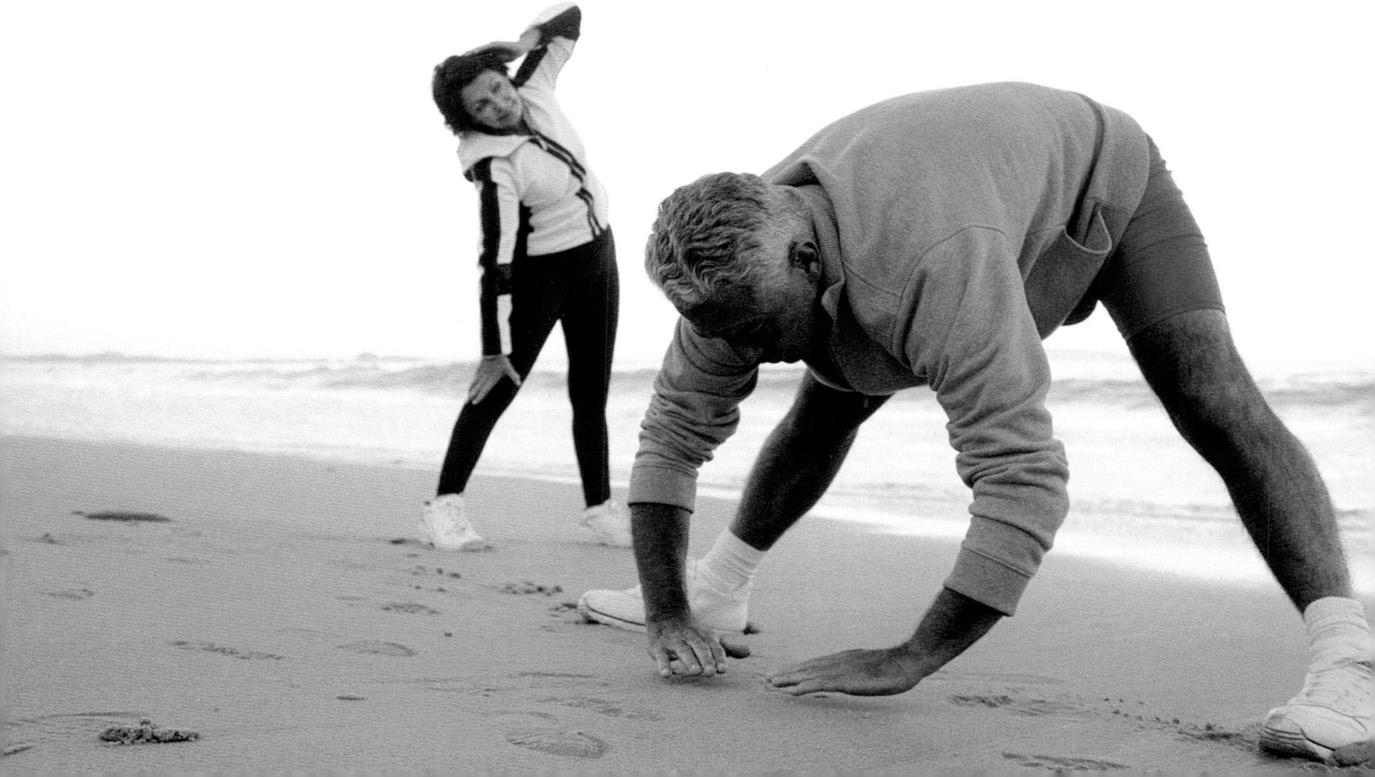

take CARE ! SAFETY FIRST

If you're starting to exercise for the first time, or if it's been a while since you were last active, or you have an underlying health condition, always consult your doctor first.

Check whether you need any medical check-ups such as a blood pressure test. If you have a chronic medical condition or a disability, ask if there are any types of exercise you shouldn't do. Exercise shouldn't hurt or make you feel unwell, although your muscles may be slightly sore afterwards. To exercise safely:

Do

- Stay hydrated – have a bottle of water to sip on before, during and after exercise, but don't overdo it.
- Wear comfortable clothing that allows you to move freely, and supportive footwear.
- Put on visible clothing if exercising outside in winter or at night.
- Do floor exercises (such as yoga) in front of a mirror to check you're doing them correctly.

Don't

- Eat a heavy meal before exercising.
- Exercise if you feel unwell or are injured.
- Undertake activity if you're overtired.
- Do any exercise if you've been drinking alcohol.
- Exercise outdoors if it's very hot or very cold.
- Do too much too soon – build up slowly.

Stop exercising immediately if ...

- You feel dizzy or short of breath, develop chest pain or pressure, palpitations and/or break out in a cold sweat – seek medical help immediately.
- A joint becomes red, swollen, painful or tender to touch – seek medical help as soon as you can.

- **FOR FLEXIBILITY: stretching** It's vital to do some stretches to lengthen tight or tense muscles and boost your circulation, improve posture and keep joints lubricated – all of which help you move more easily. You can do simple stretching exercises (*see* pages 147–151) or try yoga, Pilates or tai chi. Aim to stretch for 5 to 10 minutes daily.

- **FOR COORDINATION: balance exercises** Your stability will be improved by exercises that involve balancing. This includes any activity in which you transfer your weight from one foot to the other – walking, running, dancing, tai chi or playing hopscotch with your grandchildren. Balancing on one leg while standing improves your static or standing balance. If you have existing balance problems – such as Ménière's disease or an orthopaedic problem – check with your doctor before doing this.

8 ways to WORK OUT without realising it

Exercise is not all about spending hours on the treadmill. Normal activities can be transformed into moderate-intensity aerobic exercise simply by working hard enough so that you are slightly out of breath. Here's how to get more activity into the day:

1 GO AT IT WITH A MOP Housework – vigorous dusting, vacuuming, washing the floor or cleaning windows – can be just as good for you as a session at the gym in terms of your mental health, according to a study conducted as part of the Scottish Health Survey. But you really need to put your back into all those chores – making sure you use every opportunity to walk, lift and stretch. Exaggerate each movement – for example, when dusting a top shelf, really stretch out.

2 DITCH THE REMOTE Choose active over inactive every time. For example, rather than using the remote control, get up and switch off the TV. Doing this ten times a day burns over 15,000 kJ a year – the equivalent of half a kilo of body fat.

3 MULTI-TASK Don't sit around – do the dusting while you listen to the radio, iron standing up, walk around when you make a call. That's the message from researchers at the University of Missouri, who have found evidence that sitting adversely affects the way the body handles fat.

4 USE YOUR BUS PASS Leave your car at home and catch the bus to go shopping. According to researchers at Imperial College London, taking the bus usually involves a relatively long walk to the bus stop and more walking once you reach your destination. In addition, carrying shopping bags requires energy, meaning more kilojoules burned.

5 GET GARDENING Research from Kansas State University confirms that gardening is an effective way to exercise. Reaching for weeds, pruning tall branches, bending to deadhead flowers and extending a rake are good for flexibility, while carrying a watering can, pushing a wheelbarrow and lifting pots are all weight-bearing activities. An hour of energetic gardening can burn 3000 kJ.

6 WALK A DOG Dog walking can make you fitter than walking with a partner or friend, say researchers from the University of Missouri. In a 12-week study of 54 older adults, those who walked with a dog improved their walking speed by 28 per cent compared with just 4 per cent for those who walked with a friend or spouse.

7 BE A FIDGET Moving around – what scientists refer to as 'incidental physical activity' – can boost your cardiovascular fitness and also make a difference to whether you're fat or thin. So instead of just sitting there, jiggle your legs, get up and down from your chair, tap your toes, drum your fingers or pace up and down.

8 COOK UP A STORM Peeling, chopping, stirring, whisking and beating all burn more kilojoules than simply heating up a ready meal in the microwave. And if you really want to work up a sweat, try making your own bread – kneading dough is good hard work, and therapeutic, too.

HOW MUCH IS ENOUGH?

The amount of physical activity you need depends on your age, health and level of fitness. The National Health and Medical Research Council's exercise guidelines are the same for healthy people over 60 as they are for adults of any age, but you obviously need to take into account your starting level of fitness and any illness or disability you may have. Seek medical advice before embarking on a new fitness program if you are at all unsure.

Take a flexible approach and vary the type of activity, as you need to keep challenging yourself to maintain your fitness gains. If you do the same exercise all the time, you'll plateau and eventually become less fit. You can do it:

The easy way

- **Aim to be active every day and do:** At least 30 minutes of moderate-intensity aerobic exercise on most days (*see* below).
- **Two or more days a week do:** Muscle-strengthening activities. Aim to work all your major muscle groups: legs, buttocks, back, abdomen, chest, shoulders and arms.

Or the harder way

- **Aim to be active every day and do:** At least 75 minutes a week of vigorous-intensity activity (*see* below).
- **Two or more days a week do:** Muscle-strengthening activities, as above.

You can swap these around, so that you combine some shorter sessions of vigorous activities such as running with some more moderate ones, such as brisk walking. Just make sure you take some exercise every day.

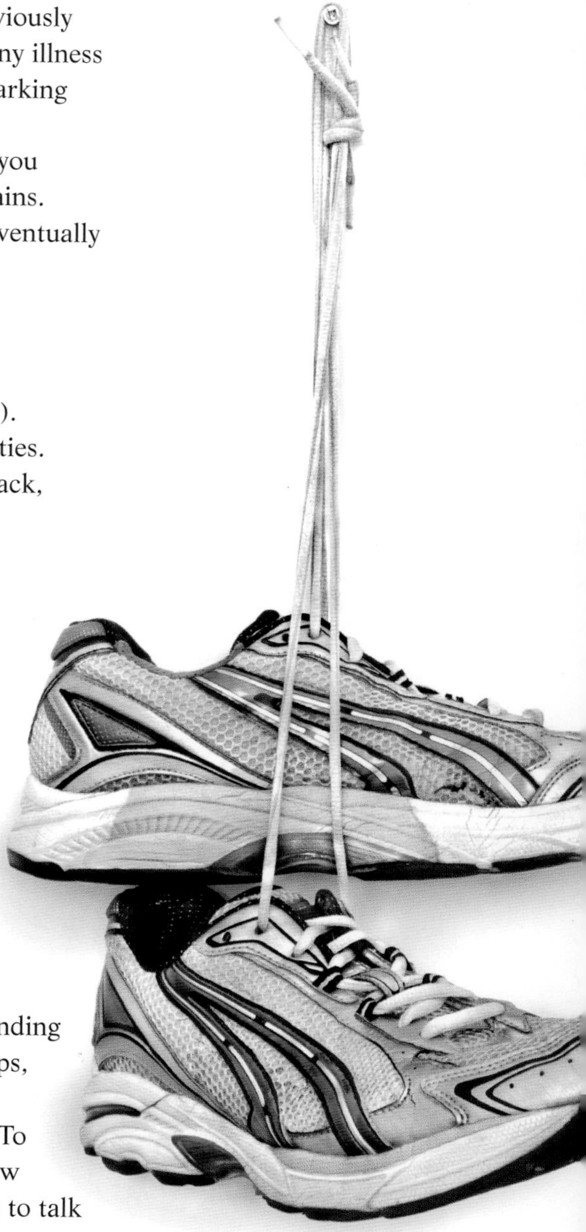

Mild, moderate or vigorous

Activities can be defined as mild, moderate or vigorous depending on how much effort you put into them. While every little helps, mild (light) exercise – going for a stroll, washing up, gentle stretching – is unlikely to have many benefits for your heart. To make it work harder, you need to sweat. How can you tell how hard you're working? As a rule of thumb, you should be able to talk but not sing while exercising moderately, whereas talking is hard if you're exercising vigorously. Moderate exercise includes golf, fast walking and a concerted bout of housework while vigorous activity is running, fast dancing (Zumba or salsa), singles' tennis or skipping. If you find it too hard to exercise moderately or vigorously at first, intersperse intervals of moderate to vigorous exercise with slower sessions – for instance, walk for a minute/jog for a minute.

If you have chronic health problems ...

Becoming more active will still bring rewards, so when you feel well enough, do try to take some exercise, even if it's less than the guidelines. Check with your doctor before you start so that he or she can advise you on the best ways to exercise and whether there are any special precautions you need to take.

- Weightlifting, stretching and 'chairobics' (*see* pages 147–148) can all help increase your range of motion, tone up your muscles and enhance the health of your heart and lungs.
- Look out for specialist classes aimed at people with mobility problems – your family doctor may be able to advise you (or *see* Resources).
- Check that any class you attend is run by a qualified instructor with specialist knowledge of your condition. Speak out if there are moves you find difficult – there may be easier variations.
- Don't exercise if you're feeling unwell. Remember that little and often is best.

DID YOU KNOW?

Nordic walking, in which you use poles to help propel you along, is a good way to increase the benefits as you exercise more muscles and burn more kilojoules than you do with standard walking. A randomised controlled trial from the University of Jyväskylä, in Finland, of a group of sedentary individuals in their late 60s, found that a nine-week, twice-weekly program of Nordic walking significantly improved the participants' ability to function in everyday life.

KEEP ON TRACK

Many of us struggle to keep up an exercise regimen, however much we want to get fit. Here are three ways to help you keep going:

1 **Make a note** Keep a record of your exercise sessions in your diary or use one of the many online trackers that are now available (for example, 'MapMyRUN' at www.mapmyrun.com). Or try fitting sensors to your running shoes, which not only helps ensure you stick to your exercise plan but also shows you how far you've progressed.

2 **Find a friend** It's easier to stick to your regimen if you feel you're accountable to someone else – so why not exercise with your partner, a friend or a fitness buddy? Or sign up to a group class.

3 **Read up** Subscribing to a fitness or sports magazine or even following sports or dance competitions on TV can help you stay motivated and give you fresh ideas.

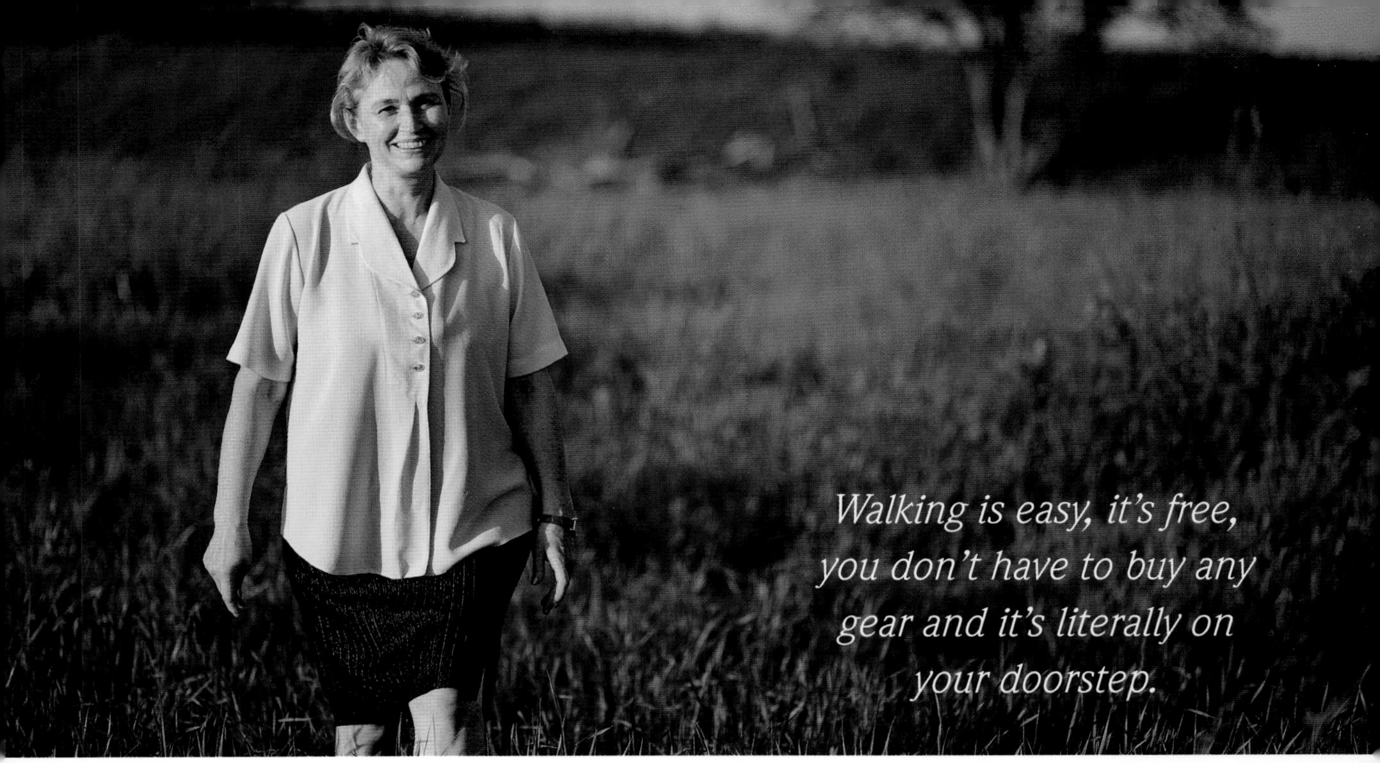

Enemies of motivation

Here are some of the excuses people make to avoid exercise – and why you shouldn't make them.

- **My health is poor** This is the most common reason older people give for not exercising, according to research by Florida Atlantic University. But being ill is usually no reason to avoid exercise and, in fact, being more active can help alleviate pain and many symptoms.
- **It takes too much time** The secret is to fit exercise into your everyday life as much as possible (*see* page 136). If you join a gym or a formal class, go for one that is close to your home or on your way to somewhere you go regularly. And prioritise exercise – think of it as being as essential as cleaning your teeth.
- **I find it uncomfortable** According to an American review looking at what stops older people from exercising, many dislike sweating, heavy breathing and muscle soreness, and imagine (wrongly) that these are harmful. Learn to welcome the signs of physical exertion as proof that you're getting fitter.
- **I'm too fat to be fit** You can still be fit if you're carrying extra kilograms. That's what Dr Steven Blair, Professor of Exercise Science at the University of South Carolina, found when he studied what he calls 'the obesity paradox'. He says that low cardiorespiratory fitness and inactivity are a greater health threat than obesity, and that being moderately fit and fat is healthier than being unfit and slim.

7 ways exercise **KEEPS YOU** young

Being active brings rewards for practically every part of the body. Here are seven of the best benefits that exercise provides.

1 YOU FEND OFF MUSCLE LOSS In 2010, the Japanese Nakanojo Study of exercise in older people found that walking 7000 to 8000 steps a day helped to preserve muscle mass in a group of 175 people aged 65 to 84.

2 YOU SLEEP BETTER In tests carried out at Chicago's Northwestern University, a 16-week program of walking, cycling or treadmill training for 40 minutes four times a week, together with tips on sleep hygiene, helped break the sleepless cycle of people aged 55-plus who were suffering from chronic insomnia.

3 YOUR CONFIDENCE IS BOOSTED Exercise makes you feel better about yourself, which motivates you to carry on, according to research on older people that was carried out at Stanford University, California.

4 YOUR BONES ARE STRONGER When Finnish researchers put 149 women aged 70 to 78 through an all-round exercise program, combining balance, agility, jumping and weights work, they found their bones became stronger – protecting against osteoporosis.

5 YOU ARE CALMER In 2011, scientists at the University Institute of Geriatrics of Sherbrooke, Quebec, found a chemical link between exercise and mood. In a study of men aged 57 to 70, an hour on the treadmill boosted their absorption of tryptophan, an amino acid associated with relaxed mood and found in foods such as turkey, lettuce and milk.

6 YOU LIVE LONGER An active lifestyle after the age of 50 can add four and a half years to your life, according to the Framingham Heart Study, which has been following the health of 5209 residents of Framingham, Massachusetts, since 1948.

7 YOU KEEP YOUR BRAIN SHARP A growing body of research suggests that being physically active can help preserve mental function. One 2011 study conducted in Paris found that just half an hour's brisk walking daily could slow cognitive decline by five to seven years. Physical activity is also linked to lower levels of protein plaques, a hallmark of Alzheimer's disease.

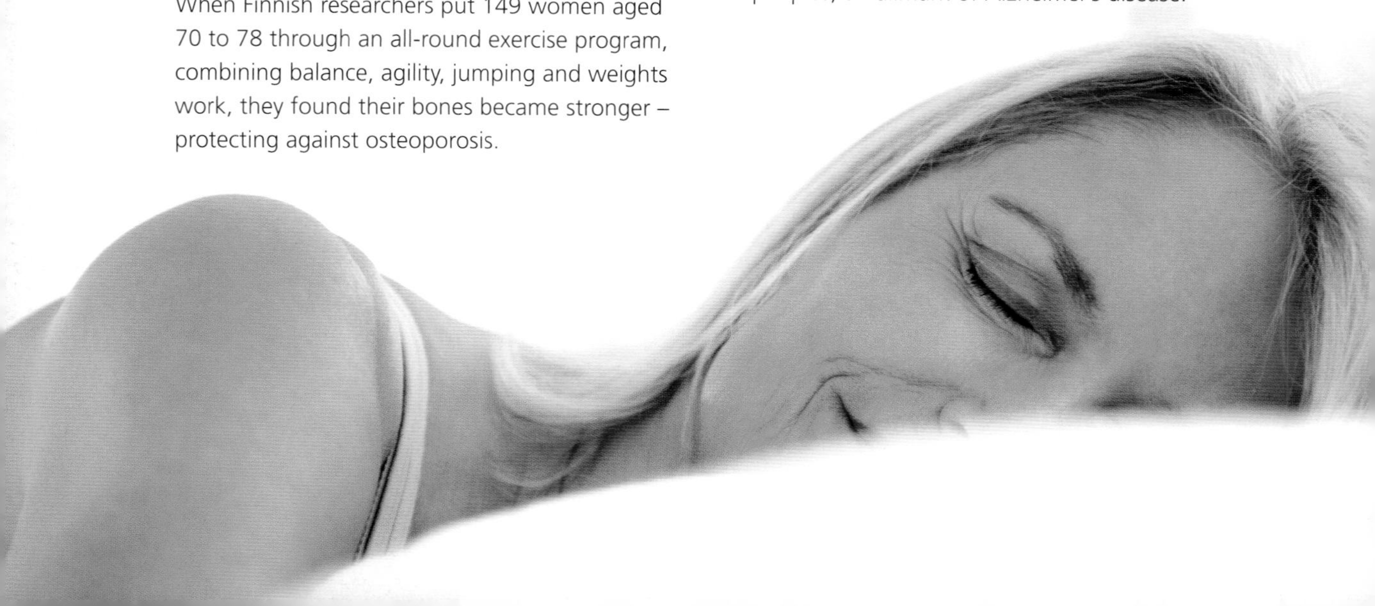

BUILDING MUSCLES
for a stronger body

Muscles are vital for everything from carrying a bag of shopping to walking, and getting up from a chair. Your muscles shrink as you grow older, but there's a lot you can do to slow the process and stay strong.

You will lose more than 8 per cent of muscle mass between the ages of 40 and 50, and this shrinkage speeds up to more than 15 per cent a decade after you hit 75. But change doesn't have to be all one way. Resistance training, also known as strength training, can help you to build muscle at any age, even if you have already lost muscle tissue.

There are plenty of good reasons for working on your muscles. For one, it boosts your metabolism, making you less likely to lay down fat. At the same time, it reduces insulin resistance (when the body makes but doesn't respond as well to insulin), lessening your risk of type 2 diabetes. It also increases stamina: a US study of 62 men and women aged 60 to 83 found that six months' resistance training improved their aerobic capacity by a fifth and their ability to run on a treadmill by a quarter.

You don't necessarily need weights to weight train – many strength exercises use the weight of your own body to provide resistance and thus increase the effort your muscles need to put in.

Six top tips

- Warm up before exercising by walking on the spot for 2 minutes, swinging your arms as you do so; gently stretch afterwards.
- Wear joggers or flat shoes with a good grip if using weights.
- Maintain good posture and remember to breathe evenly – holding your breath can increase blood pressure. Perform movements slowly.
- Build in recovery time. Your body builds new muscle in the 48 hours after resistance exercise, so take a day off between sessions.
- If anything hurts, stop straight away and get yourself checked out.
- Do check with your doctor or physiotherapist before starting a resistance training program if you have a chronic condition, have not exercised for a while or have high blood pressure.

DID **you** KNOW?

Protein is a powerful nutrient. Eating small amounts of high-protein foods such as meat, poultry, cheese and eggs throughout the day – and always after exercise – is the best way to boost muscle, according to researchers at McMaster University in Ontario. Why? As you get older, muscle breaks down at a faster rate and new muscle cells are synthesised at a slower rate, leading to age-related muscle wastage (sarcopenia). To combat this, try to include some protein with every meal and have a little after you exercise.

WORK OUT: exercises for strength

Do resistance exercise two or three times a week to build strength and stave off muscle loss. This set of exercises works all the main muscle groups. Start gently and build up to repeating each exercise ten times.

Some of the exercises in this chapter use equipment, such as small weights, resistance bands and exercise balls. If you want to invest in any of these, make sure you get the right size or type for you – ask a shop assistant for advice. These are a good way of targeting particular muscle groups or increasing the resistance required to do specific exercises. But you don't have to buy equipment to get a good workout – you can stick to the exercises that don't use equipment at all if you prefer. Do make sure you're comfortable, though, to avoid back strain. It's best to use a mat rather than a hard floor – either a yoga mat or a thicker exercise mat.

● **A STRONG CENTRE** Having strong core muscles – the deep abdominal and back muscles attached to your spine and pelvis – is essential for good posture, and they give you the stability and balance you need to respond to the demands of everyday life. Balance balls give your core muscles a good workout, but if you are unsteady, have someone standing behind you to lend a hand.

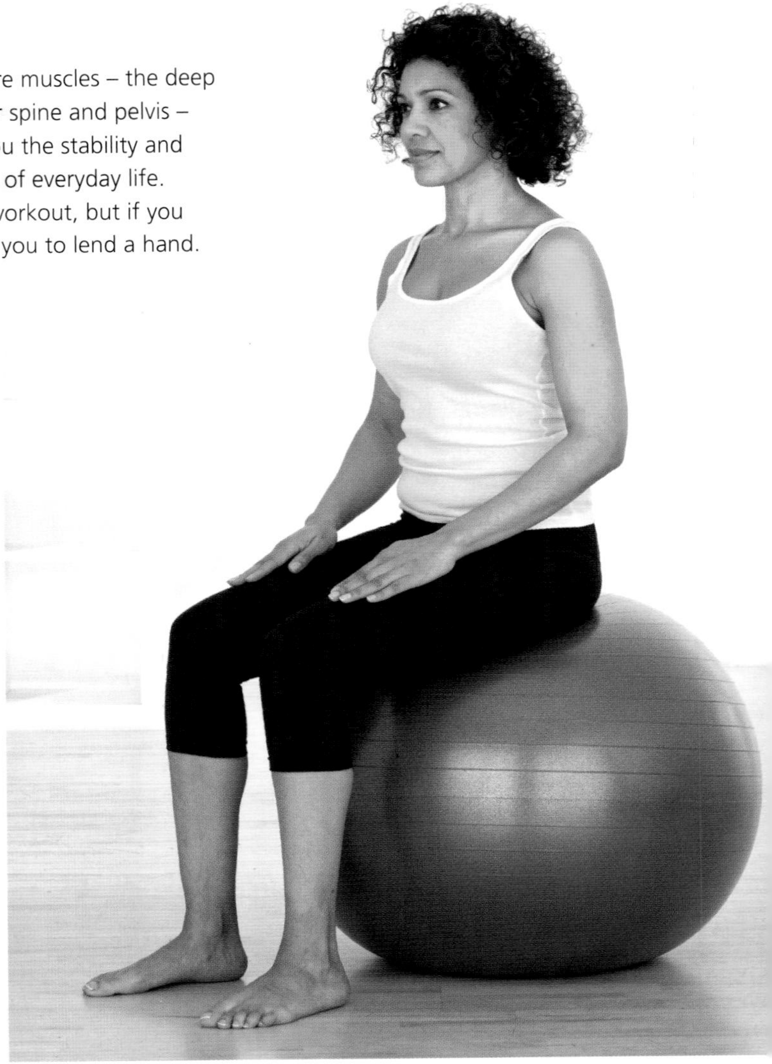

1 CORE MUSCLES ON THE BALL

Sit on the centre of the ball, feet shoulder-width apart. Slowly roll your bottom backwards and forwards. As you roll forward, sit tall, extending your spine and neck. As you roll back, curl your lower back, flexing your spine.

Now move your bottom in small circles, holding your arms out to the sides. Circle for 1 minute, then change direction. You should be able to feel your abdominal muscles working.

2 CORE STRENGTH FLOOR TWIST

Lie on your back on a firm surface with your knees bent up, and your arms and hands by your sides. Rest your head on a pillow. Place your feet on the floor and, keeping your knees together, slowly lower them as far as you can to the left, return to the midline, then roll them to the right. Return your knees to the middle.

- As well as working on your abdominal muscles, this exercise helps to keep the back mobile. and improves your ability to turn (*see* page 149).

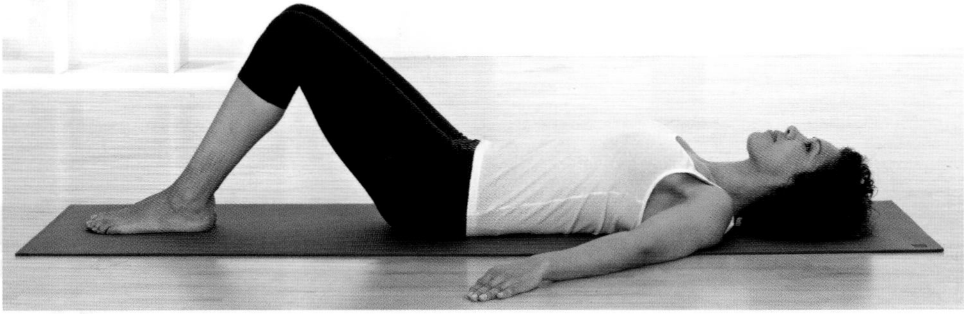

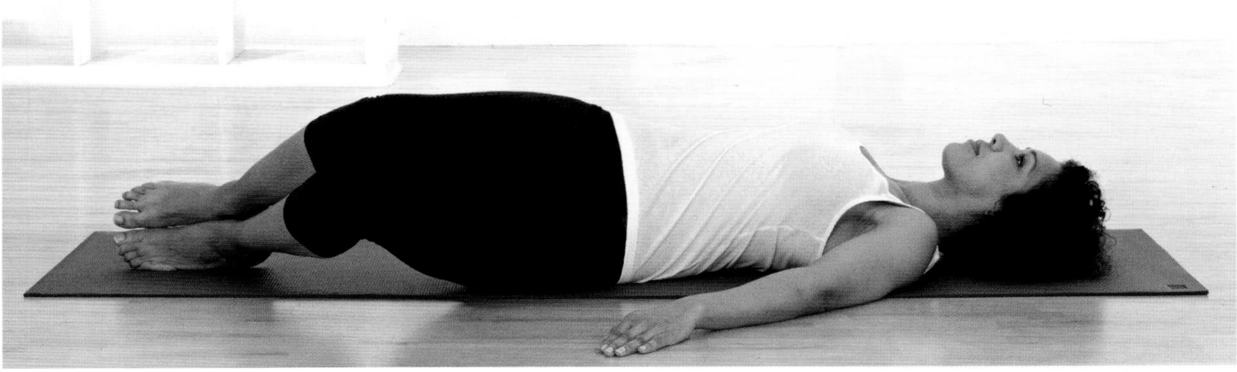

3 TWIST ON A BALL

You can also try exercise 2 using a ball. Lie on your back with your lower legs on the ball. Roll the ball 15 cm to the left slowly, return to the centre, then roll to the right.

- This exercise works a surprising number of muscles. You will probably feel the hamstrings at the back of your thigh, your hip muscles, and the side and front of your trunk working.

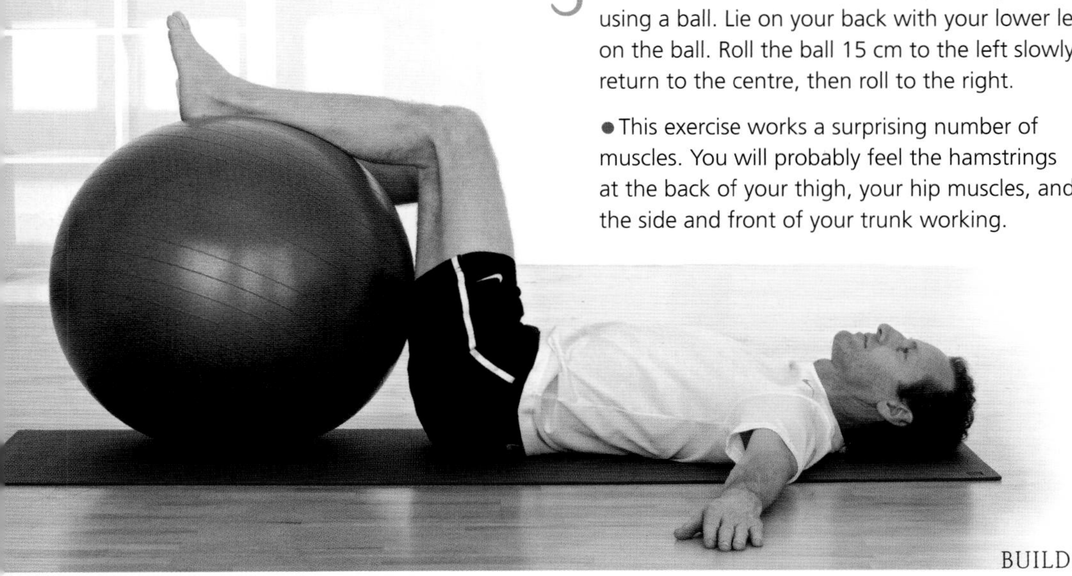

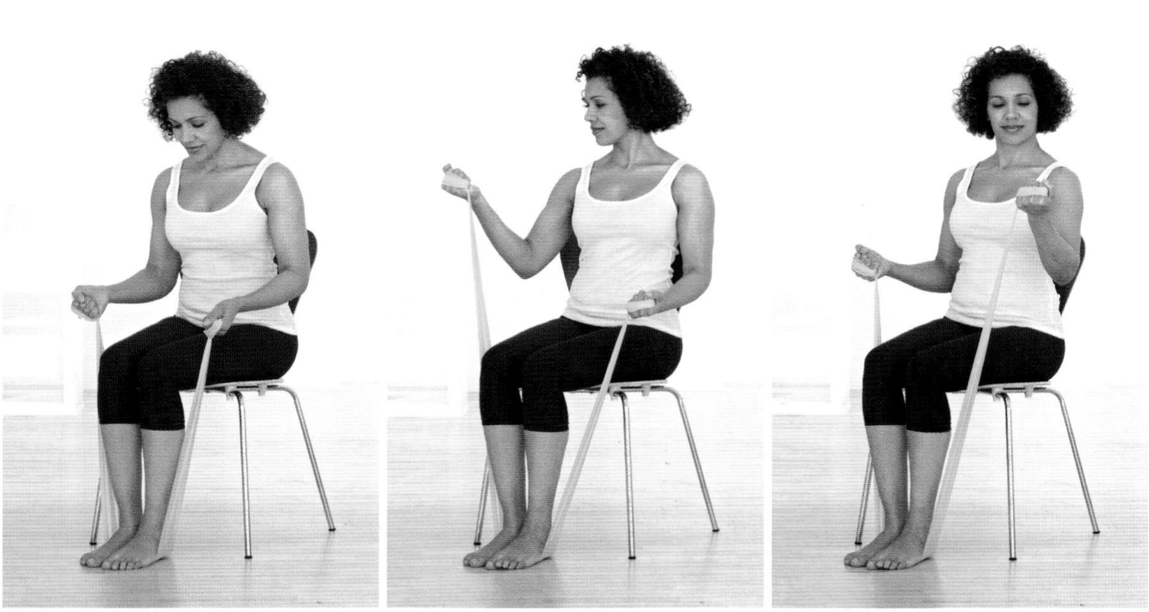

● **CHOOSING A RESISTANCE BAND** These exercises use a broad latex band (latex-free versions are also available), which is easy to hold and provides the necessary resistance to make the exercises effective. As you get older, it's generally better to use a lighter resistance band and increase the number of times you do the exercise.

4 **BICEP CURL** Wrap the ends of the band round your fingers and hook the band under your feet. Slowly bend and straighten your elbows alternately, pulling against the resistance band. Keep your wrists straight, and your back and neck held upright.

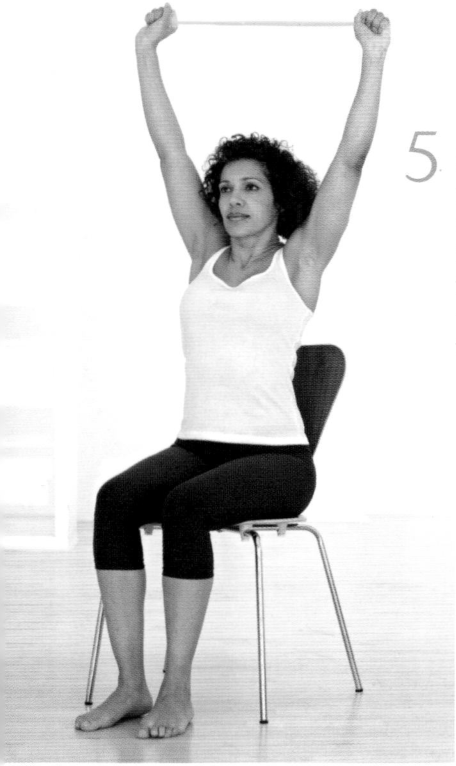

5 **SHOULDER ADDUCTION** Raising your arms above your head and with your elbows straight, see if you can stretch the band to double its original length. Control the slow return to the start position. Then repeat the movement with your arms in front of you at shoulder height.

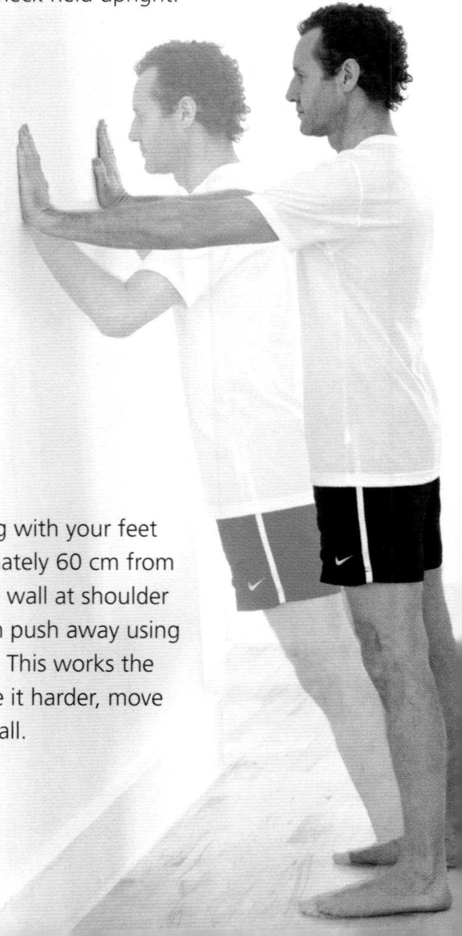

6 **STANDING PUSH-UP** Standing with your feet shoulder-width apart and approximately 60 cm from a wall, place your hands flat on the wall at shoulder height. Lean towards the wall, then push away using your arms, like a standing push-up. This works the shoulders, chest and arms. To make it harder, move your feet a little farther from the wall.

7 **QUADRICEPS EXTENSION** Lie on the floor (or on a firm bed) with your legs straight out in front of you. If you're uncomfortable lying flat, place a few pillows under your head or support yourself on your arms. Bend your right knee. Tighten your left quadriceps (on the front of your thigh) and push your left knee down, onto the floor. At the same time, pull your toes up towards you, then lift your left heel 15 cm off the surface. Hold for a count of five, then lower your leg, making sure the calf touches down before your heel. Repeat with the other leg.

- Maintaining strength in the quadriceps muscle is essential for standing up, going up and down stairs and walking.

Take care Never lift both legs at the same time as this can hurt your back.

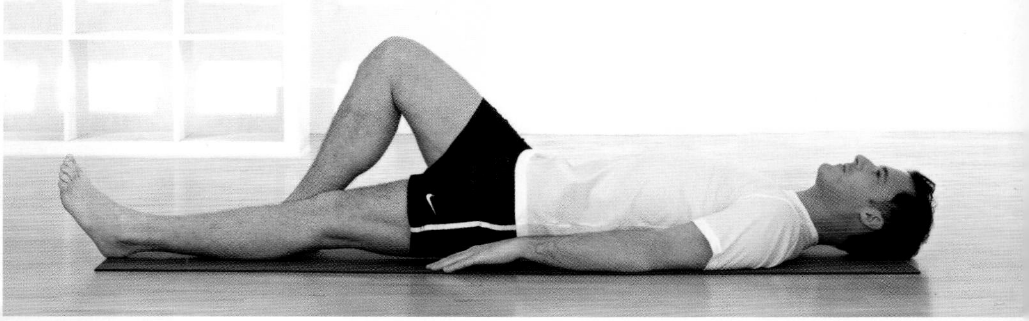

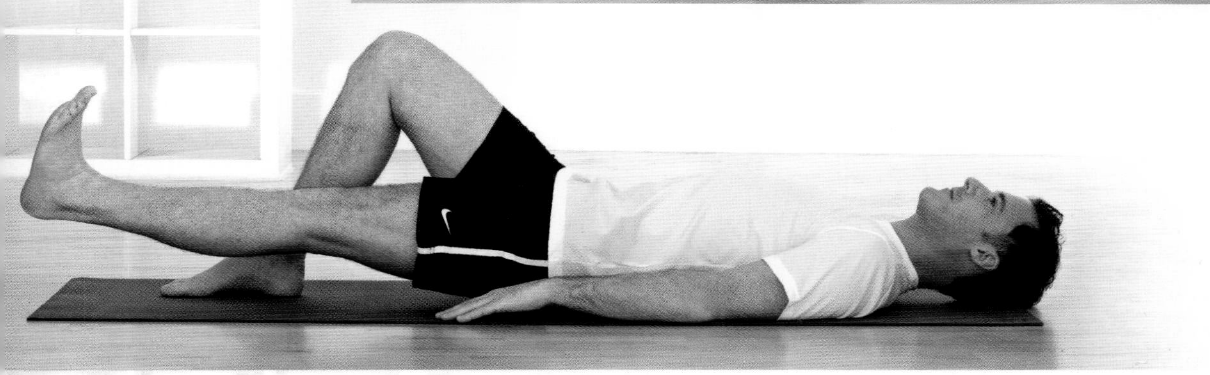

8 **INNER THIGH LIFT** Lie on your left side with your left foot under a padded dining chair (you can place a folded towel on an ordinary chair). Lift your right leg and rest your right foot on the front of the seat. Tighten your left quadriceps muscle (on the front of your thigh), pull your toes towards you, then lift your left leg towards your right. Hold for a count of five, then slowly lower your left leg. Turn over and repeat with your right leg.

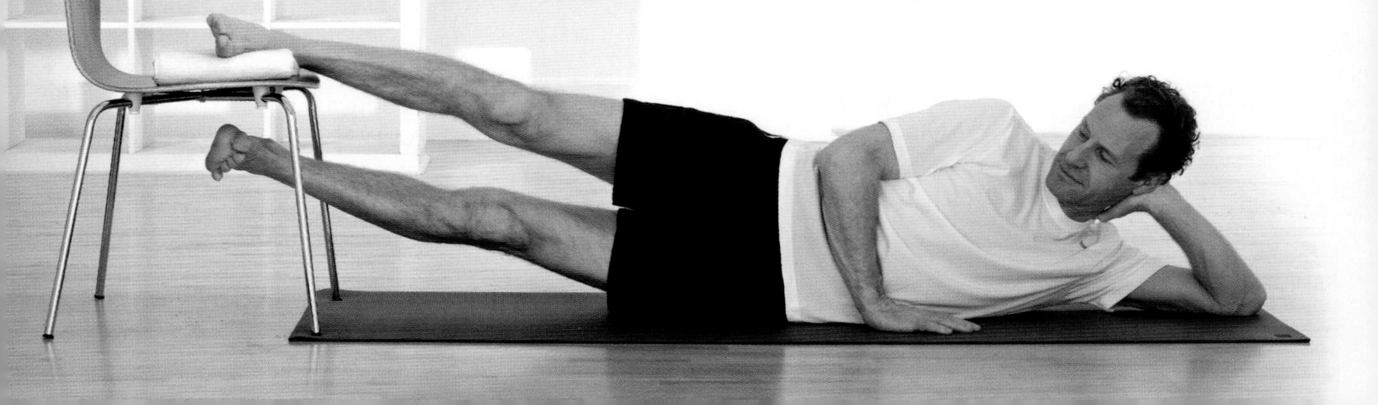

Flexibility is a neglected aspect of fitness; marathon runners often can't touch their toes.

STRETCH YOURSELF
keeping supple

Being as flexible as possible is essential if you want to retain freedom of movement throughout your life, and stretching is the best way to keep your joints and muscles supple.

As you age, you may get stiffer and the range of motion in your joints may decrease, making it harder to do everyday things. There are many reasons for this: loss of muscle strength, changes in the ratio of elastin and collagen (proteins found in connective tissue that give it stretch and strength), an increased build-up of fibrous scar tissue (adhesions), deposits of calcium in the tissues, and changes in your nervous system. But all of these changes can be helped by regular stretching – just 10 minutes a day is enough to increase your suppleness. You'll also find that with regular stretching, your posture will improve (rounded shoulders and a hunched back are often linked to inflexible muscles). Stretching relaxes and eases muscular tension – such tension can raise blood pressure, decrease sensory awareness and reduce the amounts of oxygen and nutrients going to the cells, which in turn can lead to fatigue, aches and pains.

You can do stretching exercises, such as the ones in this book, at home – even while sitting down or watching TV. Or you may prefer to join a stretch-based exercise class such as yoga, Pilates or tai chi – many people find it easier to stay motivated if they are in a group.

Before you start ...

Here's how to make the most of stretchwork:

- Check with your family doctor or physiotherapist before doing any stretching exercises to make sure they're suitable for you.
- Breathe slowly and evenly throughout the exercise.
- Try to warm up your muscles before stretching. Warmth increases the elastic properties of collagen within your muscles and tendons, allowing for a greater stretch and protecting against injury. Stretch when you've been active or after warming up by walking on the spot for at least 2 minutes, swinging your arms as you do so.

- Stretch the muscle until you feel a slight pull. Pause and hold the stretch for 10 to 20 seconds. Don't bounce at the end of the movement, and take care not to stretch farther than you can comfortably manage. A stretch should not feel painful, although it may be mildly uncomfortable – yoga practitioners call this sensation 'sweet pain'.
- Be patient. You can increase your flexibility at any age, but it takes longer when you are older.

WORK OUT: flexibility exercises

Make time for stretching at least twice a week. These exercises include stretches for all the main parts of the body. Repeat each exercise three times.

- **NECK STRETCHES** help to keep the mobility in your neck. If you have signs of cervical spondylosis – wear and tear in the neck (with pain and stiffness) – it's usually good to keep the neck moving. But check with your doctor before doing the exercises. Stop if you feel any pain or other symptoms, and seek medical advice.

1 **NECK TURN** Sit up straight, look ahead, relax the shoulders. Turn your head towards your right shoulder as far as you can comfortably go, hold for a count of five, then return to centre. Repeat twice more. From the centre, repeat to the left.

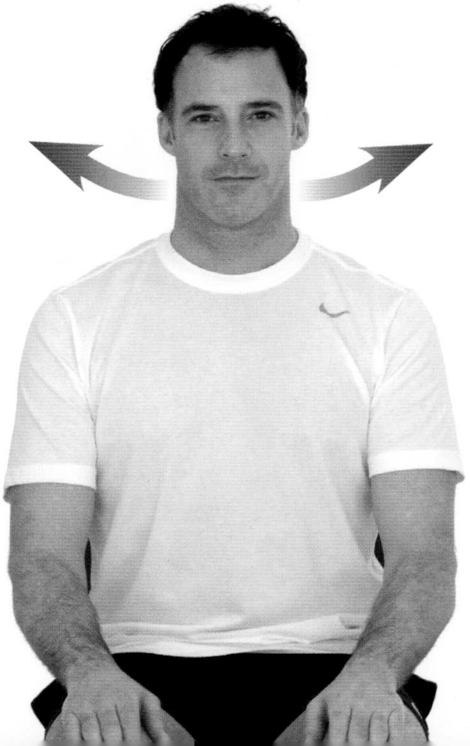

2 **NECK DROP** Sit up straight, look ahead and relax your shoulders. Place your left hand on your right shoulder, then slowly tilt your head to the left (hold your shoulder down). Hold for a count of five, and then bring your head back up. Do this a total of three times, then repeat on the other side.

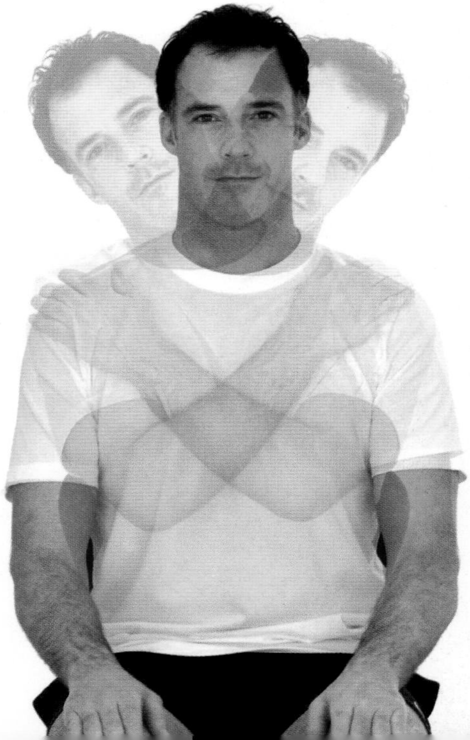

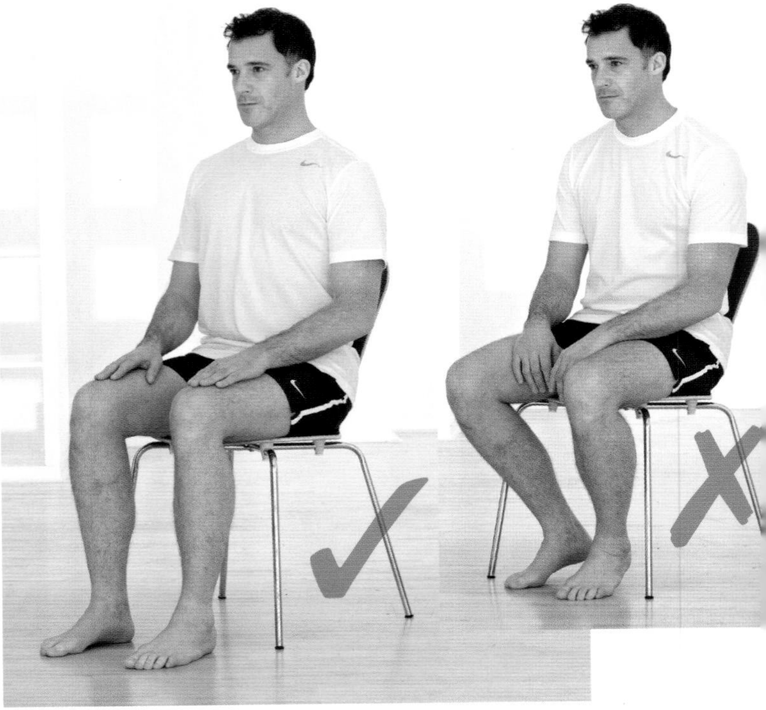

3 **SEATED STRETCH** Sit on a firm chair, feet flat on the floor. Sit up as tall as you can. Feel your pelvis rock forward, pull your tummy in, let your shoulders drop and most importantly pull your chin in (you should have a double chin now). Avoid tipping your head as you pull your chin in and keep your eyes pointing forward.

● This is a good exercise to do whenever you sit down (especially if you spend time in front of a computer, sitting with your back curved and chin poking forward). Poor spinal posture (*see* far right) is often responsible for neck pain, back pain and headaches. As you sit tall, feel the soft tissues at the back of your neck stretch.

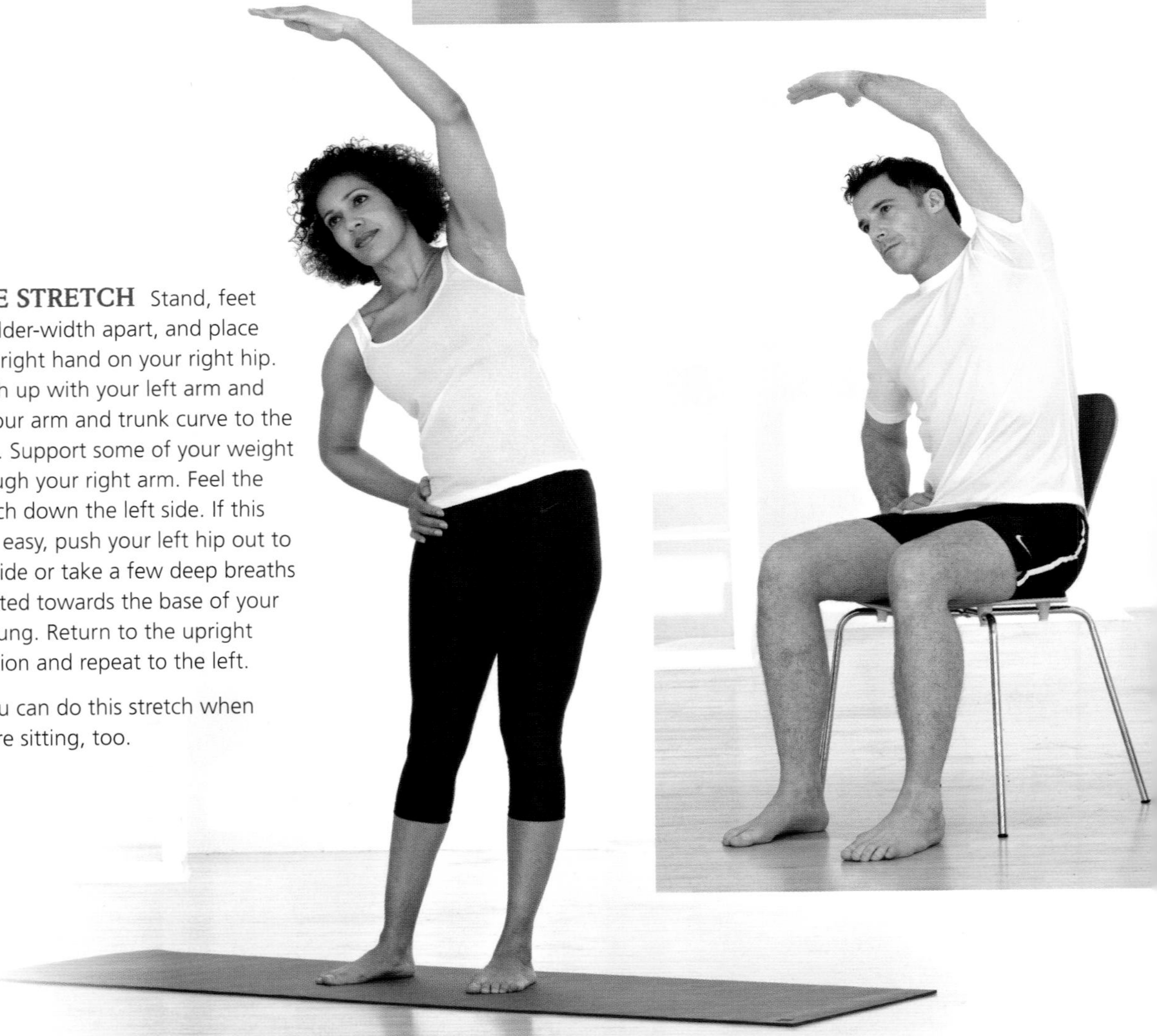

4 **SIDE STRETCH** Stand, feet shoulder-width apart, and place your right hand on your right hip. Reach up with your left arm and let your arm and trunk curve to the right. Support some of your weight through your right arm. Feel the stretch down the left side. If this feels easy, push your left hip out to the side or take a few deep breaths directed towards the base of your left lung. Return to the upright position and repeat to the left.

● You can do this stretch when you're sitting, too.

5 **BACK CURL** Lie on your back on a firm surface, bend your legs and place both feet flat on the floor. Lift your left leg up towards your chest. Hold your knee with your left hand. Bring the right leg up to join it. Gently pull your knees towards your chest, curling and stretching your lower back. If you find this position comfortable, you can rock slightly backwards and forwards.

- From your starting position for this exercise, you could also repeat the core strength floor twist exercise (2) described on page 143. This provides a good stretch and helps to retain your spine's ability to rotate so that you can turn easily when you need to reverse the car or look behind you. It can also be good for lower back pain.

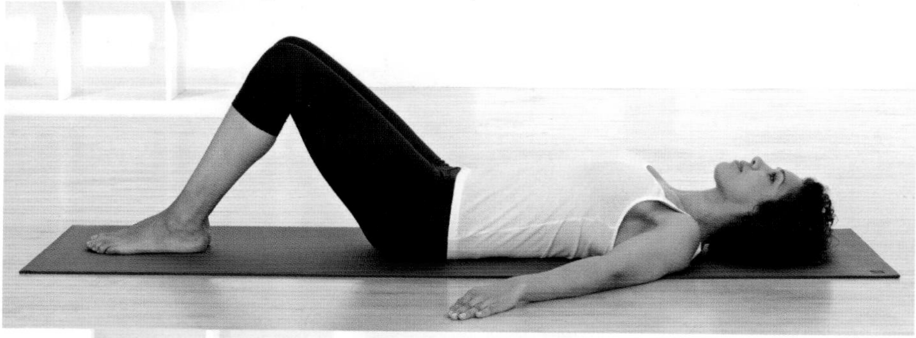

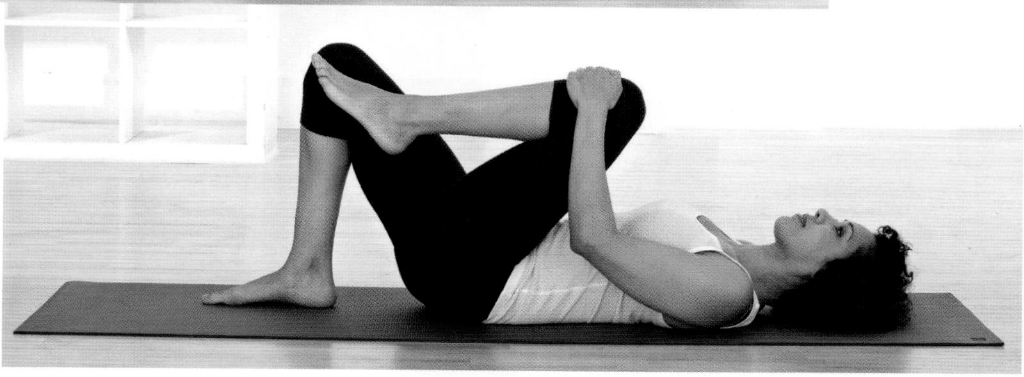

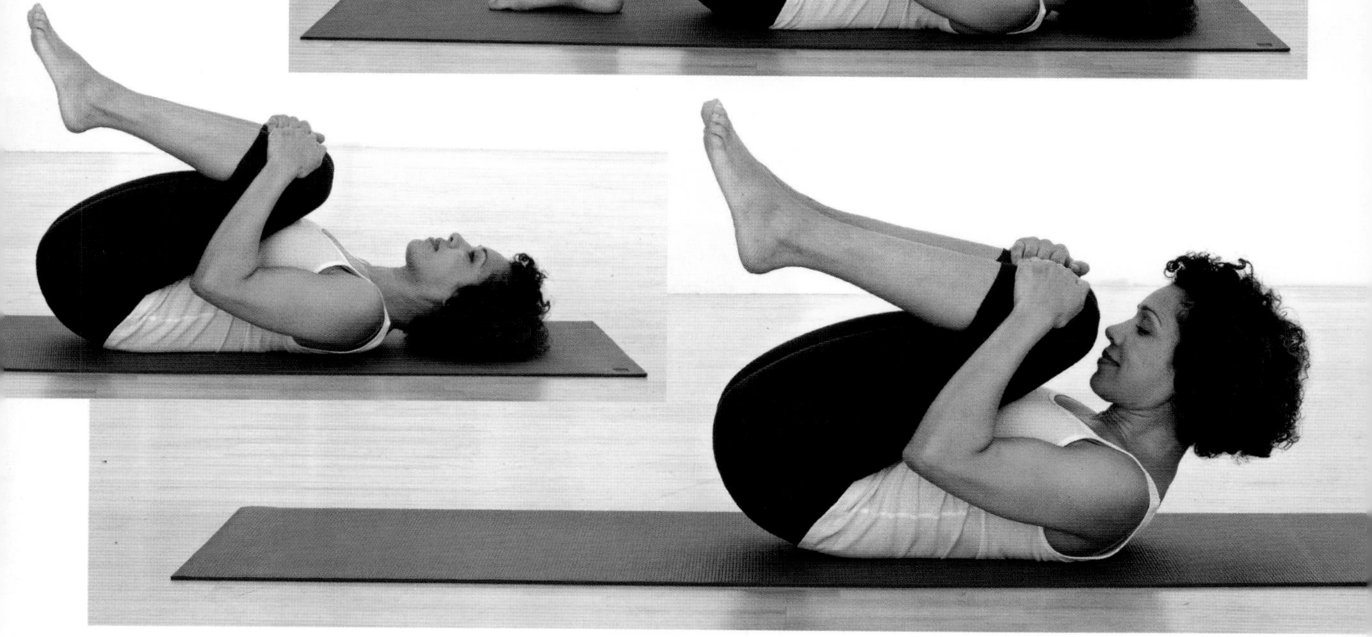

6 **LOWER BACK STRETCH** Lie on your front on a firm surface. Raise your upper body by coming up onto your elbows. If it feels comfortable, move your hands back and straighten your arms.

- This exercise helps maintain the flexibility of your back in an extended position – it's particularly useful if you spend much of the day sitting.

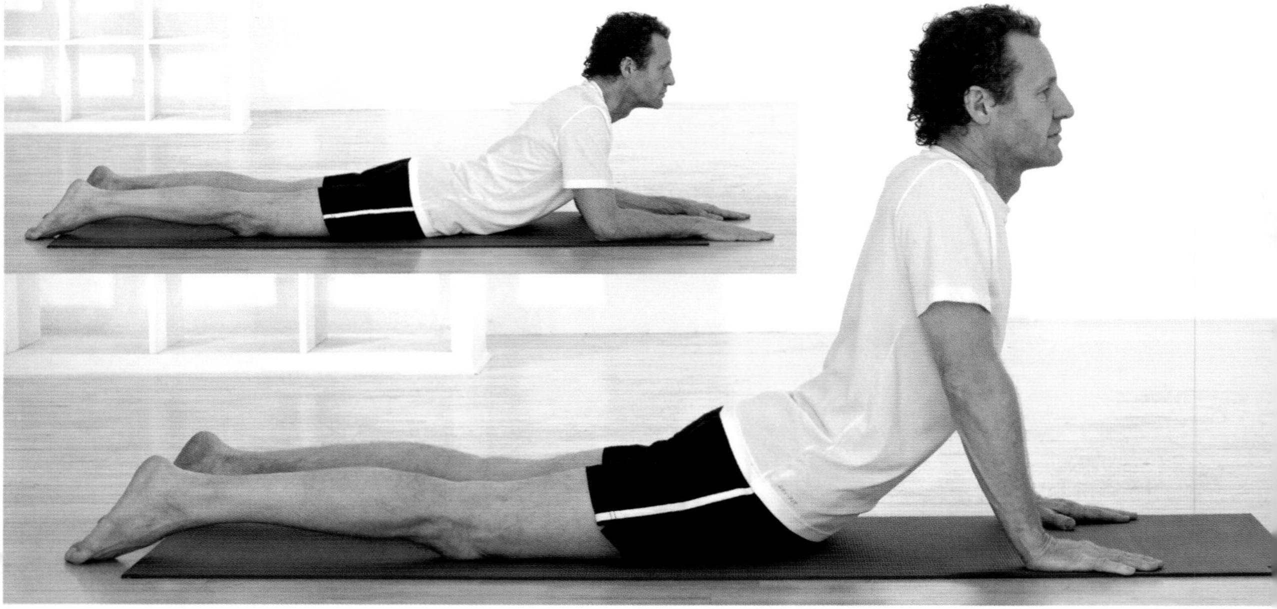

7 **HAMSTRING STRETCH** Sit on a firm surface with your legs out in front of you and place your hands on your shins. Reach towards your feet. You should feel a pull in the centre of your hamstring muscles – most people don't need to reach very far to feel this.

- This is a good stretch if you are fairly fit already; if you have back or sciatic pain, do the lying-down stretch with a resistance band (exercise 8) instead.

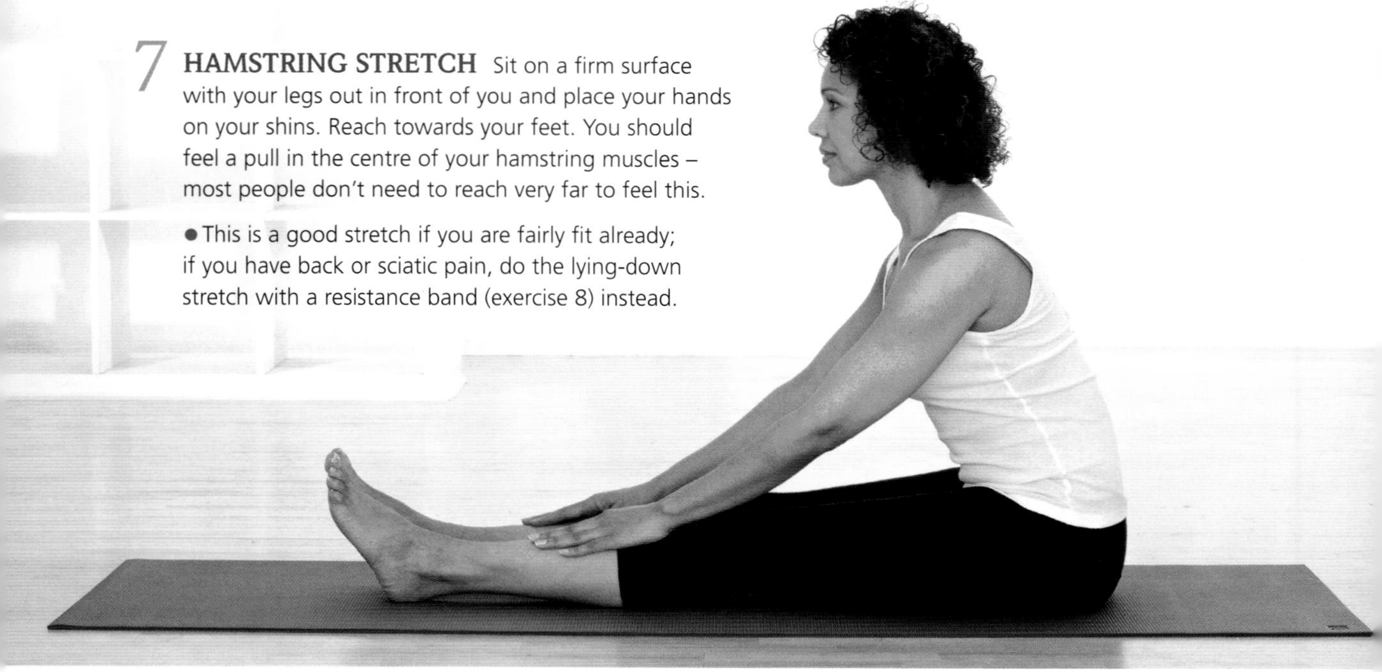

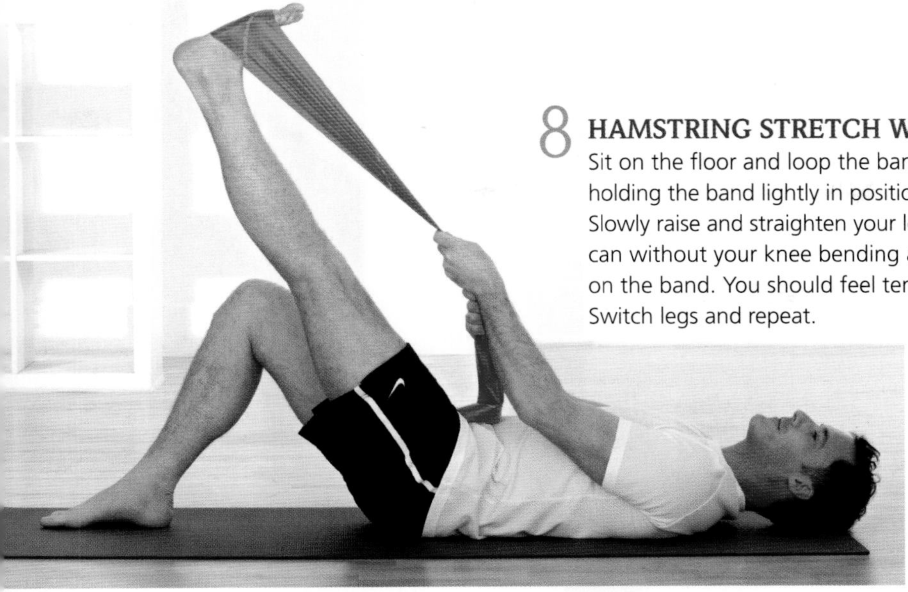

8 HAMSTRING STRETCH WITH A RESISTANCE BAND

Sit on the floor and loop the band round your left foot. Lie back holding the band lightly in position. Bend your right knee for stability. Slowly raise and straighten your left leg. Raise your leg as high as you can without your knee bending and apply a gentle stretch by pulling on the band. You should feel tension in the back of your left thigh. Switch legs and repeat.

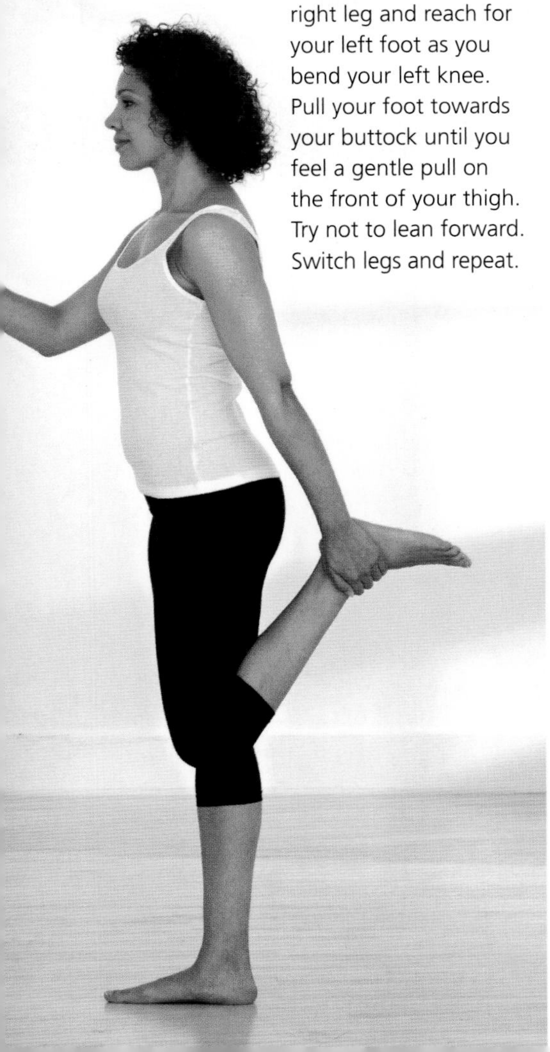

9 QUADS STRETCH

Holding on to a stable surface, stand on your right leg and reach for your left foot as you bend your left knee. Pull your foot towards your buttock until you feel a gentle pull on the front of your thigh. Try not to lean forward. Switch legs and repeat.

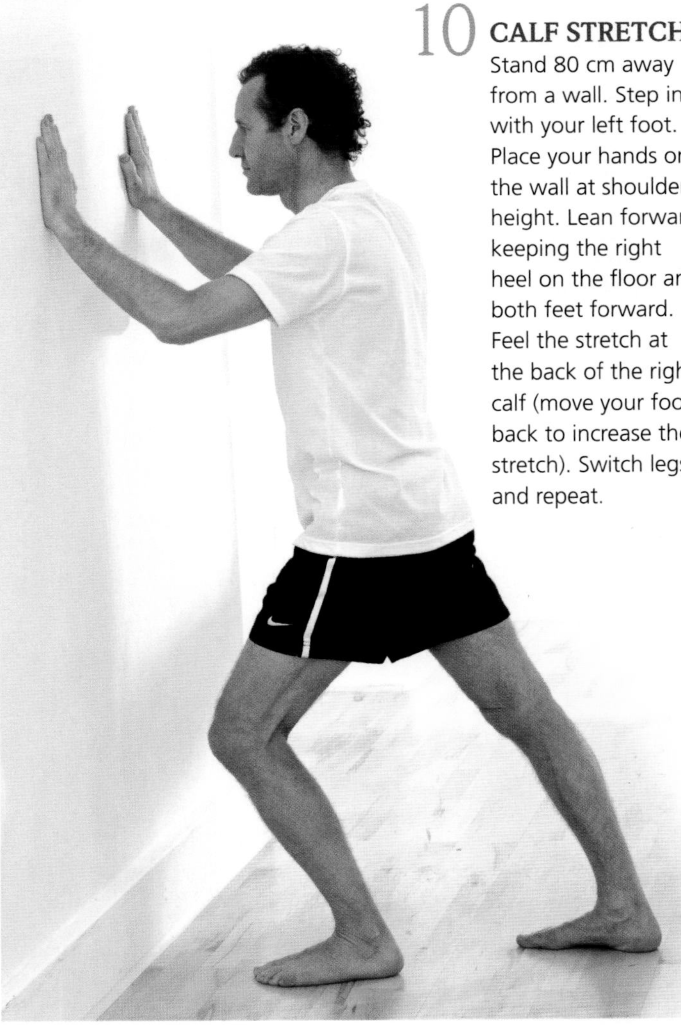

10 CALF STRETCH

Stand 80 cm away from a wall. Step in with your left foot. Place your hands on the wall at shoulder height. Lean forward, keeping the right heel on the floor and both feet forward. Feel the stretch at the back of the right calf (move your foot back to increase the stretch). Switch legs and repeat.

KEEPING YOURSELF well balanced

The mental and physical changes that occur with the passing of time can upset your innate sense of balance. Keeping generally active and doing some specific balancing exercises will help you stay steady for years to come.

When you were young, you took your balance for granted. But your body's sense of equilibrium is more complicated than it may seem. It involves a constant, minutely regulated set of physical adjustments based on a stream of mental data about your spatial circumstances; which way is up, and the nature of the ground beneath your feet. Get this slightly wrong – as you are more prone to do as you get older – and you might end up taking a tumble. One in three people over the age of 65 experiences at least one fall each year, 10 to 15 per cent of which are linked with serious injury.

What is it about age that makes falls more likely? It is a combination of factors: poorer muscle power and a reduced range of motion in your joints; a deterioration in your eyesight and other senses; inner ear problems; changes in your nervous system's mechanisms for controlling movement. Taken together, these make it trickier to maintain balance effortlessly, and less easy to stabilise your body before you perform any movement. Meanwhile, your reaction times may become slower, and this means that it is harder to save yourself by, say, grabbing a doorhandle.

Beat the effects of ageing

There are plenty of ways to prevent falls and keep yourself safe:

- **Step out** Walking is one of the best ways to maintain good balance. Why? Walking is actually a series of controlled falls. You fall forward and put one foot out in front to check yourself; as you push yourself past that foot you begin to fall again, so put your other foot forward – and so it goes on. Practising heel-to-toe walking – in which you place one foot in front of the other along an imaginary line – is a simple way to improve your balance skills.

DID **you** KNOW?

There are two main types of balance:

- **Static balance** is what you need to stay steady when you stand still, for example, at a stove to cook dinner, waiting in a queue or doing some yoga poses such as the Tree.
- **Dynamic balance** – the ability not to topple when you're moving – is actually more important for day-to-day life. It's the sort of balance needed for any movement from simply walking to turning a corner.

take CARE! SAFE BALANCING

When you do exercises that work on balance, start slowly, taking plenty of time to move from one position to the next. Most of us balance better on one side than the other – it's important to train your weaker side, too.

- If you have any medical condition that may affect your balance, such as ear or eye problems or a stroke, check with your doctor or physiotherapist before doing any of these exercises.
- If you're at all wobbly, hold on to a sturdy table or chair at elbow height, or ask someone to help you. Make sure any surface you hold is non-slip and dry.
- Wear flat, well-fitting supportive shoes. Avoid heels and slingbacks, thongs, slippers and slippery soles.
- Be patient. Every small movement or shift of your body weight changes your body's centre of gravity. It takes time for your body to adjust.
- To aid your balance, fix your eyes on a single spot and maintain your gaze as you perform the movement. At first this should be on the ground a couple of feet in front of you. As you get used to the exercises, lift your eyes and chin and look at a spot straight in front of you level with your eyes. The higher your gaze, the more difficult it is to maintain stability.
- Aim to build up the time you hold static balance poses – ideally you are aiming to stay steady for up to 20 seconds.
- Do each pose once or twice on each side.

- **Do tai chi** There's evidence to suggest that tai chi can help improve balance and confidence, according to researchers at Oregon Research Institute, USA. And a Hong Kong study involving 40 people over the age of 70 found that practising tai chi improved body awareness and balance in people with visual impairment. Seek out an experienced teacher and go to a class – it's impossible to learn tai chi correctly from a book.
- **Get tangoed** Dancing involves both static and dynamic balance, and tango in particular may help to improve balance, increase confidence and prevent falls, according to a ten-week study carried out at McGill University in Montreal, Canada.
- **Try Pilates** The Pilates system involves strengthening your core muscles, and can help improve both static and dynamic balance – as measured by participants' ability to stand on a foam cushion with their eyes closed without swaying. That was the conclusion of a 16-week study from the University of Tasmania, Australia.

DID **you** KNOW?

A study of 23 older people carried out at the University of Northridge in California in 2009 found that a three-month activity program incorporating specific balance training helped to improve muscle strength, gait and balance, and significantly reduced the risk of falls.

WORK OUT: balance exercises

Start with the easiest variation of the exercise and move on only if you're steady during the previous exercise. Repeat each exercise as frequently as you want to throughout the day. Lightly rest your fingertips on a sturdy chair or have someone nearby, depending on how steady you are. If your balance is good, try the exercises freestanding and/or with your eyes closed. The key to balance exercises is control. Perform each exercise slowly; the more slowly you do them, the more you'll benefit.

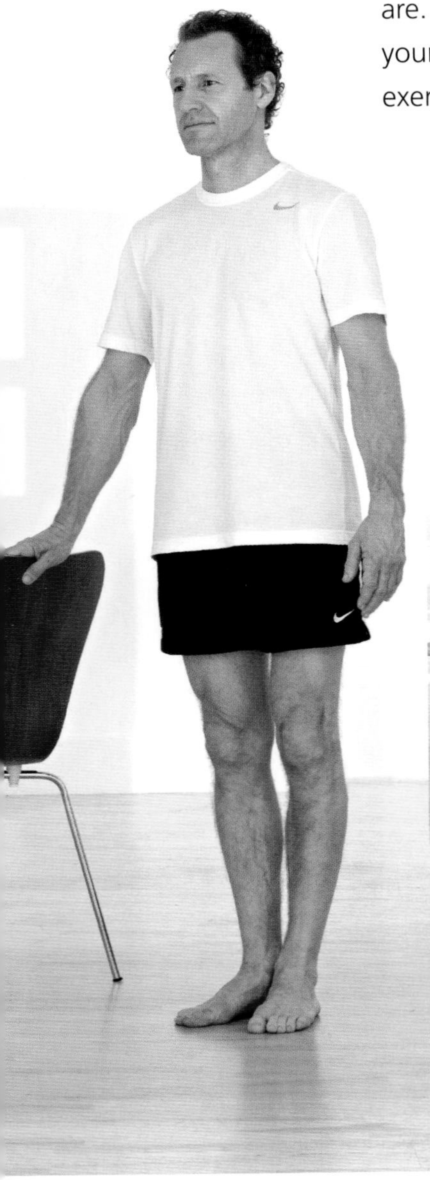

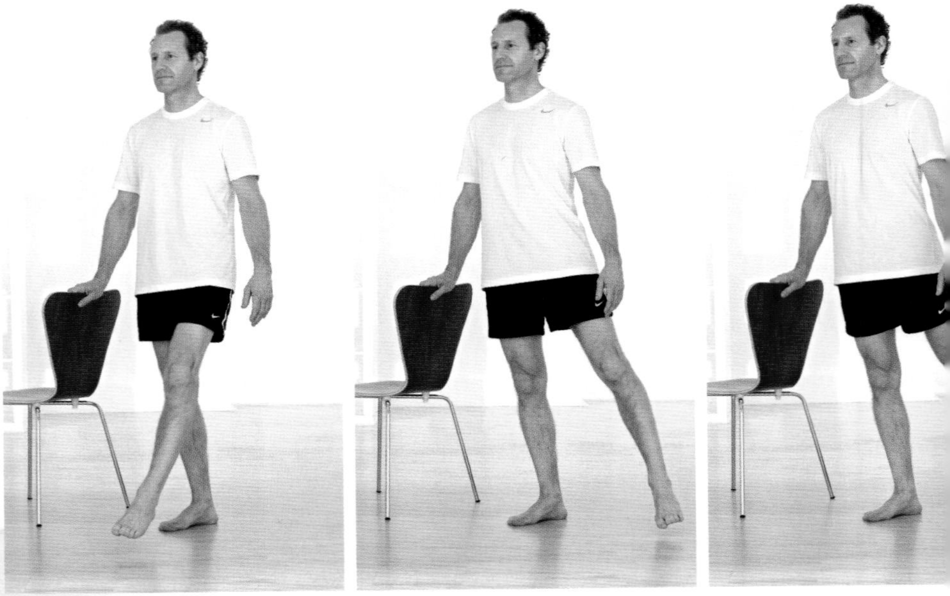

1 **LEG SWINGS** Stand with a chair or other support to your right side and hold on with your right hand. Swing your left leg forward by about 30 cm to 40 cm, depending on what feels comfortable. Keep it straight then move it out to the side by about the same amount, then behind you. Remain upright with your shoulders and hips facing forward and move your leg fluidly in a semi-circle. Turn around and hold the support with your left hand, then repeat the exercise with your right leg.

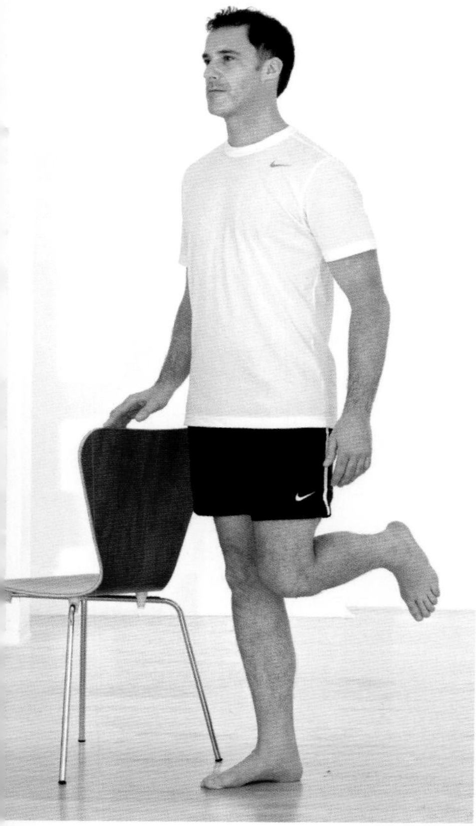

2 KICK BACKS Stand tall with your right hand on the back of a chair; tighten your abdominal muscles by pulling in your belly button. Lift your left foot behind you and hold for a count of ten. Repeat standing on your left leg. Most people balance better on one side than the other. See which leg you favour. If you still feel steady, do the exercise again with your eyes closed.

3 CHAIR SQUATS Stand in front of a sturdy chair. Keep your back and neck straight and your feet hip-width apart and flat on the floor. Lean forward and slowly bend your knees until you feel the seat touch the back of your thighs (don't let your knees come farther forward than your toes). Then rise up again to standing. If you're steady, hold your arms out in front of you. Repeat ten times without sitting.

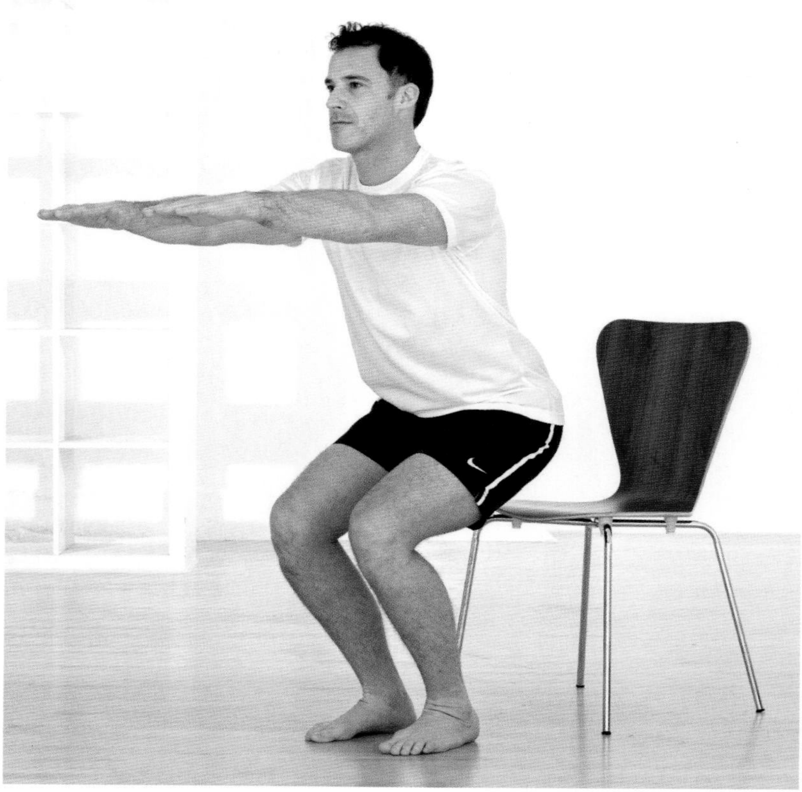

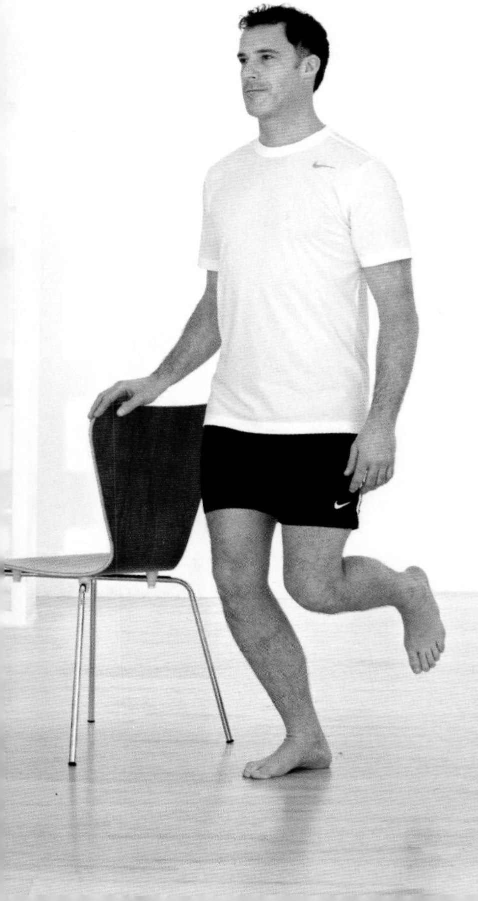

4 ONE-LEG SQUATS Standing on your right leg, bend your right knee a few degrees as if starting to squat, and lift your left leg behind you as shown; hold the position for a count of ten then straighten up. Make sure that you keep your knee over your foot and if you find your knee wobbles, straighten up. You do not need to bend your knee very far to find this quite challenging. Repeat with your other leg.

BACK TO BACK
be structurally strong

A strong back is key to a healthy, active life. Your spine is the pillar that supports the edifice of your body. It is also a conduit that contains your spinal cord, the bundle of nerve fibres that carries messages and instructions from your brain to your limbs and organs.

Prevention is better than cure. To protect your back, work at having good posture. It is vital to maintain strength and suppleness in your spine as well as keeping the whole body working well. Good posture helps you look younger, keeps your bones and joints aligned, prevents the strain that can lead to arthritis and ensures that your muscles work efficiently. All this helps you avoid backache and muscle pain, saves energy and prevents fatigue. And it can protect you against fractures caused by bone overload, according to research at the University of California, USA. Pilates and yoga are good for improving posture. Here are four essential spine-protecting tips:

- **Be back-aware** Make good posture central to everything you do. Do the posture exercise on page 148 – every day, whenever you sit down. Pay attention to how you are sitting and standing.
- **Learn to lift** When bending or lifting, bend at your hips and knees and keep the object close to your torso – don't bend your back.
- **Get up safely** Never push yourself up from a prone position. To get out of bed, roll onto your side, then push yourself up.
- **Don't hunch** Check you're wearing the correct glasses if working at a computer, as poor eyesight can cause you to hunch forward.

DID you KNOW?

Developed in the 19th century, the Alexander Technique (AT) is not so much a therapy as a way of re-educating your body to function more naturally. It involves learning new, more efficient ways to sit, stand and move. Research carried out at the Neurological Sciences Institute in Oregon shows that AT training reduces back pain and stiffness of the trunk and hips as well as improving participants' posture.

A PAIN IN THE BACK

If you develop back pain – which is more likely with age due to strained muscles and ligaments or general wear and tear – there are ways to reduce the likelihood of the discomfort lasting long, or becoming chronic (note that persistent back pain or pain that wakes you at night should be investigated by your doctor, while back pain with other symptoms such as incontinence, fever or leg weakness

focus ON ... HYPERKYPHOSIS

Hyperkyphosis, an exaggerated humping of the back, which causes stooped posture, affects between 20 and 40 per cent of people over the age of 60. It's widely known as dowager's hump, but men as well as women can develop the condition.

The most common causes of hyperkyphosis in older people are osteoporosis, fractures in the midback region and degeneration of the discs between the spinal vertebrae. Certain forms of arthritis, connective tissue disorders and tumours in the spine are also sometimes responsible.

As your back becomes more hunched, you may experience muscle fatigue and pain in your neck and shoulders and your abdomen may protrude. It's worth trying different strategies to mitigate the condition – as more severe hyperkyphosis can begin to interfere with daily life, affecting your mobility, digestion and breathing.

Stretching, walking, practising special posture exercises and specific techniques with a physiotherapist – for example, lying on your back on a foam roller – can be helpful, as can doing breathing exercises. Other measures include wearing a special brace and 'taping' – in which special adhesive tape stimulates you to hold your spine in a better position. In severe cases, you may need surgery.

Help yourself

- Try to maintain a good posture at all times (*see* Be back-aware, opposite).
- If you can, practise balance exercises regularly (such as the ones on pages 154–155). Kyphosis can upset your stability.
- Work on improving your spinal flexibility. Try yoga, Pilates or tai chi, and try the lower back stretch on page 150.
- Strengthen your core muscles – have a go at the ball and floor exercises on pages 142–143.
- Always check with a physiotherapist before trying any exercises.

calls for a visit to the emergency department). Contrary to what was once advised, physical activity is good for most types of back pain. All expert guidelines recommend that initial treatment should be exercise, plus pain management and manual therapies (such as physiotherapy) or complementary therapies such as acupuncture. Yet older people are often offered only painkillers and/or other medication by their doctors.

If you're not offered further help and advice by your doctor, ask what exercises you can do and whether you should be referred to a physiotherapist or other specialist. And once the initial pain wears off, try the exercises that follow: they're just as useful if you're recovering from a bad back as they are if you're trying to avert problems.

WORK OUT: back recovery exercises

These gentle exercises will help you regain mobility and strength in the back after injury; they are also good for general back support. Do them once your back is recovering, rather than when you are in pain; check with your physio or doctor first.

1 **PELVIC TILT** This is one of the most versatile back exercises you can do; it moves the joints and strengthens the muscles that support the spine. Lie on your back with knees bent and feet flat on the floor. See if you can slip your hand between your lower back and the floor. Rock your pelvis back and try to squash your hand. Once you can feel the correct movement, remove your hand and flatten your lower back against the floor. Hold for 5 seconds then relax and let your lower back come off the floor.

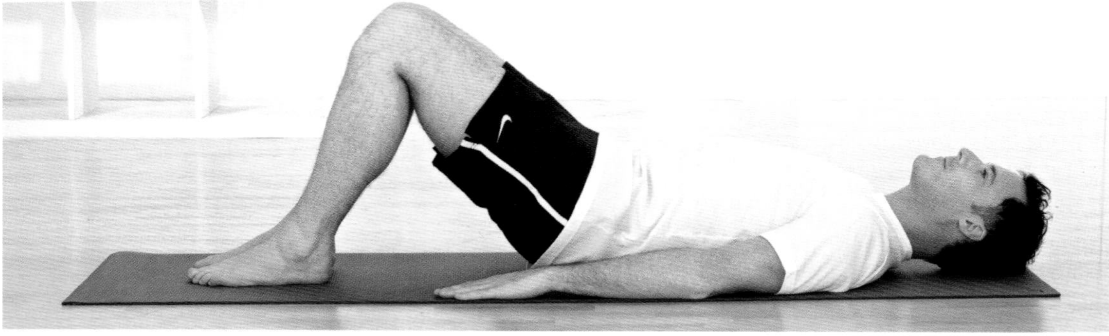

2 **THE CAT** Kneel on all fours, knees hip-width apart, hands shoulder-width apart. Let your head drop and raise your back in an arch (go as far as is comfortable; don't push yourself). Feel your abdominals tighten and your pelvis rock backwards, and hold for a count of five. Then lift your head and hollow your lumbar spine, relaxing your abdominals and feeling your pelvis tilt forward. Hold for a count of five.

- Ease your weight forward or back to feel different parts of the spine move. Do the movements rhythmically, without holding them, to ease stiffness after sitting all day.

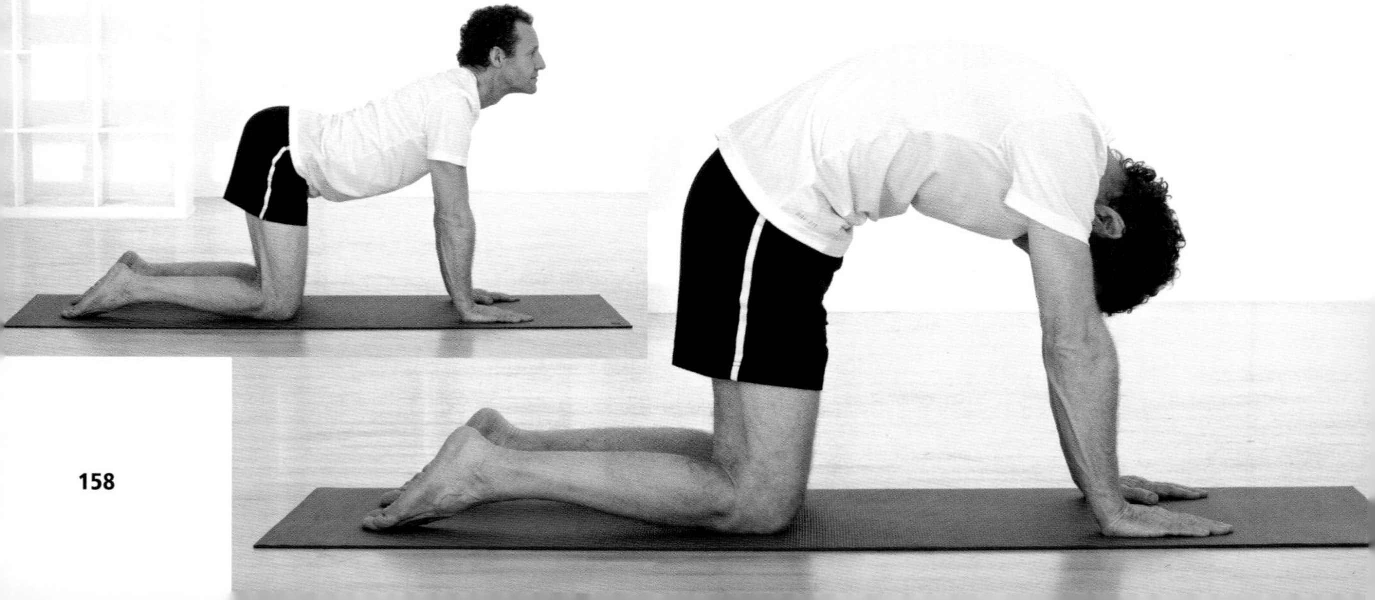

WORK OUT: in bed

If your back is stiff in the morning, here is a simple workout that you can do before you get up. It's also a good way of keeping the body moving if you are laid up for any length of time. Get the OK from your doctor or physio if you are ill, injured or suffering from back pain.

Exercising may be uncomfortable if you have tight tissues or weakness from lying in bed. But if you feel no sense of stretch, you may not be doing enough. As a general rule, discomfort that is short-lived and settles quickly is probably harmless, but pain that lasts longer and doesn't settle may mean that you have overdone your exercises. If in doubt, ask your doctor or physiotherapist.

- Do the exercises slowly and steadily.
- Aim to reach the end of each movement.
- Try to do at least five repetitions of each exercise, three times per day.

1 **BRIDGING** Lie on your back and bend both knees so that your feet rest on the bed. Slowly lift your buttocks off the bed so that your body is straight. Hold the position for 5 seconds then slowly lower your buttocks to the bed. This is good for your gluteus maximus (buttock) and hamstring muscles.

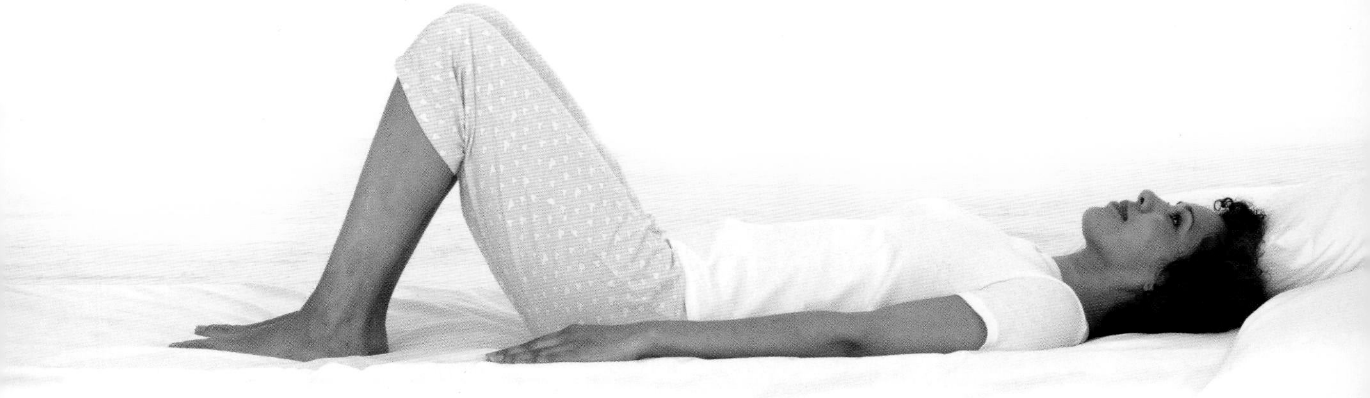

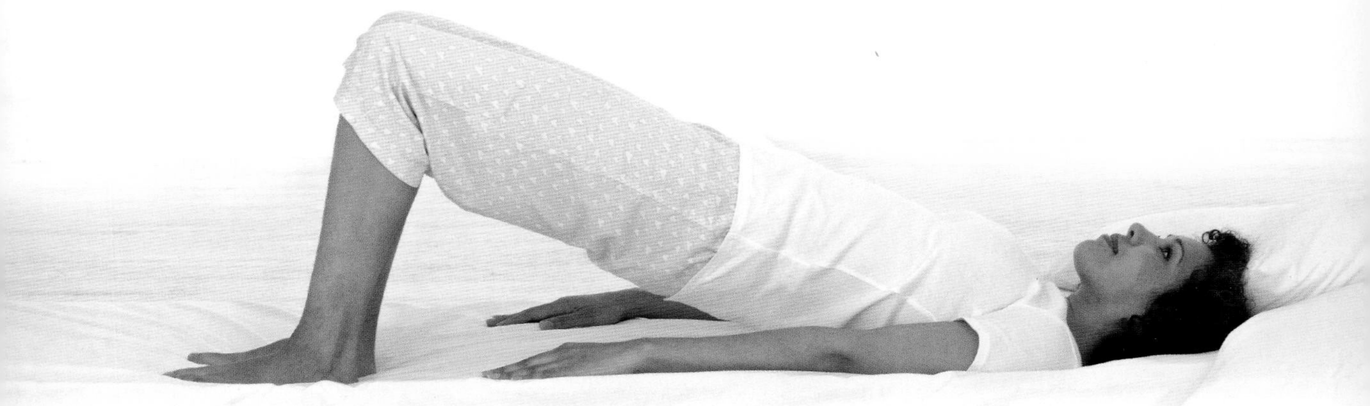

2 **NECK RETRACTION AND ROTATION** Lie on your back and stretch the length of your spine as far as possible. Tuck your chin in, but keep your head on the pillow. Rotate your head slowly to the left until your left ear touches the pillow. Return to the middle then repeat to the same side. Once you have done five repetitions to the left, repeat five times to the right. Do not move alternately from side to side.

Take care If you feel dizzy, stop this exercise and seek advice.

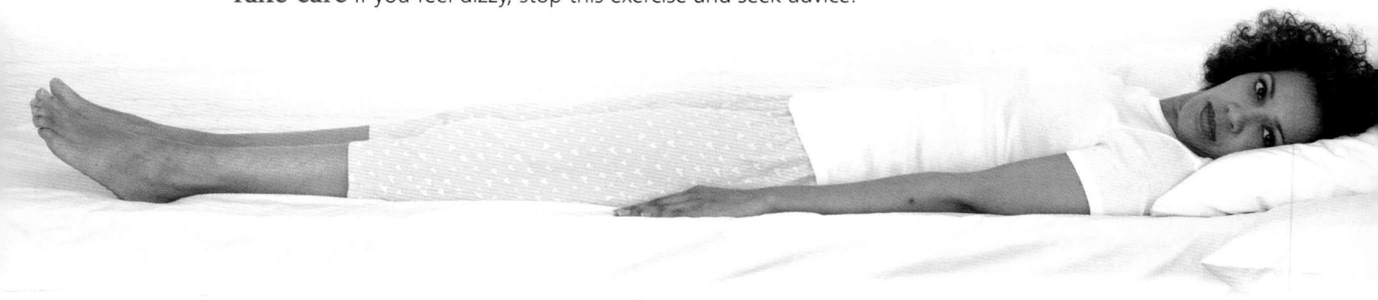

3 **SPINE ROTATION** Lie on your left side and, keeping your left leg straight, let your right knee drop down onto the bed. If this is comfortable, roll the top half of your trunk back so that your shoulders are flat on the bed. Return your shoulders to midline so you are lying on your side. Do this five times, then turn onto your right side and repeat the exercise.

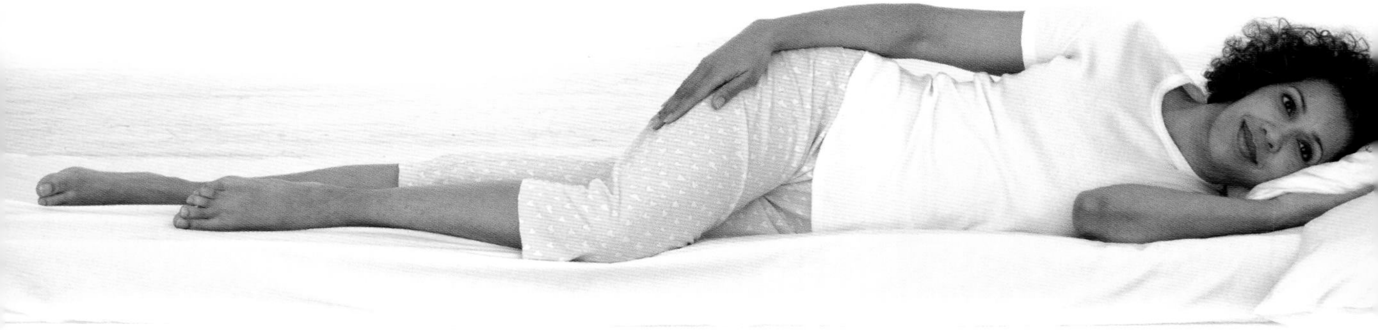

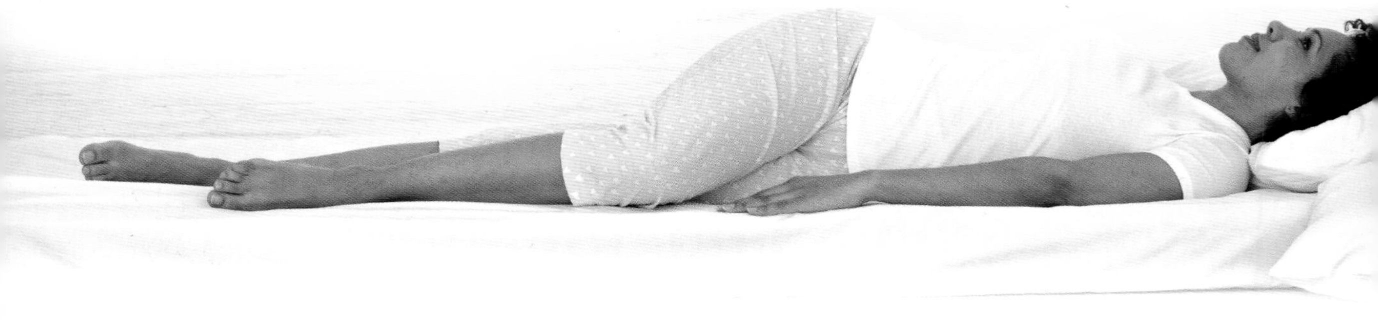

4 **QUADRICEPS STRETCH** Place a rolled-up towel or small firm pillow under your left knee and rest your heel on the bed. Bend your right knee, and tighten your left quadriceps (on the front of your thigh) so that your heel lifts off the bed. Hold the knee straight for 10 seconds, then slowly lower your heel. Repeat five times for each leg.

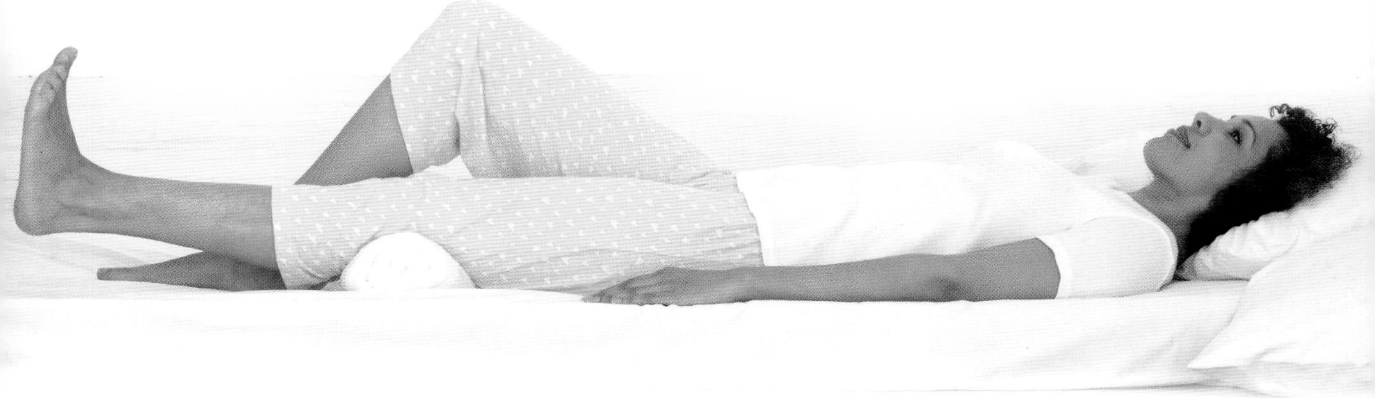

5 **ANKLE STRETCHES** This exercise will keep your ankles moving and the muscles in your calves working. Most importantly, it will stimulate the circulation in your lower legs and help prevent deep vein thrombosis. Lying on your back, point your toes downwards, then pull them up towards you. Move your ankles through their full range so that you can feel the muscles in your calves contract (toes pointing) and stretch (toes pulled up). Repeat ten times on as many occasions as you can throughout the day.

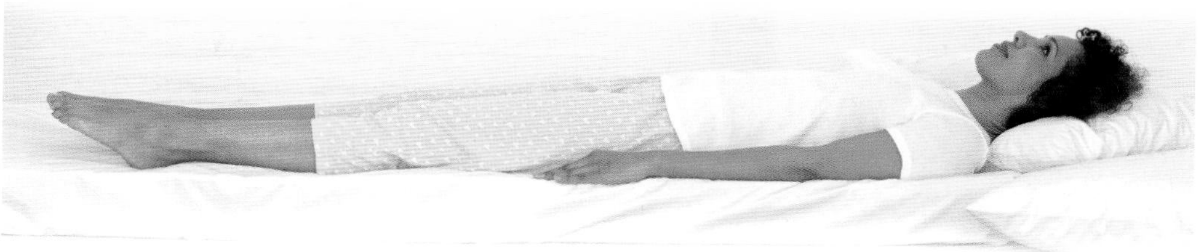

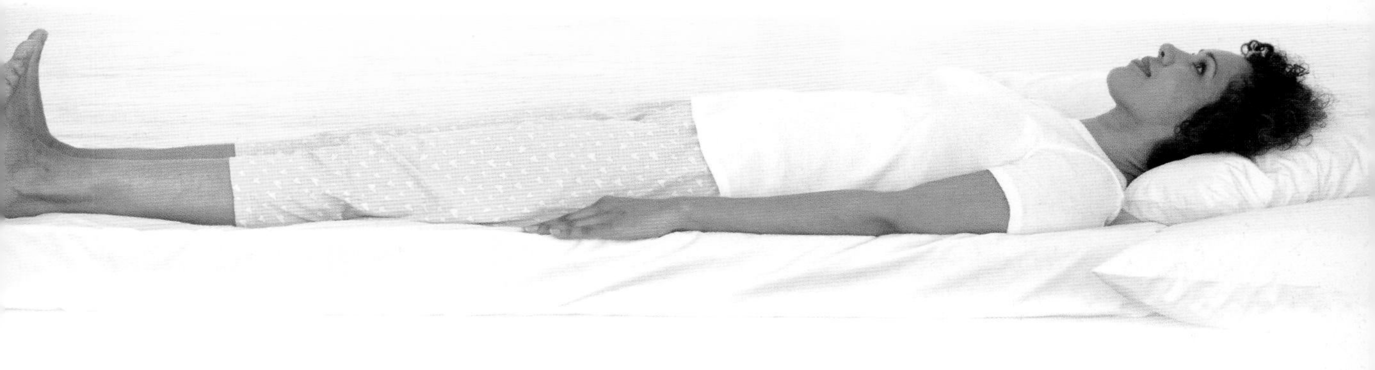

Walking, weight work and supplements can increase thigh bone density by over 10 per cent.

TAKING CHARGE OF joint and bone problems

Keeping your joints, muscles, bones, tendons and ligaments in the best of health is vital as you get older. Staying active can prevent problems and help you to manage symptoms.

Bone is living tissue that is constantly being built then broken down. After the age of 30 or so, bone loss outstrips the amount of bone building, and both men and women lose about 1 per cent of bone each year. In women, the pace of bone loss accelerates to around 4 to 5 per cent a year for several years after the menopause. This means that by the age of 65, both men and women will have lost at least 30 per cent of their bone mass and women may have lost considerably more.

STRESS YOUR BONES

Regular exercise can help restore bone density. A Florida study found that women aged 66 to 72 who underwent an exercise program that included strength training and walking – and who were given vitamin D and calcium supplements – increased the bone density of the neck of their thigh bone (femur) by 11 per cent.

Stressing your bones, as you do when you undertake any kind of weight-bearing activity, helps to encourage new bone cells to form. To be effective, though, it must stress your bones over and above what's normal. A gentle 30-minute walk, for example, does wonders for your heart but not a great deal for your bones as it doesn't stress them enough. To counter that, if you're fit and have good balance, add in an uphill and downhill hike over rough ground wearing a backpack, or do weight work. Dancing, jogging, running, skipping, jumping and activities that involve changing direction – games such as tennis or squash – where the muscles pull in different ways can also help strengthen bones. Of course, if you haven't exercised recently, are overweight or have underlying health concerns, or if you have reason to believe you may already have weak bones, you should consult your doctor first.

5 effective ways to **FEED** your bones

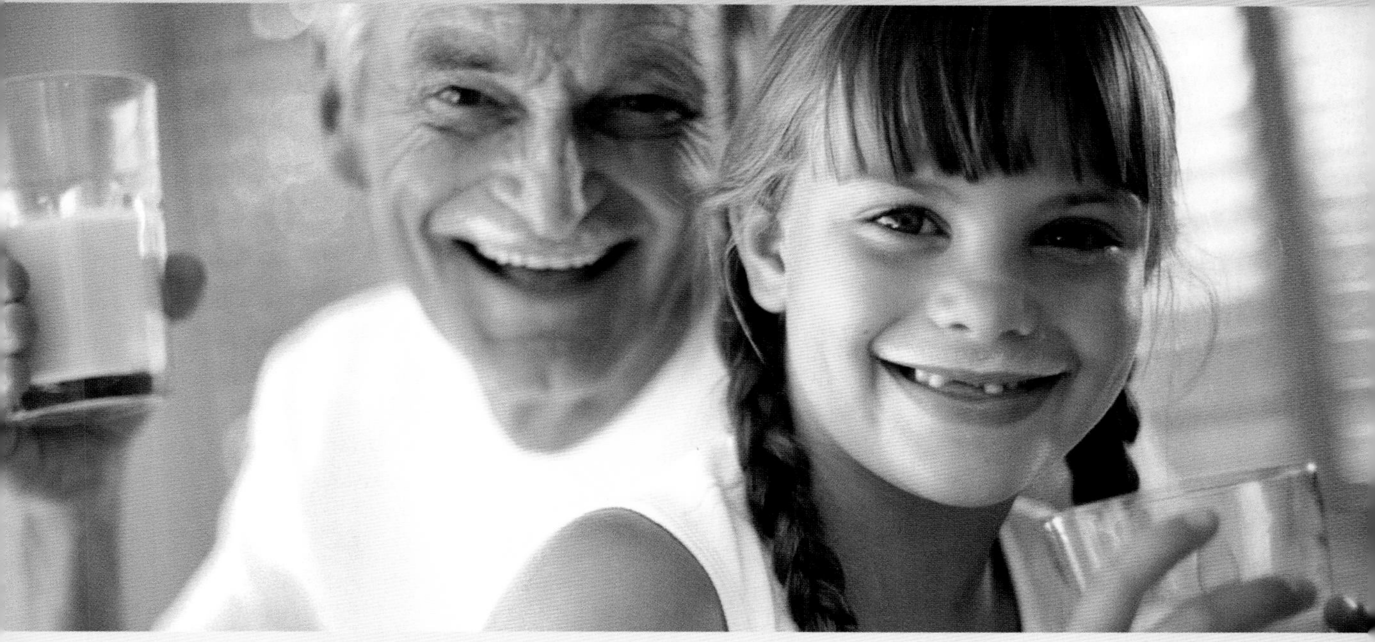

Your bones need good nutrition to stay strong and healthy. Here are some ways to ensure that what you eat benefits your bones:

1 PILE ON THE PROTEIN Contrary to popular opinion, a higher protein intake results in less bone loss over time, so include some protein at every meal.

2 GET YOUR SEVEN Fresh fruit and vegetables contain the minerals magnesium and potassium, both vital for healthy bones. Leafy green vegetables are also a source of vitamin K, which researchers at Tufts University, Boston, found reduces the risk of hip fracture by two-thirds.

3 AVOID PROCESSED FOODS A diet high in processed foods, coffee, tea, sweets and alcohol leads to calcium loss – and so weaker bones. Excess sodium (salt) also leaches calcium from your bones.

4 CALCIUM COUNTS Calcium helps to strengthen bone. It's best consumed in dairy foods such as milk and yogurt rather than alternative sources because then it comes with other important nutrients, including protein, potassium and magnesium, which all help the body to process the calcium.

5 GET IN THE RED Red-coloured foods, including watermelon, tomatoes and tomato products such as tomato paste and tomato sauce, contain lycopene, a member of the carotenoid family of nutrients that protect against inflammation, a cause of bone loss. Consuming five or more serves of lycopene-rich foods a week is linked to a significantly lower risk of fracture.

OSTEOPOROSIS

If your bones become significantly less dense and are so thin and brittle they are liable to break, you may have osteoporosis. It's sometimes called the 'silent disease', because symptoms are not experienced until you have lost a considerable amount of bone. One clue, however, is if you lose more than 4 cm in height a year, as this can be a sign of a spinal compression (one of the main consequences of osteoporosis, caused by weakened bones). Other symptoms include stooped posture and back pain due to collapsed or fractured vertebrae, plus fractures elsewhere, especially the hip, with minimal cause.

Risk factors for osteoporosis include age (both sexes), being post-menopausal (women) and taking corticosteroids in the long term (your doctor may give you osteoporosis medicine to counteract this if it applies to you). You're also more likely to develop osteoporosis if you have a family history of the condition or are small-boned. Other lifestyle issues that lower bone density are being sedentary, not eating much calcium, drinking too much alcohol or fizzy cola-type drinks and smoking.

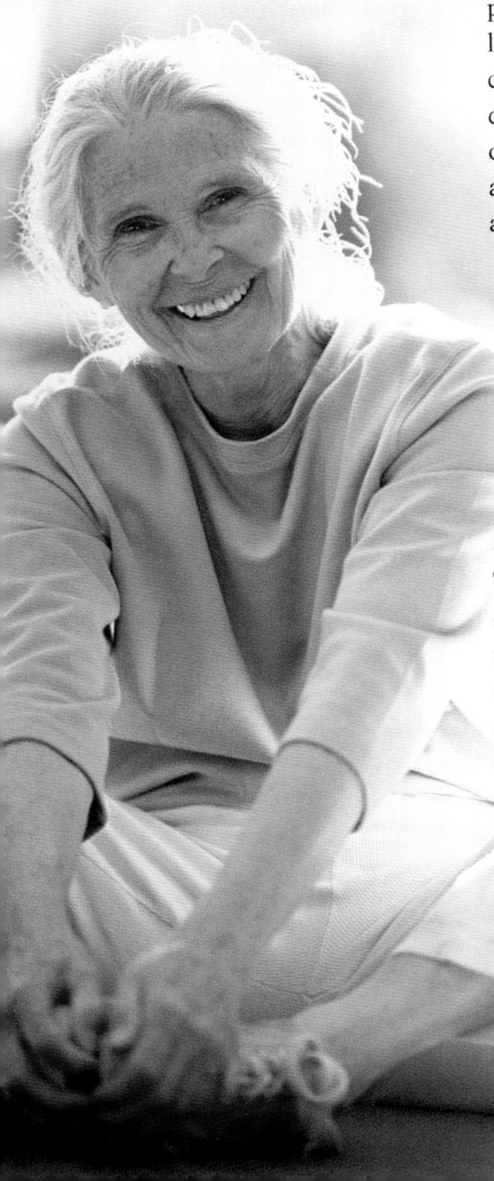

Exercise is good for bones, but the wrong type can cause fractures if you already have osteoporosis.

Reversing the damage

The good news is that it's possible to reverse the stage before osteoporosis, osteopenia (when you have lower than normal bone mass) through lifestyle changes – such as doing more weight-bearing exercise and eating a bone-friendly diet (*see* page 163) – as well as taking medication. If you have osteoporosis, medicine (and calcium and vitamin D supplements) help to keep the condition under control.

- **Softly, softly** Exercise is good for bones, but the wrong type can cause fractures if you already have osteoporosis. Avoid high-impact exercises such as running, jogging, skipping, aerobics, football and activities that involve bending forward at the waist.

focus ON ... FRACTURES

Your risk of fractures increases as you get older – half of women and a quarter of men over the age of 50 have an age-related fracture at some point in their lives.

Older people are more likely to suffer a fracture if they fall because the bones become less dense with age (*see* opposite). But recent research suggests that changes in bone toughness – how well a bone's structure resists fracture – could also be to blame. In other words, bone quality may play a role in fractures as well as bone quantity.

- Improve your bone health through exercise and diet (*see* pages 162–163). And cut your risk of falls by taking sensible safety precautions and by working on your balance (*see* pages 152–155).

Heal faster

Bone healing is slower as you get older. There are four distinct stages of healing, which can't be hurried – inflammation, soft callus, hard callus and bone remodelling. Age also brings a greater risk of complications and failure or delay in the bones knitting together, but you can take action. Here are four ways to help ensure that your bones heal well:

- **DON'T SMOKE** Smoking restricts circulation to the bone, depriving it of healing nutrients and cells.

- **BALANCE YOUR DIET** To heal, bone needs high-quality nutrients such as calcium, found in dairy foods, nuts, sesame seeds and green leafy vegetables, and vitamin E. In a Baltimore study of 148 women aged 65-plus who had sustained a hip fracture, those with higher blood levels of vitamin E healed better and recovered function more quickly.

- **BE PATIENT** Your doctor may recommend various forms of treatment, including a plaster cast, crutches or a walker. Follow medical advice – removing a plaster cast or walking on a broken bone too soon can delay healing.

- **ASK ABOUT SURGERY** Some surgeons recommend that older people have surgery to fix the bone in place during the prolonged healing process.

- **Sun yourself** Exercise outdoors when you can. Vitamin D, which is made in your skin on exposure to sunlight, enhances bone formation and calcium absorption as well as boosting muscle, and this helps to protect you against falls and fractures. How much sunlight your body needs each day to make an adequate amount of vitamin D depends on where you live and how dark your skin is. Ask your doctor for individualised advice. People who can't get enough sun or who are already vitamin D deficient should talk to the doctor about the best dose of supplement (*see* pages 120 and 122).

it's a **MYTH** ...

... that exercise **RAISES YOUR RISK OF OSTEOARTHRITIS**

The fact that footballers and other top athletes are sometimes plagued with osteoarthritis (OA) in later life has led to suggestions that regular exercise can be harmful to the joints and increases the risk of the condition. A review of studies carried out in 2009 at the New England Baptist Hospital in Boston concluded that this was a myth. 'Despite the common misconception that exercise is deleterious to one's joints, in the absence of joint injury there is no evidence to support this,' said the researchers. 'Rather it would appear that exercise has positive benefits for joint tissues in addition to its other health benefits.'

OSTEOARTHRITIS

Osteoarthritis (OA) is the single most common cause of disability in older people. Around 85 per cent of knee and hip replacements worldwide are performed as a result of the condition. Initially, symptoms such as pain, swelling, stiffness and creaking joints tend to be most troublesome when you move, but as time goes on they can start to affect you at rest and disturb your sleep. The joints most often affected are the hands, hips and knees.

Your age, genes, gender and lifestyle can all play a part. Women tend to suffer from more severe OA than men, especially in the hands and knees. If you are overweight you are far more likely to get the condition. Other risk factors are previous joint injury, having suffered sports injuries when younger, and having done jobs involving repetitive thumb use, such as computer-based deskwork. A number of gene mutations also contribute.

Help yourself ...

Here are some steps you can take to make life easier if you have OA:

- **Do your research** Learn as much as you can about managing the disease – get in touch with the national arthritis organisations, which can provide support and advice. Exercise, physiotherapy and medical devices such as splints and shoe inserts can help.
- **Lose weight** Shedding excess kilograms is a good first step to managing your condition.
- **Target pain** Try simple painkillers such as paracetamol and/or non-steroidal anti-inflammatory medications (NSAIDs). Cortisone injections can help if the pain comes on suddenly and severely, but there's a limit to how many shots you can have each year, as too much cortisone can cause joint damage. A sensory wrap – which will keep the muscles warm and relaxed – can help to ease knee pain.
- **Further measures** If the pain becomes debilitating and is having a substantial impact on your daily life, joint-replacement surgery (arthroplasty) is worth considering.

WORK OUT: keeping moving

Osteoarthritic joints can lose movement and strength and this in turn can cause pain and further limitation. Exercise will ease stiffness, increase the flexibility of your joints and strengthen the supporting muscles.

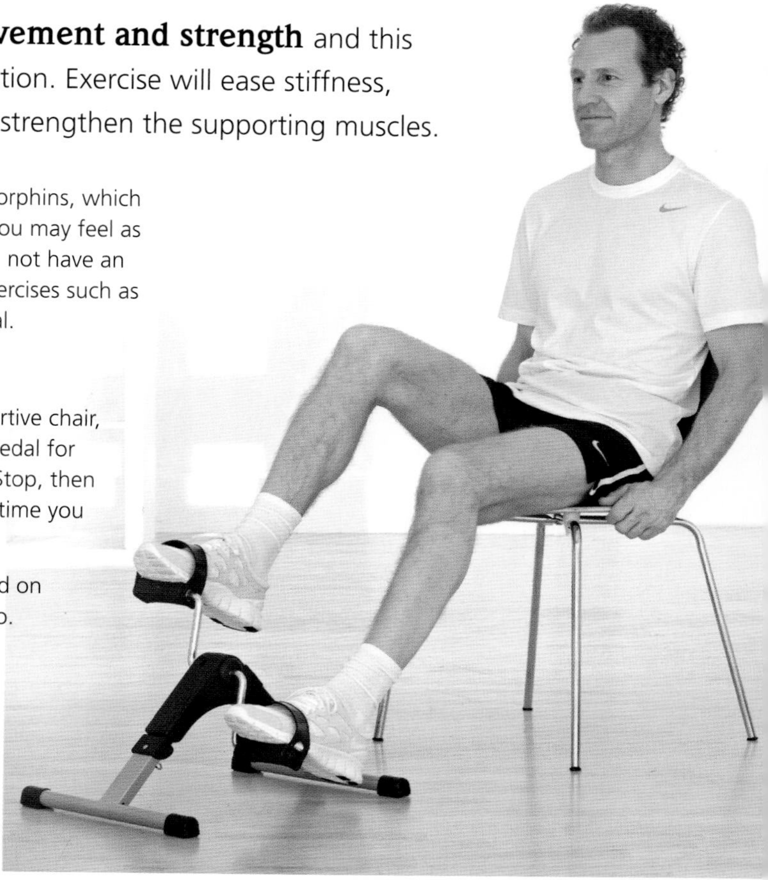

Exercise has the added advantage of releasing endorphins, which are the body's natural painkillers. After exercising you may feel as if your muscles have been working, but you should not have an increase in pain. Rhythmic, non–weight-bearing exercises such as swimming or static cycling are particularly beneficial.

1 **USING A PEDAL EXERCISER** Sit in a supportive chair, arms by your sides and feet on the pedals. Gently pedal for 2 minutes ensuring that both legs share the work. Stop, then reverse pedal for 2 minutes. Gradually increase the time you are pedalling or increase the resistance to progress.

- Pedal exercisers are not expensive and can be used on a table or other stable surface to work the arms, too.

2 **HIP ABDUCTION** Lie on your left side and support your head on your hand. Keep the right knee straight and the ankle in a neutral position (the left leg can be bent). Raise the right leg, hold for 5 seconds, then lower it gently. Repeat five times, then turn and repeat with your left leg.

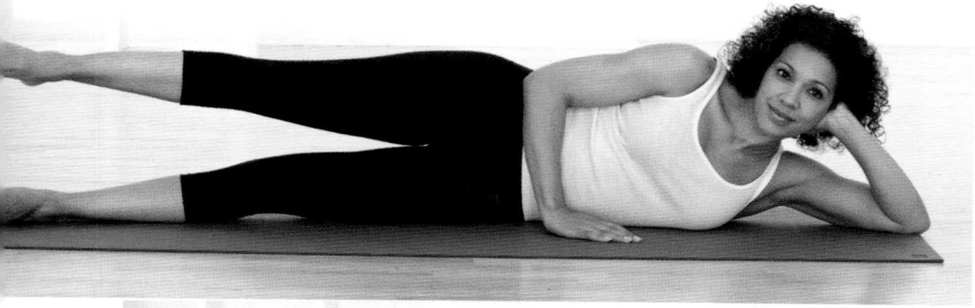

- Strengthening the hip abduction muscle, which can be affected by OA, is important for good balance and walking.

To enhance this exercise, hold the lift for longer or use a resistance band (*see below*) or a small weight such as a beanbag over your ankle.

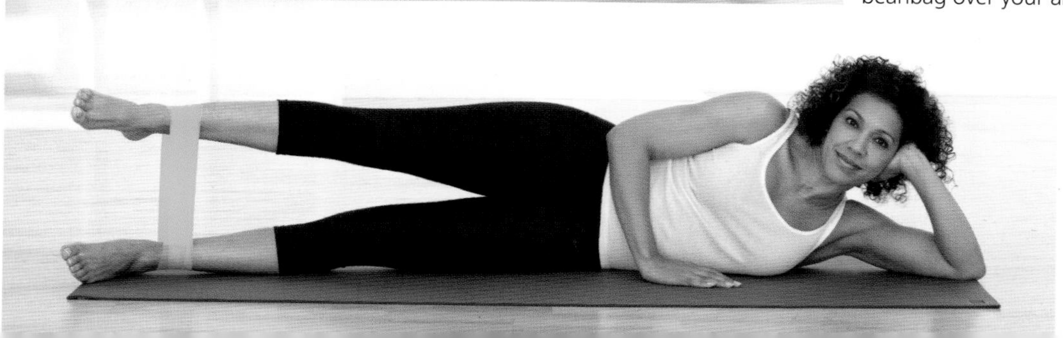

BEATING PAIN

Pain is not an inevitable part of ageing, but many conditions that cause pain become more common as you get older. According to one study conducted in Philadelphia, 80 to 85 per cent of over-65s experience pain as a result of problems such as osteoarthritis, rheumatoid arthritis, osteoporosis or diabetes. Meanwhile, Australian research suggests that about one in three people over 65 have some sort of chronic pain.

Moving can help

Left untreated, pain can rob you of your vitality and make it hard to sleep, walk or go about daily life. It can be tempting to rest, but moving around is often the best thing you can do to alleviate discomfort. Conversely, lack of activity can exacerbate the pain because your muscles weaken, your joints stiffen and you put on weight – all of which increase inflammation and worsen the pain. Consider a program of gentle movement specifically targeted at problem areas. Start with something such as walking, swimming, dancing or simple stretches and build up gradually to something more demanding. Your doctor or physiotherapist can help you choose an exercise regimen to suit you.

Good pain, bad pain

Some muscle discomfort and/or stiffness is normal if you haven't moved much for a while, but it shouldn't be excruciating or prolonged. Sharp, burning pain or a sore joint could be a sign of inflamed tendons or damage to cartilage, while pain on or in the bone without an obvious cause, such as a fall or a blow, could indicate a stress fracture, a small breakage due to overuse. Seek medical help if your pain persists for more than a day, or if it is sharp or burning and seems to be in the joint rather than the muscle. See your doctor also if you have pain that limits movement, or comes with numbness, weakness or joint swelling.

what's NEW

DO IT WITH MIRRORS A technique called visual mirror therapy can ease chronic pain. Here's how it works. If you have, say, a painful arthritic right hand you place it on a table and a mirror is positioned so that your forearm and hand can't be seen. Someone with a healthy right hand stands behind you and puts their left hand down on the table so you can see this and its reflection in the mirror. He or she opens and closes their left hand and you mimic the movement with your hidden hand while looking at theirs. Astonishingly the optical illusion tricks the brain into perceiving your own hand as healthy. The therapy has been used in the UK, USA and Australia to help a host of painful conditions.

9 healing ways to manage **PAIN**

1 DON'T SUFFER IN SILENCE The mistaken belief that pain is an unavoidable part of ageing can deprive you of effective treatment. Telling your doctor does not make you a 'moaner' or a 'bad patient'.

2 CROSS YOUR WIRES Crossing your arms when you feel pain confuses your brain and may reduce the intensity of the pain, according to researchers at University College London.

3 GIVE PAIN THE NEEDLE Acupuncture and acupressure have been used for centuries in China and other eastern countries to help with pain relief. A host of small studies have been published showing that these therapies can indeed help alleviate pain.

4 BE MINDFUL Mindfulness meditation involves concentrating on the here-and-now, and being aware of your surroundings. Research from the University of Pittsburgh looked at older adults with chronic low back pain, and reported that those who learned to meditate experienced less pain and had improved attention, better sleep and enhanced wellbeing.

5 USE YOUR IMAGINATION Using guided imagery or visualisation – for example, imagining chilling out in a pool of healing blue water – helped reduce symptoms and use of medication in a group of OA sufferers, according to one American study.

6 WATCH YOUR DIET Some research suggests that the food we eat has a part to play in rheumatoid arthritis symptoms. A study published in the journal *Rheumatology* found that following a vegan diet and cutting out gluten can help relieve the joint pain associated with the disorder.

7 PRACTISE DEEP BREATHING A study from Arizona State University of two groups of women with fibromyalgia found that slow breathing reduced their ratings of pain intensity.

8 GET MANIPULATED If your doctor thinks it may help, try physiotherapy, chiropractic or massage therapy. Always go to a reputable practitioner, who belongs to the recognised regulatory body.

9 ASK ABOUT PAIN CLINICS If you get no relief, ask to be referred to a pain clinic; a team of experts will help you work out a comprehensive program of management.

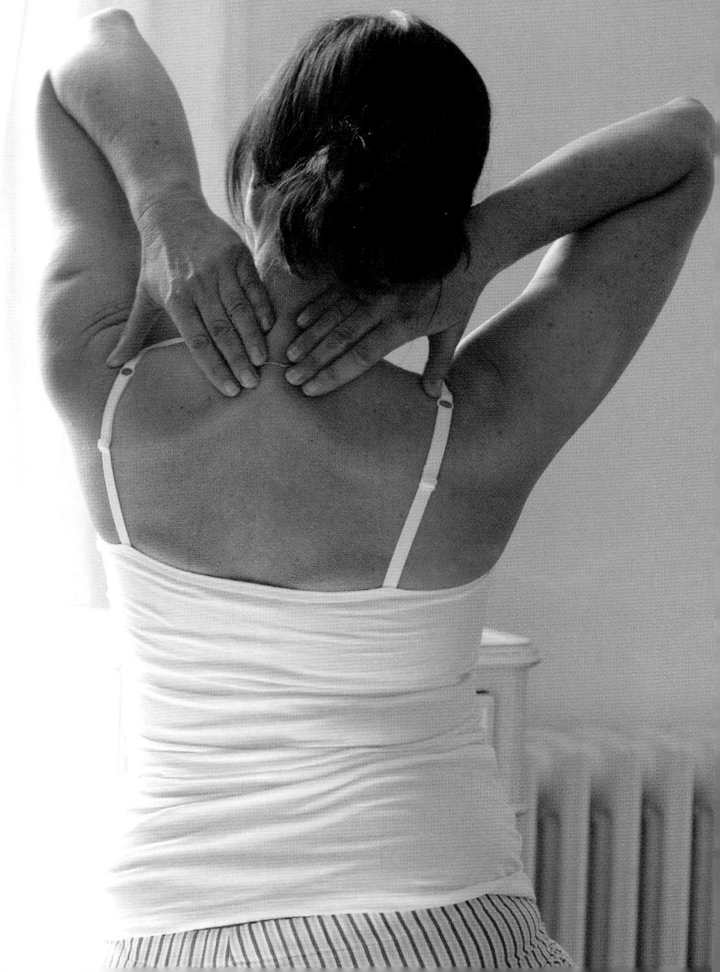

See a chiropodist for foot pain – 75 per cent of people over 65 suffer from it, often needlessly.

GET TO GRIPS
healthy hands and feet

You need strong, healthy feet and dextrous hands for just about every daily activity – both are key to staying independent as you get older. Here's what to do to finetune the movement in yours.

As you get older, you may find it harder to do small movements such as getting change out of a purse or writing a note. This may be because of loss of muscle tissue, changes in your tendons, bones, nerves and blood supply and in the parts of the brain that control fine movement; or it may be due to an underlying condition such as osteoporosis, osteoarthritis, arthritis or Parkinson's disease. Exercise can help. Researchers at the Department of Biomedical Engineering at the Cleveland Clinic Foundation in the USA found that older people who exercised their fingers improved the strength of their pinch and had increased steadiness and speed of movement.

● **CARPAL TUNNEL SYNDROME** If fluid builds up in your carpal tunnel – the small passage running from the base of your wrist to your lower palm – it can lead to carpal tunnel syndrome (CTS). This painful condition is more common between the ages of 75 and 84. Typical symptoms include tingling, numbness and weakness, and CTS can cause nerve damage if left untreated. Moving your hand or shaking your wrist can alleviate the symptoms temporarily as can hanging your affected arm over the side of the bed at night. Non-steroidal anti-inflammatory medication (NSAIDs), wrist splints, cortisone injections or, in around 50 per cent of cases, surgery can help.

FEET FIRST

Foot pain is common as you get older – in one study by New York University, more than three-quarters of people aged over 65 complained of pain associated with a foot problem. Underlying diseases such as osteoarthritis, osteoporosis, peripheral arterial disease and diabetes can all affect your feet, leading to pain, stiffness, poor blood flow, abnormal sensations – such as burning, tingling, itching and reduced sensitivity to heat and cold – as well as changes in skin colour. Other complaints include corns, bunions, metatarsalgia (pain in the ball of the foot) and plantar fasciitis (pain and inflammation of the thick band of tissue that connects your heelbone to your toes).

- **Respect your feet** Wear well-fitting shoes and examine your feet regularly for problems. Do daily foot exercises to maintain mobility.
- **Check it out** See a podiatrist at least once a year for a foot check – more often if you have a medical problem affecting your feet such as diabetes. Seek medical advice for pain or other symptoms.

WORK OUT: hands and feet

Below and on the following pages you'll find a short selection of exercises to help keep your hands and feet mobile. Be sure they are appropriate for you – if you have any pain or a medical condition affecting your hands and feet, seek advice from a healthcare professional. The exercises should not hurt – stop straight away and seek medical advice if they do. Do each exercise five to ten times, three times a day.

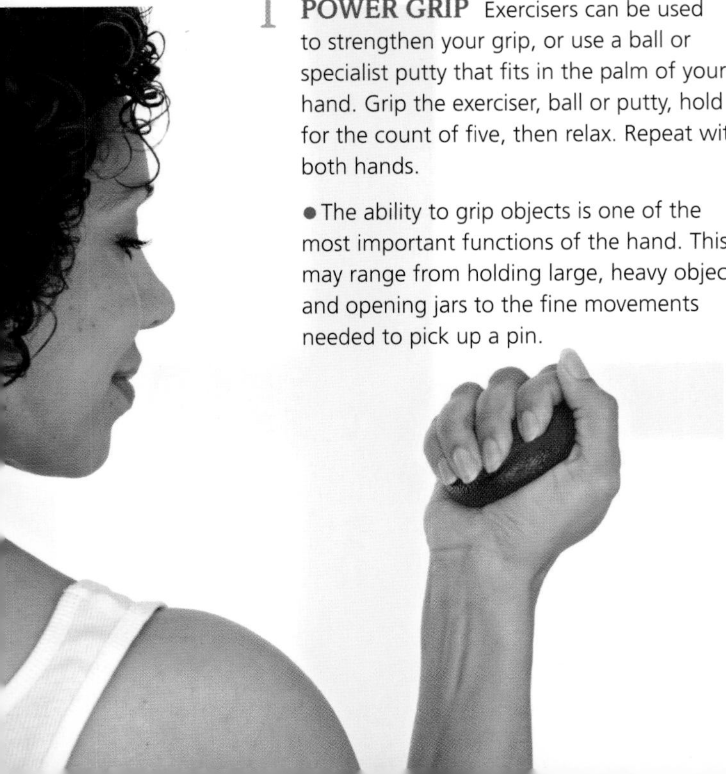

1 **POWER GRIP** Exercisers can be used to strengthen your grip, or use a ball or specialist putty that fits in the palm of your hand. Grip the exerciser, ball or putty, hold for the count of five, then relax. Repeat with both hands.

- The ability to grip objects is one of the most important functions of the hand. This may range from holding large, heavy objects and opening jars to the fine movements needed to pick up a pin.

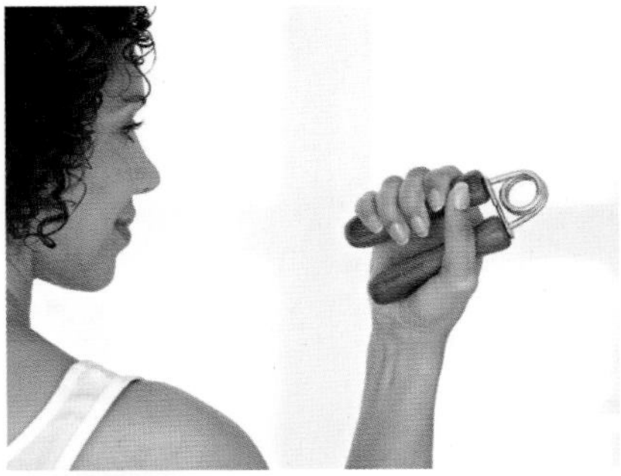

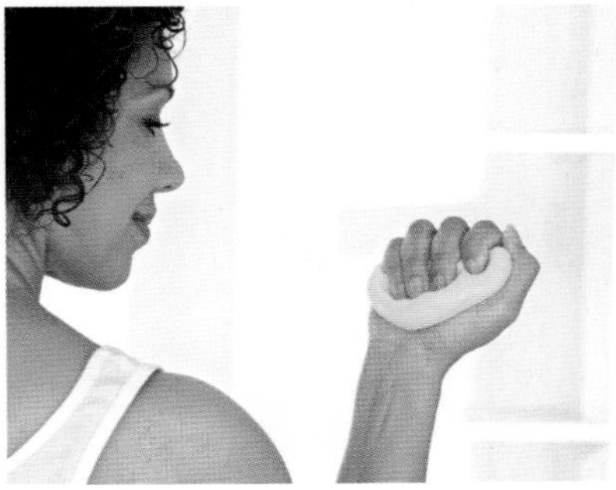

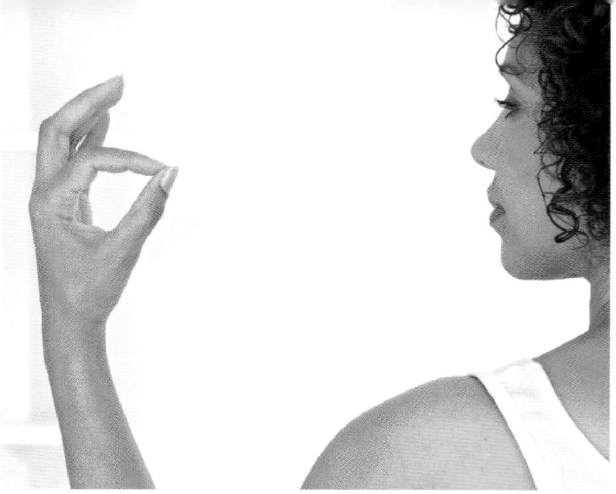

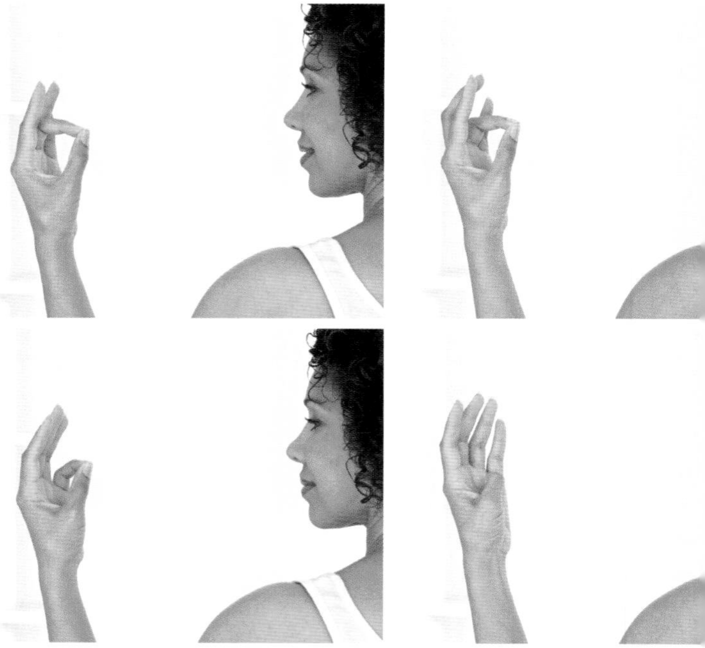

2 PINCH GRIP

PINCH GRIP Touch each fingertip in turn with your thumb then touch the base of the little finger. Move back and forth across the fingertips and base of the little finger as quickly as you can. Repeat with both hands.

- Opposition grip is important for many fine-movement tasks that you do with your hands.

3 EXTENDING WRISTS

EXTENDING WRISTS Put your hands together in front of your face and slowly move your elbows apart while keeping the heels of your hands together. Then move back into the starting position.

- This exercise stretches the soft tissue of the wrists and hands and helps keep your wrists and fingers flexible.

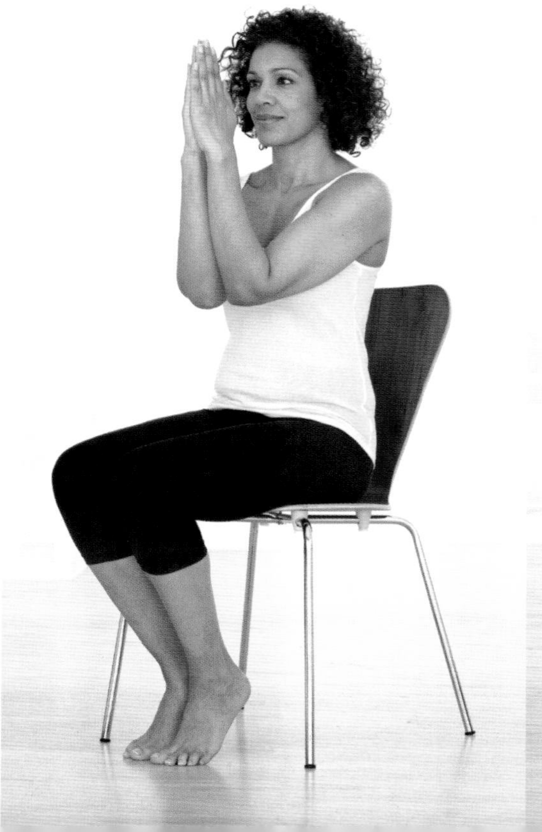

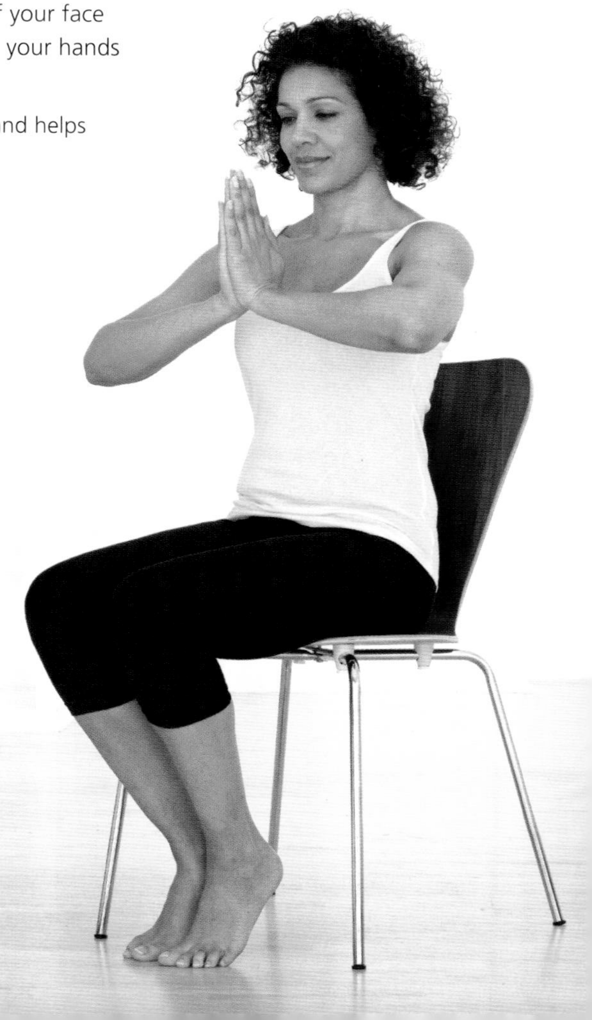

4 **TOE RISE** Stand with your feet together and hold on to a stable surface for balance (do the exercise freestanding if you find it easy). Rise up onto your toes to the count of five, pause, then lower yourself down to the count of five.

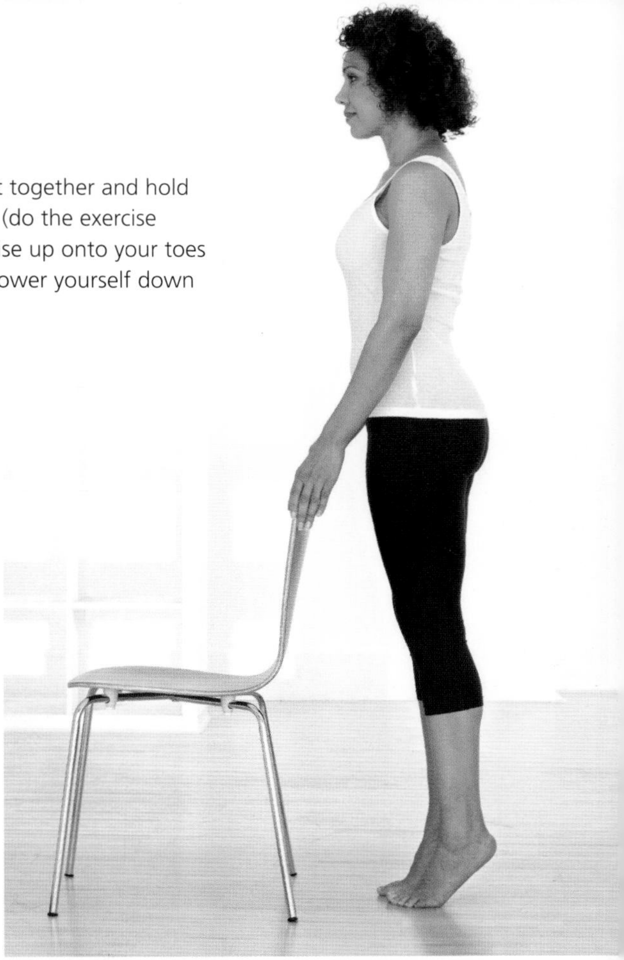

5 **TOE PICK-UPS** Make a pile of small objects on the floor, such as marbles, pebbles or die. Pick them up, one at a time, with your toes and move to make a separate pile. Use different toes to pick them up. Then use the other foot to move them back.

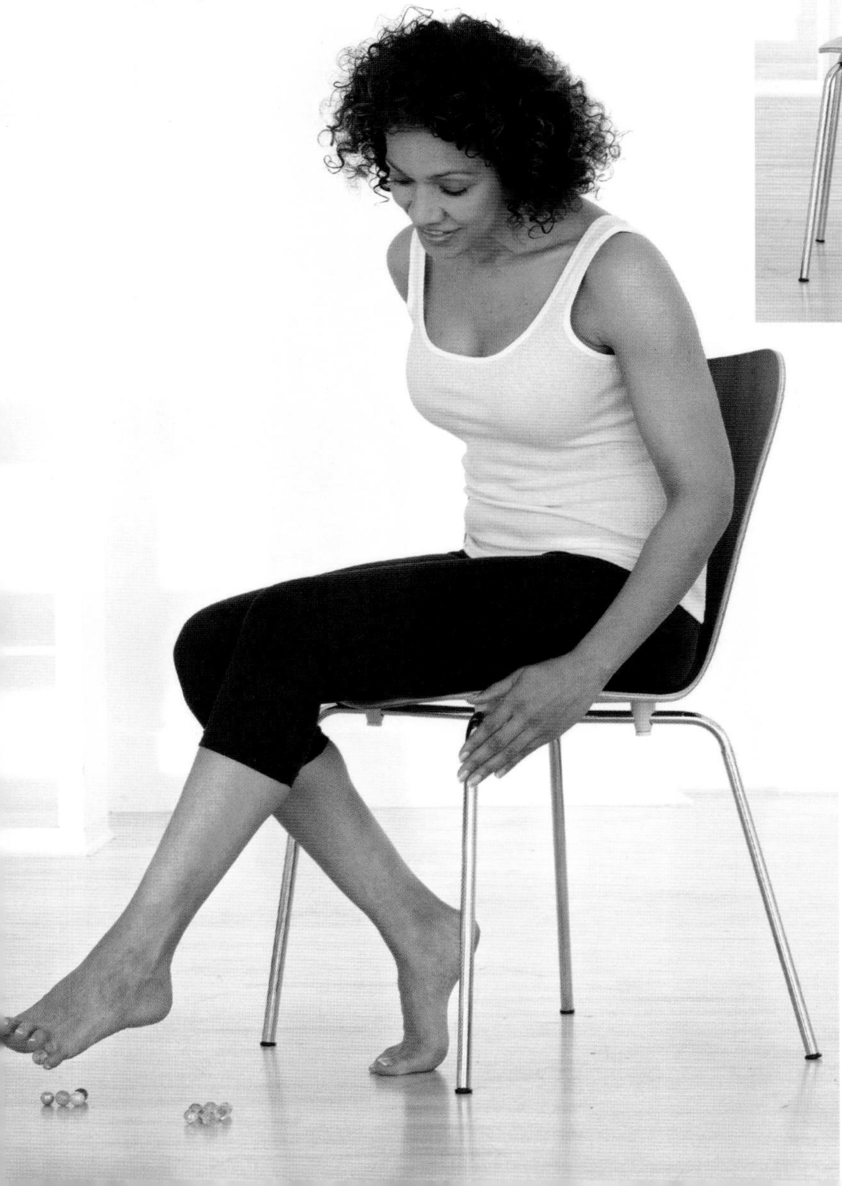

6 **ANKLE CIRCLES** To keep your ankles flexible, move your feet in large circles. Circle outwards for five rotations, then circle inwards. Accentuate every movement so that your foot moves up, points outwards, moves down and points inwards as far as you can.

- Your ankle joints also help you to balance, so practise the exercises on pages 154–155 to improve this function, too.

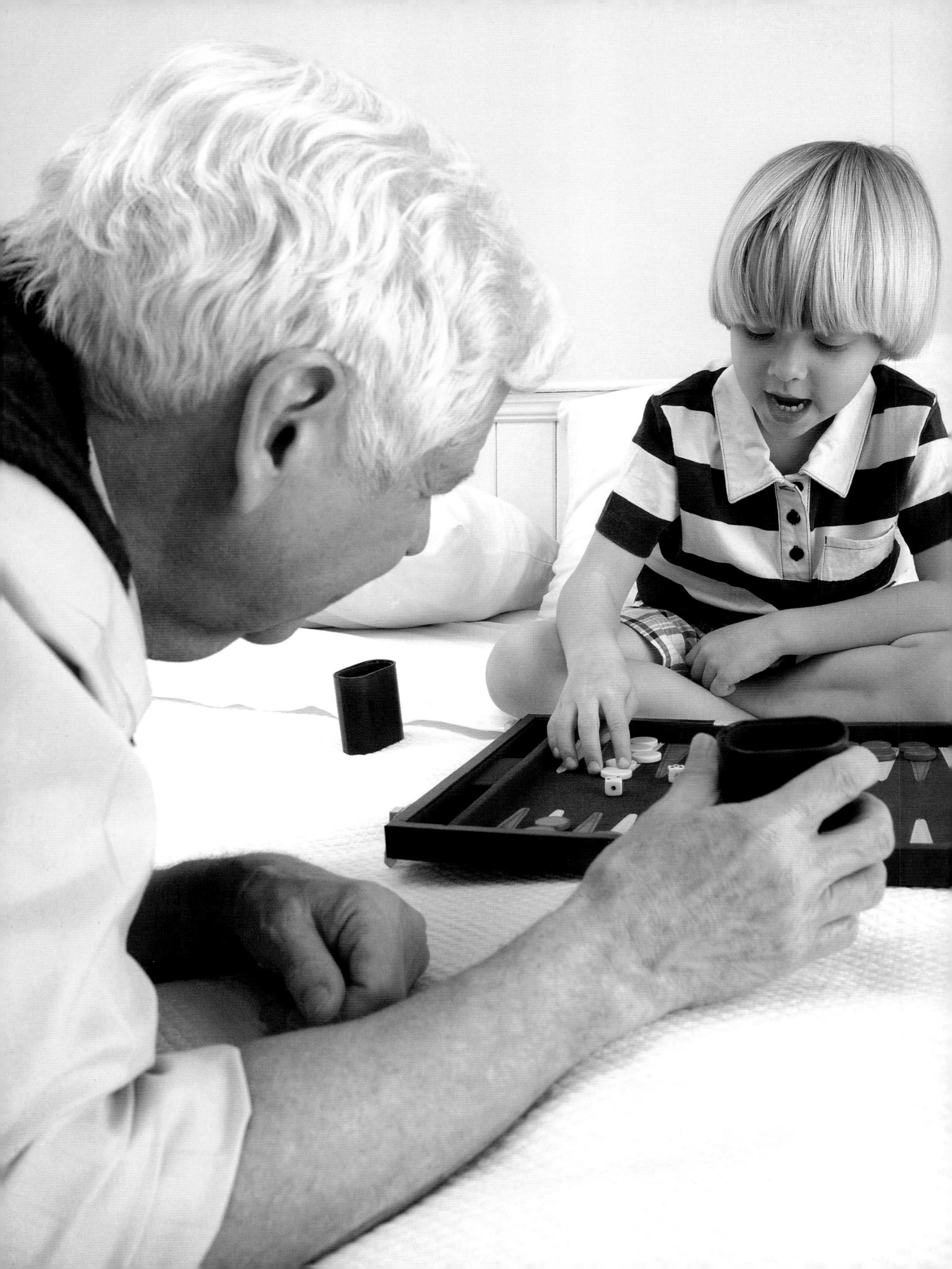

7

All in the MIND

Are you one of those people who tend to think of themselves as much younger than their chronological age? If so, all power to you. Some physical aspects of ageing are inevitable, but there is no reason to assume that your brain must lose its potency as you grow older. If you exercise your mind and look after it, you can carry on learning and growing mentally and intellectually, and you will be better equipped to deal with cognitive problems if they do occur.

Halve your risk of cognitive decline: strengthen and nurture your relationships.

YOUR AMAZING BRAIN
what makes it tick

Your brain is your body's most intriguing and mysterious organ: the most complex entity in the known universe. This strange object – to look at, not very different from a large bowl of cold porridge – is capable of astounding things, and throughout a person's lifetime it is more resilient, adaptable and powerful than anyone suspected even a few years ago.

Take a moment to stop and think about what your brain does. You may never have paused to consider its peculiar dual role. On the one hand, it is the control centre of the physiological organism that is you. Silently, automatically, without you ever having consciously to consider it, your brain manages the myriad processes that keep you functioning normally: breathing, blinking, balancing, sleeping, your reactions to physical stimuli such as cold and pressure, early-warning systems such as your awareness of hunger or thirst or pain or fear, your involuntary emotional and social responses such as the urge to cry or smile – and also your sexual appetite. While this happens on autopilot, so to speak, your brain processes the constant torrent of information that you receive from the outside world, through your eyes and ears and other organs, and turns it instantly into coherent information that you can act on and respond to.

AS THE BRAIN AGES

Research over the past few decades has uncovered some incredible facts about the ageing brain. It turns out that, although age-related changes do take place, your brain appears to be far more flexible than was previously thought. The really good news is that your ability to process information remains intact into your 80s, so long as your brain remains healthy. Many of the changes once attributed to ageing are now believed to be due to other factors such as depression, stroke, underactive thyroid and dementia.

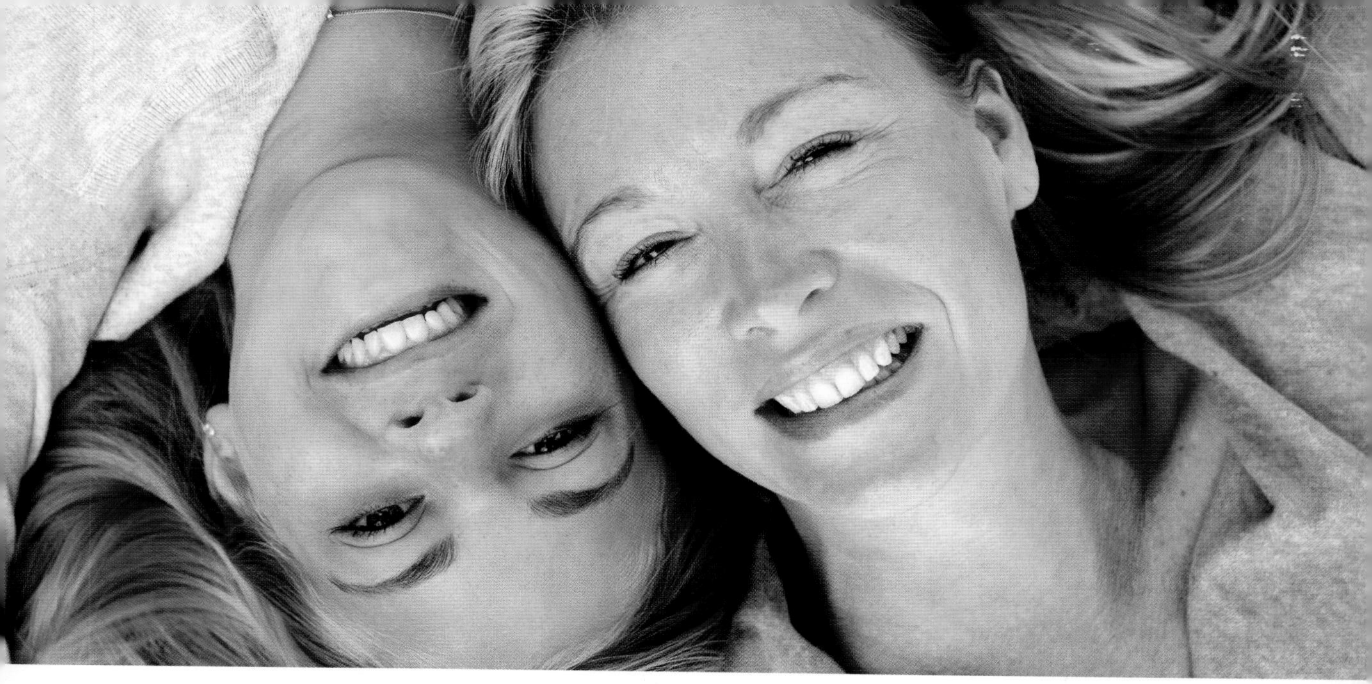

Some changes to the brain are simply a natural part of ageing. Loss of nerve cells and natural shrinkage of certain areas – notably your prefrontal cortex and hippocampus – and a decrease in some chemicals can affect the communication system of your brain. This is the cause of those so-called senior moments that we all experience at some point, when you forget particular words, for example, or go into a room to get something, only to forget what it was you wanted.

Your adaptable brain

This is nothing to fret about overmuch: it can actually be the source of many a wry chuckle to yourself. It is a fact that short-term memory ceases to be razor-sharp as you grow older, and that your concentration and focus become less clear. You may also find it harder to do more than one thing at a time, and your reaction times may be more sluggish because nerve impulses are transmitted more slowly. But your brain possesses several compensatory mechanisms that make up for age-related losses.

For example, your innate intelligence and your life experience both contribute to your 'cognitive reserve', the spare capacity your brain has that can help to offset loss of neurons and enable your brain to operate effectively even if its normal function is disrupted. Cognitive reserve differs from one person to the next, but your genes, education, career, lifestyle, what you do in your spare time and your other life experiences all have a part to play.

DID **you** KNOW?

With age, your verbal reasoning may improve, and your general outlook may well become more balanced. That's according to a University of California study, which looked at the brain scans of 3000 men and women aged 60 to 100 and found that the capacity to ride out emotional storms grows as you get older. Why so? Your brain produces less of the chemical dopamine, which fuels emotion and impulse. So your slower responses really are wiser. What you lose in reaction time you make up for in better decision making.

BOOST YOUR BRAINPOWER

There is every incentive to develop your mental muscle. Scientists speculate that the more cognitive reserve you have, the more resilient your brain is to damage. After reviewing 22 studies on the subject, Australian researchers at the Prince of Wales Hospital in Sydney concluded that a high cognitive reserve cut the odds of being diagnosed with Alzheimer's disease by 46 per cent. You can increase your reserve at any age by:

- Staying mentally active.
- Taking regular exercise.
- Eating a healthy diet.
- Being sociable.

Making connections

Another exciting discovery is that your brain cells continue to forge new connections with each other throughout your life. This means you never stop being able to learn and form new memories. What's more, some parts of your brain – notably the hippocampus – can actually form new cells. And the best news of all is that this regrowth and rewiring is something that's under your control, as a now-famous study of London taxi drivers proves.

The original study, which used magnetic resonance imaging (MRI) scans to look at the drivers' brains, found that they have an enlarged area in the part of the hippocampus used for navigating in three-dimensional space. What's now becoming clear, thanks to even newer research from University College London, is that the brain changes as it undergoes the intensive learning process. This proves that stimulating your brain by doing complex tasks can actually help it to grow – even in older age.

● **MAKE IT WORK** The growth effect is not just about rehearsing what you know, like a taxi going down the same old routes and back roads. Research shows that novelty helps to reshape your brain,

what's **NEW**

EAVESDROPPING ON THOUGHT

US scientists have used a computer to tap into patients' brains and identify which areas were activated when they played them certain words. A computer program was able to read these electrical impulses, and turn them back into recognisable sounds. The experiment suggests that it may one day be feasible to decode the electrical signals in the brain that normally manifest as speech, and so help people, such as victims of stroke or trauma, who have lost the ability to talk. But that breakthrough – if it ever happens – is years or (more likely) decades away.

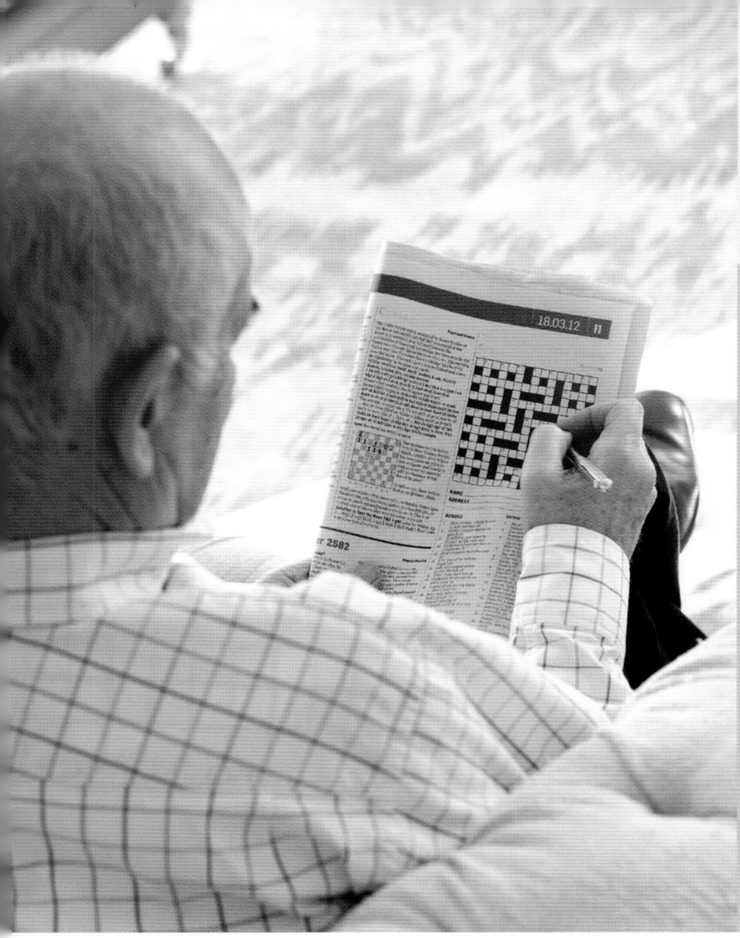

it's a **MYTH ...**

... that just doing **CROSSWORDS** reduces your **DEMENTIA RISK**

You may be a demon at crosswords but don't rely on that alone to protect yourself against the onset of dementia. True, if you have been a crossword addict all your life, you might have a lower statistical risk of developing dementia. But that may be because people with higher baseline intelligence seem to be less at risk – precisely the kind of people who tend to be crossword addicts. The daily crossword may stimulate your mind, but this won't necessarily protect you against cognitive decline. To keep your brain fit, it's important to keep stimulating it by learning to do new things, which means tackling all sorts of mental challenges.

which in turn can help create new brain cells and lower your risk of memory-related problems. Learning a new game, such as chess or others that require memory and strategy, will help to build bridges between your brain cells. You don't even have to go to that much effort to do this. Simply doing familiar everyday activities in a new way – for example, taking a different route to the local shop, eating or brushing your teeth using your 'wrong' hand – will make your brain work harder.

● **GET ONLINE** According to a 2009 study at the UCLA Center on Aging in the USA, surfing the internet can help to sharpen up your brain. Using MRI scans, researchers measured the intensity of brain activity in adults aged 55 to 76 while they looked up something on the internet. Half of the participants had experience of using the internet while the other half had not. Although the whole group showed an increase in activity in the areas of the brain that control language, reading memory and visual ability, only those with previous experience showed a marked boost in the regions related

it's a **MYTH ...**

... that you **CAN'T TEACH** an old dog **NEW TRICKS**

It's not just younger people who can learn new skills – older adults can, too, according to research. And one of the best ways to ensure that information sticks is by rewarding yourself, according to a University of California study. Researchers who studied both younger (aged 18 to 33) and older (aged 66 to 92) adults found that both groups were much more likely to remember when promised a financial reward. Try promising yourself a present in return for learning something new and see how well you succeed.

to decision making and complex reasoning. And even those who rarely used the internet were able to trigger these centres after only one week of surfing for an hour each day.

Movement helps your brain

If you want to fire up your ageing brain, get active. It's long been known that exercise boosts levels of endorphins, the feel-good hormones in the brain that help us to feel relaxed and happy. Studies suggest that it also increases the availability of key brain messenger chemicals, such as serotonin and dopamine, levels of which start to decline with age.

● **UP THE PACE** For optimum brain benefit – and specifically to protect against the shrinkage of brain tissue that happens as you get older – aerobic exercise (any activity that gets you slightly out of breath and sweaty but enables you still to carry on a conversation) wins every time. That's because our brain cells, like all our cells, need oxygen, and aerobic exercise helps to increase oxygen-carrying blood flow. A study carried out at the University of Illinois and published in the journal *Nature* reported that a group of 124 relatively unfit people over the age of 60 performed much better at complex tests, especially those that involved task switching, after they'd walked rapidly for 45 minutes three days a week. They were also better at focusing, and ignoring irrelevant information.

Staying in touch

Maintaining good relationships seems to have a protective effect on the brain. Research carried out at the Rush Alzheimer's Disease Center in Chicago found that lonely people may be twice as likely to develop Alzheimer's disease. The reason? Those who are persistently lonely seemed to be more vulnerable to the changes in the brain that occur alongside dementia.

And a study done at the University of Chicago in 2009 shows just how much loneliness can affect how our brains operate and how we behave. A team led by neuroscientist Professor John Cacioppo,

7 ways to keep your **BRAIN SHARP**

1 GO MED There's growing evidence that a Mediterranean diet (*see* pages 79–82) can help protect against the effects of ageing, including some forms of dementia. A review carried out in 2010 by researchers from the University of Florence found that eating the Mediterranean way was linked with a 13 per cent lower risk of brain diseases.

2 BE GAME Playing video games can help enhance your memory and speed up your reaction time. In a study at the University of Illinois, USA, a group of over-60s who played a computer game called Rise of Nations for eight weeks scored higher in tests of what scientists call executive function – the ability to plan, reason, problem solve and multi-task – than those who simply looked on.

3 EMBRACE STILLNESS Meditation is good for your brain. In a 2011 study carried out in the USA and Germany, participants were given brain scans before and after a program of weekly meetings and daily meditation exercises. The results showed changes in their brain structure, such as increased grey-matter density in the hippocampus, the brain area used for learning and memory.

4 LEARN THE LINGO You'll stimulate the frontal lobes of your cerebrum – the part of your brain associated with short-term memory. Research at Tel Aviv University shows that adults have great potential for learning new languages – although they learn them differently from children. Try learning the language used at your favourite holiday destination.

5 CALMLY DOES IT Constant stress can impair your brain health and mental performance. Studies show that high levels of cortisol, one of the body's main stress hormones, can damage the hippocampus and dent memory and learning.

6 CHUCKLE AWAY The old saying that laughter is the best medicine holds true for the brain as well as the body, according to researchers in South Korea. Why? It helps to activate areas associated with creativity and learning.

7 SLEEP ON IT Getting enough shut-eye helps to fix your memories. And a 2010 US study showed that as well as consolidating our memories during sleep, the brain is busy organising them and picking out the most salient information, which may aid creative thinking.

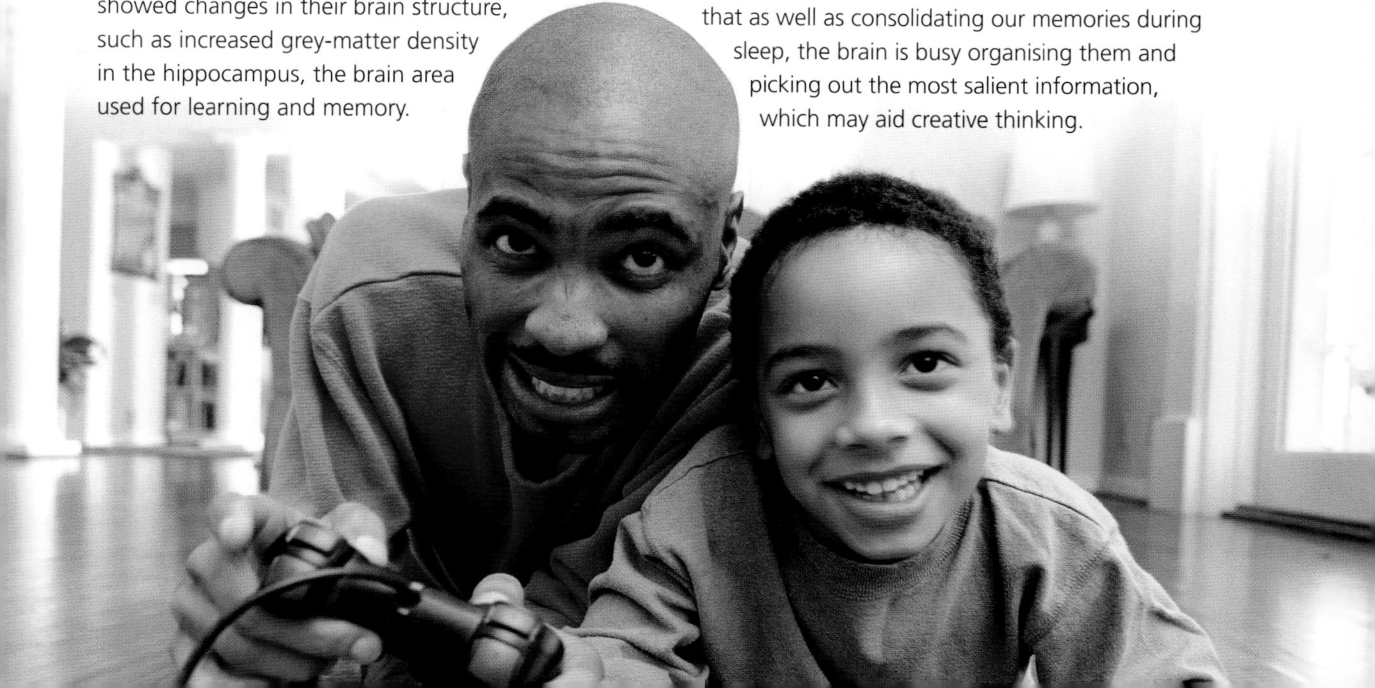

which used MRI scans to study the connections between feeling lonely and brain activity, found significant differences between the brain activity of people who perceived themselves as lonely compared with those who didn't. He suggests that persistent loneliness is linked to poorer physical and mental health.

'You can judge your age by the amount of pain you feel when you come into contact with a new idea.'

Pearl S. Buck, American writer

● **MAKE CONTACT** So all the research suggests that you should seize every opportunity that comes your way to meet friends and make new ones. One 12-year study that followed more than 1000 adults aged 65 and over found that those who had five or six social ties had less than half the risk of cognitive decline than those with none. US psychologist Elliot M. Friedman made a similar discovery. In a study of 74 women aged 61 to 90, he found a link between having good friends and low blood levels of an inflammatory chemical called interleukin-6, high levels of which are linked with a range of illnesses including Alzheimer's.

If you combine socialising with some activity, then so much the better. Join a swimming club, go to bridge or dancing classes – any kind of engagement with other people can reduce your risk of dementia. That's what the Einstein Aging Study in the USA found when it looked at the link between leisure activities and dementia risk in 469 participants aged 75-plus.

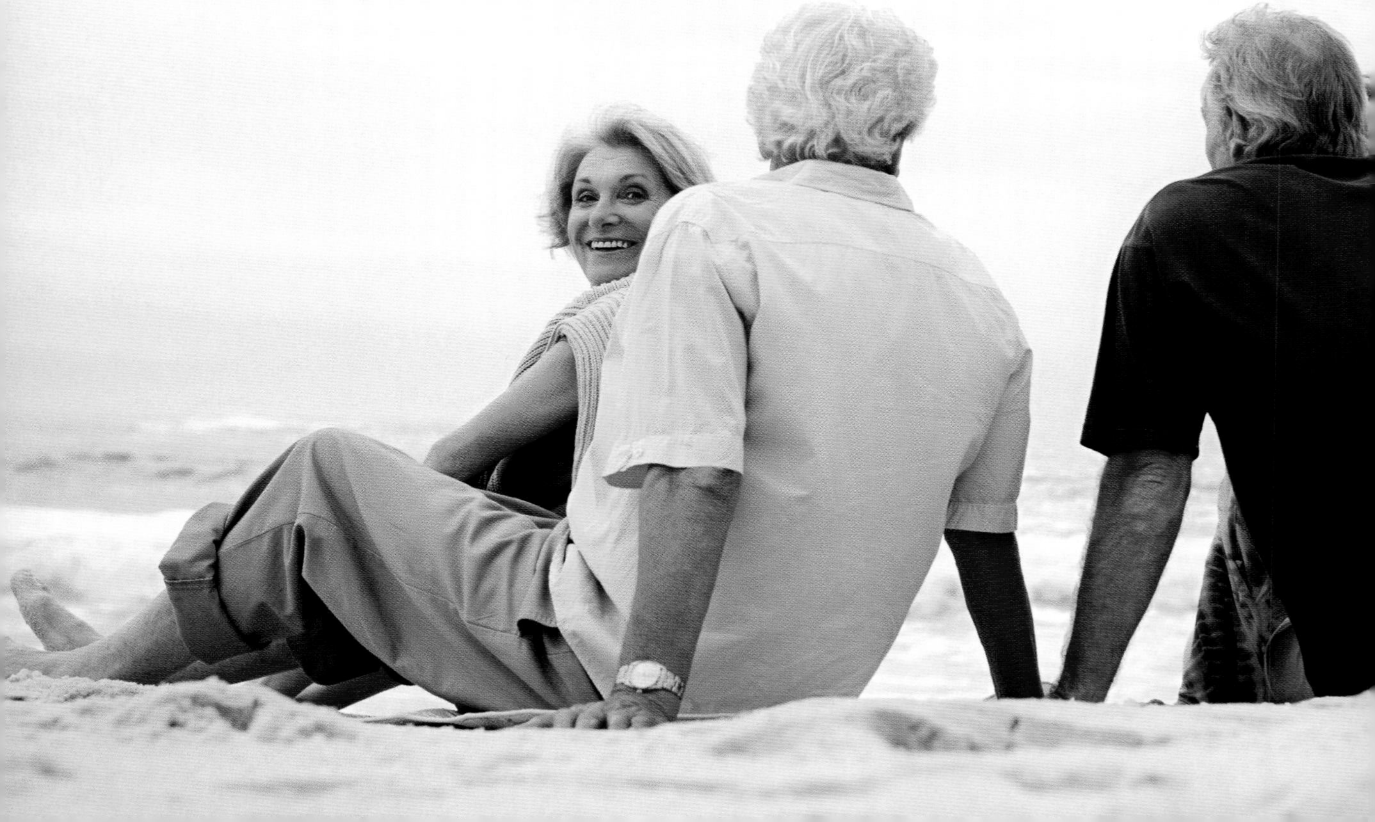

FOOD FOR THE BRAIN
lift your mood

Cut the risk of Alzheimer's by eating oily fish: omega-3 fatty acids may protect against dementia.

What you eat – and drink – can have a dramatic impact on your mood, your memory, and how well your brain works as you age.

The physical benefits of a Mediterranean diet are well documented, but a growing number of studies now suggest that eating in this way can also improve your mood and memory, and may even help to reduce your risk of dementia. The reason? The diet is packed with anti-oxidant–rich foods such as fruit and vegetables and olive oil, which help prevent attack by free radicals – harmful molecules that can damage your cells and which are involved in ageing, including brain ageing. Not only that, the diet also contains anti-inflammatory foods, such as oily fish, and these can help counter long-term inflammation, now thought to be at the root of many chronic diseases including dementia and Alzheimer's disease.

Super foods for a healthy brain

Eating a balanced diet and avoiding becoming overweight are vital for your brain and overall health, but scientists have now identified certain 'super foods' that they believe could give your brain a supercharged boost.

● **FRUIT AND VEGETABLES** Go for as many different-coloured varieties as you can to maximise your intake of anti-oxidant compounds. Blueberries, blackcurrants, carrots, pumpkins and dark leafy greens such as spinach, kale and broccoli are all good choices. Researchers at Chicago's Rush Institute for Aging found that a group of older people eating one and a half serves of vegetables a day experienced a 40 per cent slower rate of memory decline compared with a group who ate less than one serve a day.

● **CURRY** Cook up a curry. Why? The answer lies in the yellow-orange spice turmeric, a staple ingredient of curry powder. Studies show that a chemical in turmeric might help protect you against

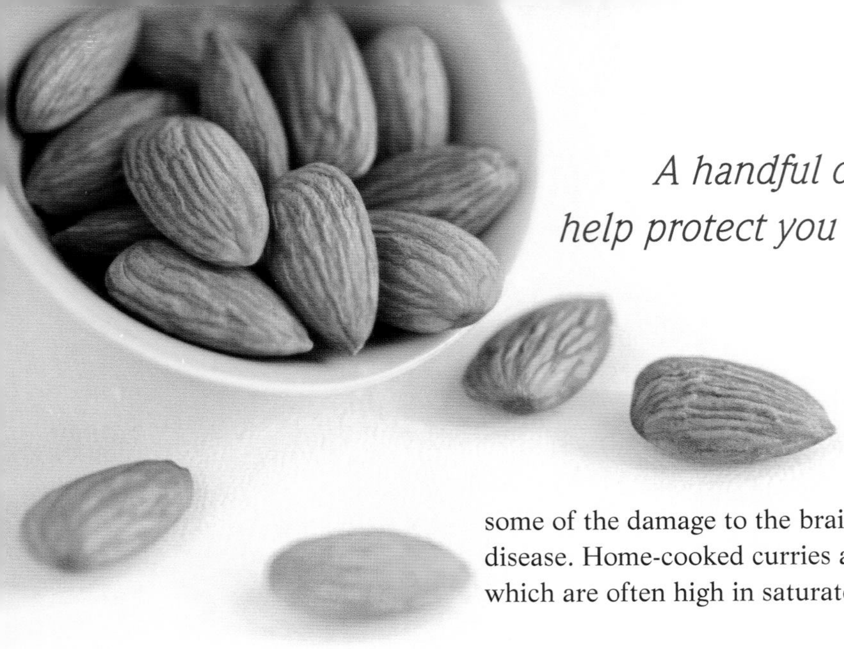

A handful of almonds a day could help protect you against memory problems.

some of the damage to the brain that is associated with Alzheimer's disease. Home-cooked curries are better for you than takeaways, which are often high in saturated and trans fats.

● **NUTS** Consuming just a handful of anti-oxidant–rich nuts every day could help to protect you against memory problems as well as filling you up and curbing any cravings for less-healthy foods. Studies, such as one carried out in India in 2010 on animals with chemically induced amnesia, show almonds to be a healthy choice for boosting memory, but other types of nut such as hazelnuts, pecans, walnuts, pistachios, Brazil nuts and macadamias are all good for you, too.

● **OILY FISH** Eat oily fish such as salmon, tuna, mackerel, sardines or herring once a week. They're rich in the omega-3 fatty acids, DHA (docosahexaenoic) and EPA (eicosapentaenoic), which are good for the brain. A study at Tufts University, USA, found people with the highest levels of DHA were 47 per cent less likely to develop dementia than those with the lowest. Walnuts and walnut oil, flax and flaxseed (linseed) oil, hempseeds and hempseed oil are other good sources.

● **EGGS** A boiled egg at breakfast can help protect your brain from the effects of ageing. A study carried out at Boston University, USA, of 1400 adults between the ages of 36 and 83 discovered that those who had a good intake of the amino acid choline, found in eggs, performed better in memory tests and were less likely to show brain changes associated with dementia than those with a lower intake. It seems that our brain cells require choline to synthesise the brain messenger acetylcholine, which decreases in the brains of those with Alzheimer's.

take CARE! Avoid ADDICTION

You may not think that the apéritif before your meal, the wine you have with it or the nightcap later on are doing you any harm. But drinking too much regularly could affect your mental as well as your physical health, and is especially dangerous if you are also taking medication. Signs that you could have an alcohol problem often include:

- Drinking alone or hiding your drinking.
- Feeling irritated if you miss your 'ritual' drink before supper.
- Loss of interest in things that used to excite you.
- Continuing to drink even though your doctor has advised against it.
- Memory problems and confusion.

Medication dependency

Medication misuse in people over 50 is a growing problem – with nicotine, alcohol and prescription medications being the main culprits, according to US research from the University of Maryland. Even a short course of anti-anxiety medications, sleeping pills or painkillers, for example, can lead to you becoming dependent. But outright dependency (addiction) usually creeps up on you.

It can be deceptively easy to start overdoing things, perhaps to ease feelings of loneliness or isolation after retirement, divorce, separation or bereavement. Or perhaps you were prescribed certain medications after a major operation or during a long stay in hospital and now find it hard to give them up.

The trouble is that dependency can be even more harmful in later life because of physical changes in your body (your liver, for example, becomes less able to deal with large quantities of alcohol) and other health problems. Mixing alcohol and medication can be especially dangerous as alcohol can increase the effects of some medications such as painkillers and sleeping tablets. Problem signs include:

- Taking sedatives or painkillers at the slightest sign of a problem.
- Being unable to get through the day without taking medications.

If any of these signs – whether alcohol or drug-related – sound familiar, talk to your doctor. There's nothing to feel guilty or ashamed about and there's plenty of effective help available. Ask if there are any services in your area specifically for older people.

Drink well

A glass or two of alcohol a day may help stave off dementia. After analysing 23 studies on people aged 65 and over, a 2011 German study concluded that small amounts of alcohol are associated with a decrease in the overall incidence rates of Alzheimer's. However, this is an association, not a definite causal link – it could be that people who drink moderate amounts of alcohol also tend to have a healthier lifestyle. And if you overdo it, up goes your risk of memory decline and neurodegenerative diseases (*see* page 107 for safe drink limits).

A UK study found non-smokers were 20 per cent better at a set memory task than smokers.

YOUR MEMORY
how to nurture it

The human brain is sometimes compared with a computer, but unlike a PC's memory, yours is potentially unlimited. There's no reason why your powers of recall shouldn't remain as sharp in later life as they ever were.

It may require a little more effort to secure your memory as you get older, but your capacity to do so does not diminish. Countless studies show that your brain has the astonishing ability to adapt and change even in old age – a process known as plasticity. More important than the number of brain cells are the connections between them. It seems that as our brain cells talk to each other, new synapses are constantly being formed or pruned away. Many experts now believe that this constant synaptic activity is what shapes our memory. And that's why challenging your brain as much as possible by doing new things is so important. The adage 'use it or lose it' is especially true for your brain. In order to forge those connections and strengthen your synapses, your brain has to stay active.

MEMORY FAILURE OR OVERLOAD?

Are you always losing your keys, forgetting your PIN number or drawing a blank on your neighbour's name? We all have moments like these, and worry about what they mean. But the latest research suggests that much of what we imagine to be memory problems are simply the result of mental clutter. We load up our brains with too much useless baggage by taking phone calls, answering emails and dealing with the demands made on us by family and friends.

These things can lead to stress, then sleeplessness, which in turn adversely affect your memory. Research suggests that relaxation exercises can help to give your mind a good clear-out. There are also lots of ways to actively improve your memory: brain-friendly lifestyle changes such as those listed on page 181 will help. You can also practise specific memory games such as the ones on pages 188–189.

Continued on page 190

take CARE! HOW FORGETFUL are you?

Occasional memory lapses are par for the course as you age, but if they start to become noticeably worse and have a knock-on effect on your daily activities, speak to your family doctor, who can give you a clinical assessment.

DON'T WORRY IF ...	SEE THE DOCTOR IF ...
You can't always remember what happened yesterday.	You find it difficult to recall recent significant events (for example, your son or daughter's wedding), although you can easily remember things that happened in the past.
You occasionally forget someone's name.	You frequently forget friends' names or what everyday objects are called.
You don't remember what you heard on the news or read in the newspaper yesterday.	You have little recall of what you've seen, heard or read recently.
You know your memory is faulty, but can laugh about it.	Others start to comment on your forgetfulness in a way that makes you feel angry or depressed.
You have to stop to remember directions, but can find your way around familiar places.	You sometimes feel confused even when you are in a familiar environment.
You sometimes find it difficult to follow stories or find the right word but can hold a normal conversation.	You forget or garble words and find yourself repeating phrases in the same conversation.

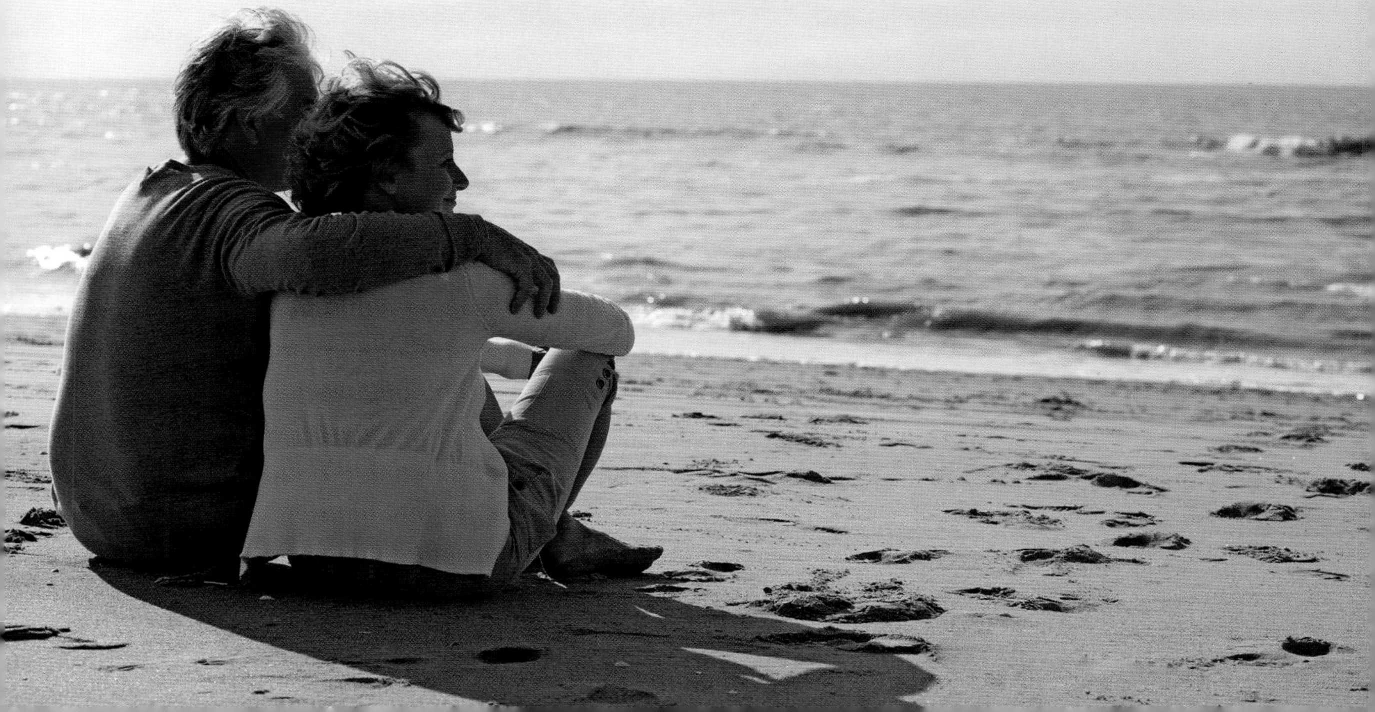

Quiz Test your **memory**

Here are ten simple ways to exercise your short-term memory. If you struggle with any of them, don't worry – the more you practise, the better your short-term memory will become. Apparent memory lapses can simply be a matter of not paying enough attention when you need to; these exercises are all designed to help you focus.

1 Read through the following numbers once only, then try to remember them all, in the same order, immediately afterwards:

6 5 1 4 3 8 7 9

2 Find an image of an unfamiliar but detailed painting online, or use an advertisement in a magazine. Study it for 2 minutes (set a timer if you need to), then try to remember ten things about it, including the colours used.

3 Look out of your window for 1 minute, absorbing as much detail as you can, then try to draw exactly what you saw – include the small details as well as any larger features.

4 Study this shopping list for 1 minute, then try to remember all of the items straight away. How many can you remember 30 minutes later?

Leeks	**Yogurt**	**Tissues**
Coffee	**Rice**	**Chillies**
Soap	**Ice cream**	**Cream**
Basil	**Butter**	**Blueberries**
Figs	**Salmon**	**Chicken**

5 Select six differently numbered playing cards and place them face down on a table. Turn them over and study them for 1 minute, then turn them all back over. Next, try to turn the cards back over in ascending order (so, lowest first). Keep practising, and once you become proficient, try with eight cards, then ten, and so on (turning over all the 1s, then the 2s etc.).

6 Watch a film you've never seen before. An hour later, write the full names of five of the characters and describe each in as much detail as you can (hairstyle and colour, clothes and accessories, any interesting features).

7 It's thought that scent is a powerful memory aid. So try this smell test: study the names of the Olympic gold medal-winning figure skaters below for 2 minutes while sniffing a scent you particularly enjoy (for example, spray your favourite perfume on a tissue). Try to recall them all 5 minutes later while sniffing the same scent. Test yourself again the following day, again sniffing the scent.

Andrée Joly	**Robert Paul**
Maxi Herber	**Irina Rodnina**
Ria Falk	**David Pelletier**
Sissy Schwarz	**Hongbo Zhao**

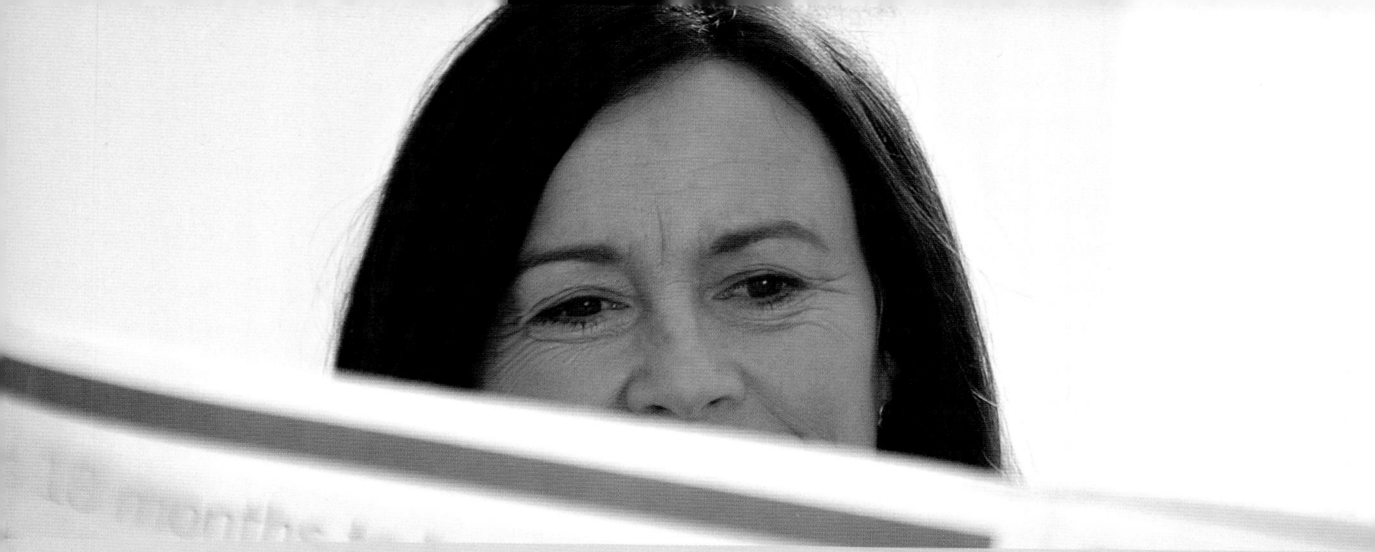

8 Find a short passage in a newspaper on a subject you know little about. Read it through twice then ask a friend or family member to ask you some questions about it. Or write down as much as you can recall yourself.

9 Study the grid of numbers below for 1 minute. Then try to recreate the grid exactly as it appears on a sheet of paper, including the white or black circles.

11	6	23
18	47	9
5	17	3

10 Read through the following list of colourful creatures three times, then try to remember them all exactly.

Angry red ant
Large blue wallaby
Smelly green otter
Hungry yellow dog
Small orange toad

The more of these you can do, the better your short-term memory is at this point. But these exercises aren't just a test, they are also a mental gym, a form of cerebral circuit training. Use them to flex your memory 'muscle' and keep it strong. Simply practising this type of activity will help you to strengthen your memory.

These exercises aren't just a test, they are also a mental gym, a form of cerebral circuit training.

what's NEW

A PILL TO REMEMBER The results of a recent study on mice could one day lead to a human memory pill. So say researchers from the Baylor College of Medicine in the United States. The scientists found that blocking the action of a molecule called PKR increased the excitability of the brain cells in the mice, and significantly enhanced their powers of learning and memory. The next step could be to develop a memory-enhancing medicine that specifically targets PKR, and so enhances memory.

Learning to remember

Being a bit forgetful isn't a disaster by any means. When people say they have what they ruefully call 'senior moments', they are usually talking about the kind of absent-mindedness described on page 187. In many instances, such lapses are not failure of memory at all, but the result of not paying attention in the first place. Can't remember the name of the person you were just introduced to – well, were you listening at the time? Did you catch it at all? Could you have asked for it to be repeated? If you get into the habit of consciously focusing on things that you know you are going to need to remember in the short term, making a point of storing them away in your mind, then you are sure to be caught out less often. Above all, don't fret: the things that your brain files in your short-term memory are *meant* to be retained briefly, then discarded.

Beat forgetfulness

If you're having trouble recalling things in the longer term, then the easiest way to mitigate the problem is to write things down. If, say, you find it hard to remember how to adjust your microwave's timer when the clocks change in spring and autumn, make a note of how to do it and leave that note somewhere you'll find it next time you need it: tape it inside the drawer underneath the microwave, say. For other things, use a planner or diary. Write reminders on sticky notes and attach them to your fridge. If your pin number constantly escapes you when you are standing at the check-out, invent a phrase with words that have the same number of letters. For instance, for 8436, try 'Withdraw cash, big splash'. Make the most of services such as direct debits and standing orders – so that occasional lapses don't cost you money. And if there is something you want to fix in your memory, say it out loud to your partner – or failing that, to the cat. It's amazing how vocalising a thought makes it stick in your mind.

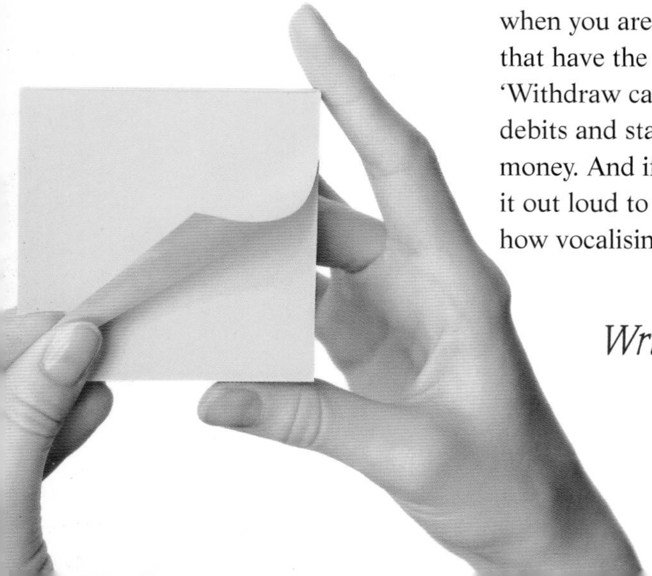

Write reminders on sticky notes ...

KEEPING YOUR MIND
healthy and happy

You have every right to be content as you grow older – and every reason to expect to be. True, life saves some of its hardest knocks for later on, but with your own inner resources, and some outside help if you need it, you can weather the emotional and mental storms.

Growing older is a happier experience than many of us might imagine. That's the conclusion of a study carried out at Queen's University Belfast. The researchers looked at people's attitudes to ageing, and discovered that, contrary to popular belief, older people are just as happy as their younger counterparts. While some young people view the prospect of old age with distaste or even dread, that negative perception tends to evaporate as the reality of it approaches. In a word, being past 60 is generally better than it's cracked up to be.

This happy truth is borne out by a study done at the University of Queensland in 2008. It measured social activities and social satisfaction in older adults (aged 66 to 91), and also in younger adults (aged 18 to 30). It found that the older we get, the more likely we are to see the good things in life and less likely to be upset by the little things that go wrong. And researchers at Warwick Medical School at the University of Warwick in the UK, who analysed the lifestyles and health of 10,000 people in Britain and the USA, concluded that our mental wellbeing continues to increase after the age of 45 – backing up previous studies which show that happiness forms a U-shaped curve.

And it's a similar story when the big things go wrong – difficult challenges such as ill health, financial strictures or bereavement. According to the British Royal College of Psychiatrists, most people cope well with the mental stresses that are attendant on growing older. Fewer than one in 30 older people become ill with depression. Studies suggest that this is because by the time we reach 60 or so, we have become pretty resilient and have developed a battery of coping strategies for dealing with life's ups and downs.

We are happiest between the ages of 65 and 80, a UK survey of 80,000 people found.

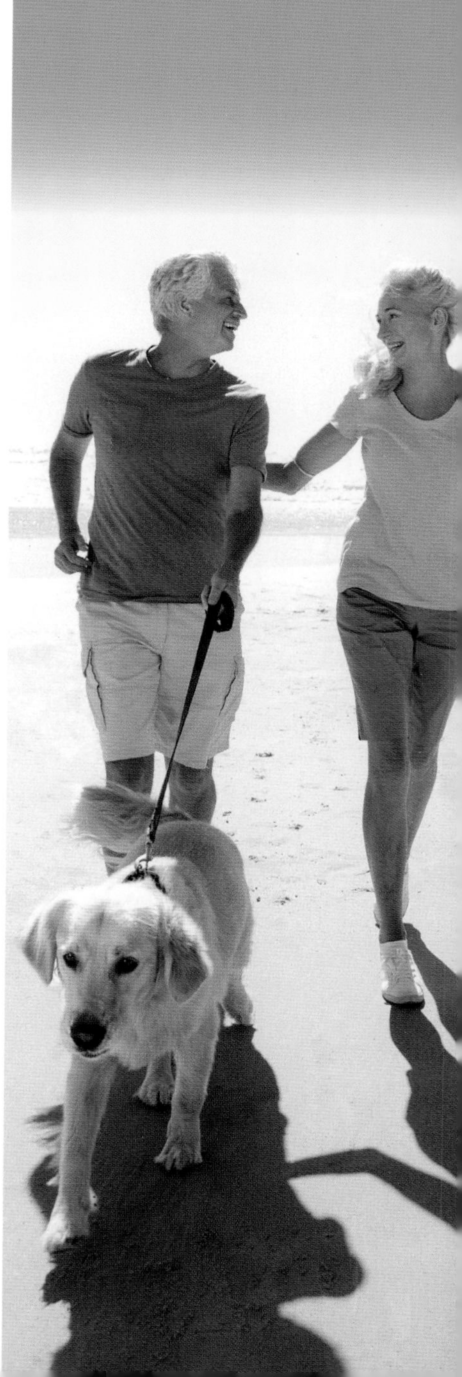

BEAT THE BLUES

That is not to say that, once you hit retirement age or thereabouts, you suddenly become immune to the blues. Every life has its share of sadness and regret, and sometimes these emotions are at the forefront of the mind. They are not the same thing as the medical condition of depression – which is something that needs to be recognised by you, and dealt with somehow.

Sometimes it's possible to get through depression without medical help by talking through your problems with a family member or close friend. If your depression persists, however, and starts to interfere with daily life, it's time to see your doctor. According to the UK's Royal College of Psychiatrists, you should seek medical help if your feelings of misery:

- Are worse than you would expect in the circumstances.
- Have gone on for several weeks.
- Are interfering with your life.
- Mean that you can't face seeing other people.
- Make you feel that life is not worth living.
- Lead you to worry you're causing concern to friends or family.
- Include thoughts of harming or killing yourself.

Do tell your doctor about any recent life changes that could be making you depressed as well, as any treatment plan needs to take these into account. If loneliness is at the root of your low mood, for example, simply taking medication is not going to solve the problem. Sometimes depression may be linked to a medical condition, such as Parkinson's disease, which also needs to be addressed.

> DID **you** KNOW?
>
> Research from the University of Essex in the UK suggests that exercising outside, surrounded by nature, is especially beneficial for boosting your mood and self-esteem. In the study, participants felt the benefits of such 'green' exercise after just 5 minutes, with light activity having the biggest effect on self-esteem, and light or vigorous activity the biggest effect on mood. Walking, cycling, boating, horse riding, gardening and 'wild swimming' in the sea or in lakes are all good options.

Effective treatments

In general, the majority of people get better most quickly using a combination of treatments: medication to relieve symptoms, and talking therapy (*see* page 195) to learn how to deal with stress, anxiety and negative thinking. If you don't feel better straight away, be patient: it can take six to 12 months to recover from a severe bout of depression. Treatment options include:

- **SUPPORT GROUPS** Joining a group can introduce you to people going through the same things, and provide a safe place to share experiences, advice and encouragement. Your doctor should have a list of what's available in your area.

focus ON ... LOW MOODS in later life

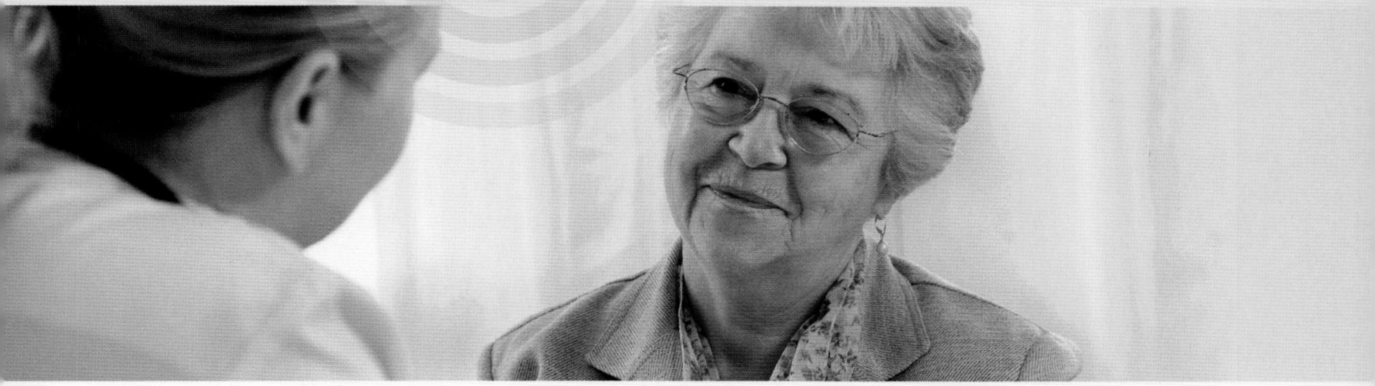

Depression when you are older differs from when you were younger. For a start, many older people imagine that feeling miserable is to be expected, although nothing could be further from the truth. And evidence suggests that depression may manifest as insomnia, weight loss, fatigue and sensitivity to physical pain rather than low mood.

Lack of focus and concentration and slowed thinking are other common signs of depression in later life. Although these symptoms are also seen in dementia, there are a few key differences:

- **DEPRESSION** is characterised by rapid mental decline, difficulty concentrating, slower speech and movement than normal and acute consciousness of any memory problems.
- **DEMENTIA** tends to involve a slow mental decline, feelings of confusion or disorientation (including getting lost in familiar places), obvious problems with writing, speech and movement, short-term memory problems and a lack of awareness of them.

Californian researchers have found evidence to suggest that some older people are prone to experience a kind of low-level misery – known as sub-syndromal depression – not quite severe enough to be classed as full-blown depression but that can make each day seem like a hard, unremitting slog.

With support and the right treatment (talking therapies and medication), you can overcome these feelings. Ways to help yourself include:

- **Getting enough sleep.**
- **Exercising regularly.**
- **Following a healthy, well-balanced diet.**

Are prescription medications to blame?

Some prescription medications can trigger depression. Culprits include blood pressure medications (beta blockers and calcium channel blockers), sleeping pills, medicines for Parkinson's disease that work on the brain chemical dopamine (for example, levodopa), heart medications, steroids, some painkillers and arthritis medications. If you've noticed that you feel more miserable after being prescribed a new medication, see your GP, who may be able to lower your dose or switch you to something that doesn't affect your mood.

With support and the right treatment you can overcome these feelings.

7 ways to KEEP SMILING

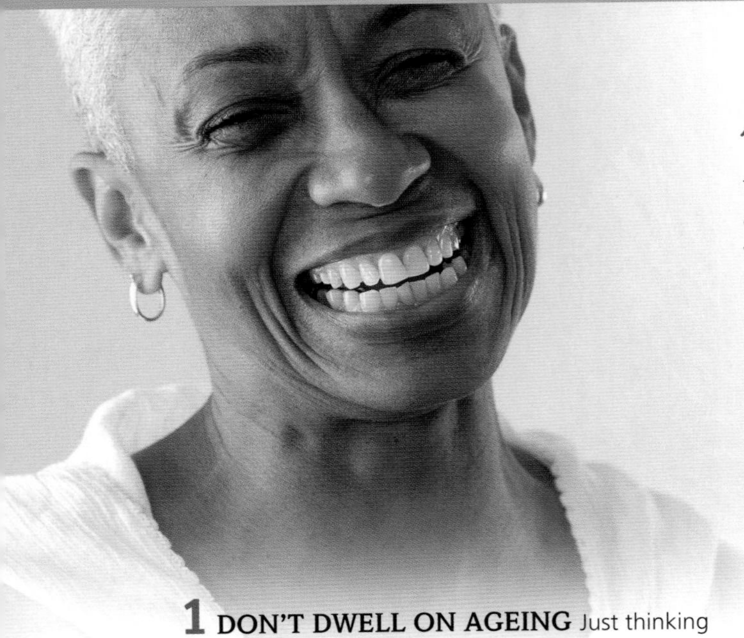

1 DON'T DWELL ON AGEING Just thinking about the clock ticking away and taking on board negative stereotypes of ageing from the media or others can lead to feelings of worthlessness and low self-esteem. So says a 2010 study on 68 older adults aged 74 and over, carried out at the University of Massachusetts.

2 BE MINDFUL Meditation practice teaches you to stand back from your thoughts and just observe them. Over time, this allows you to spot unhelpful patterns of thinking that may be contributing to a low mood. Don't force yourself to change them, just be aware and see what happens.

3 KEEP ON THE MOVE Many studies show exercise to be one of the best mood boosters. Research carried out at Sweden's University of Gothenburg, on more than 17,000 people with an average age of 64, showed a strong link between regular exercise and a lower risk of depression.

4 GIVE THE DOG A WALK Daily dog walking (borrow one if necessary) may help to ward off depression and loneliness, according to a 2008 study by the University of Portsmouth. Dog walkers reported that the daily exercise gave them a better overall sense of wellbeing, as they often met like-minded people, and this made them feel happier. Stroking a pet is also thought to help boost the feel-good brain chemicals serotonin and dopamine.

5 CATCH UP ON SLEEP A 2011 study at the Cleveland Sleep Disorders Centre in Ohio, which looked at the relationship between how long we sleep and depression, suggests that sleeping too little (6 hours or less) – or too much (more than 9 hours) – can have a negative impact on your quality of life and increase depressive symptoms.

6 TAKE UP TAI CHI A 2011 study at the University of California looked at a group of people aged over 60 who were suffering from depression. It found that a weekly tai chi class combined with a standard antidepressant helped combat the blues. Tai chi also improved quality of life, memory and other aspects of mental health, and overall energy.

7 SUPPLEMENT IT Daily omega-3 supplements may help to keep the black dog down, reveals a 2011 study from the Italian University of Pavia. When 46 depressed women aged between 66 and 95 took either omega-3 supplements or a placebo for eight weeks, both depressive symptoms and quality of life improved in the supplement-taking group.

● **MEDICATION** Taking an antidepressant can help lift your mood by changing the levels of brain chemicals thought to be a factor in depression. You may have to try several before you find what suits you best – talk to your doctor if you feel the medication is not working; don't simply stop taking it or you may suffer withdrawal symptoms.

● **TALKING THERAPY** This usually involves meeting with a trained therapist either alone or in a group, where you can talk about your problems and try to find a solution. You may be offered psychotherapy and general counselling, but most experts agree that the most promising treatment for depression is cognitive behavioural therapy (CBT), which your doctor should offer you. It shows you how to replace unhelpful negative thoughts, which could be contributing to your depression, with more realistic and balanced ones. A 2008 study carried out at the University of Pennsylvania showed that CBT could be just as effective as antidepressant medication in treating moderate to severe depression.

● **ONLINE SUPPORT** Internet-based CBT programs allow you to access help at home and in your own time. A study conducted in Sweden in 2005 suggests that treatment via the internet helps to protect against relapses. Among those with previous depression who took part in the internet program, only 10 per cent experienced a new bout of depression compared with 38 per cent who did not receive such help. Your doctor or other health professional should be able to advise you on the best program (*see also* Resources).

● **OTHER OPTIONS** Many people find complementary treatments helpful. Some, such as massage, use physical touch to get results, while others, for instance, meditation, are entirely inward, and work by helping you to refocus and by relieving anxiety.

DID **you** KNOW ?

Studies show that depression in later life can sometimes go hand in hand with an underlying problem affecting the brain, such as Alzheimer's disease. Experts are still debating whether depressive symptoms are a risk factor for Alzheimer's, whether they are an early symptom of brain deterioration, or whether they are a reaction to early signs of degeneration of the brain. But if any depressive symptoms don't go away despite treatment, go back to your doctor and ask for a check-up.

GET THE BETTER OF STRESS

It would be nice to think that most of the stress goes out of your life as you get older: work pressure is a thing of the past, the children are grown up and looking after themselves, the mortgage is paid off ... Studies from around the world, including the 2010 Stress and Generations Study from the American Psychological Association,

Work it out **RELAX, RELAX**

Try this simple exercise if you start to feel stressed or anxious. Set aside 15 minutes and go through it slowly.

- Try to find a place where you won't be disturbed.
- Lie on your back on a firm bed or mat. Let your feet flop outwards and your hands rest by your sides.
- Close your eyes and sigh to release tension. Breathe slowly five times, pausing after each exhalation.
- Release tension in your toes, feet and legs. Then do the same with your fingertips, arms and neck. Ease any tension in your shoulders by relaxing them.
- Mentally smooth out the muscles of your face.
- Be aware of the relaxation in your muscles.
- When you're ready, slowly open your eyes and stretch.
- Bend your knees and roll onto your side before slowly getting up.

have found that we get better at handling stress as we grow older. But, of course, nobody is immune to stress and apart from everyday concerns, there are some specific age-related stress factors, such as illness, immobility or bereavement, that may affect you.

Much research suggests that frequent or persistent stress is bad for the ageing brain. Researchers at Canada's McGill University followed 50 older people for five or six years. They plotted levels of cortisol (the stress hormone) against the size of the hippocampus (the brain area dealing with memory), while also measuring the degree of memory decline. They found that those with high levels of cortisol did less well in memory tests than those with low levels. Also, the hippocampus was smaller in the high-cortisol group. These results suggest that increases in cortisol secretion are linked to a higher risk of mild cognitive impairment in later life.

COPING WITH ANXIETY

There is a difference between stress and anxiety, although the words are often used interchangeably. Stress has a clearly identifiable cause such as moving house, while anxiety is more of a general worry about something that might happen in the future such as falling ill.

Anxiety can develop into a disorder in its own right (stress is never classified as a mental disorder). You may need therapy or medication to help you get over anxiety while stress is usually temporary and disappears when the cause of the stress disappears.

Research by the University of California suggests that although older people tend to be less anxious than younger people, up to a quarter suffer from some symptoms, and as we age anxiety is nearly twice as frequent as depression. Of course, it's quite normal to feel anxious about what the future might hold as you grow older, but as a 2007 review carried out by researchers at Melbourne University shows, prolonged worry can diminish your quality of life as well as increase your risk of other mental and physical health problems such as high blood pressure, depression and cognitive decline.

Ultimately, being anxious changes nothing, so it's worth doing all that you can to break the cycle. The good news is that you can. Here are some calm-down strategies to help you stay on an even keel.

- **Get it out** Sharing your feelings with family and friends can help to put things in perspective. Support groups offer a chance for you to discuss your problems with others and develop coping strategies together.
- **List it** If your brain is cluttered with anxious thoughts, make a 'to-do' list, do one thing at a time, and tick it off as you go. This will help to reduce anxiety as well as keep you motivated.

DID **you** KNOW?

According to the 2010 Stress Survey conducted by the American Psychological Centre, older adults are generally less stressed than younger age groups and are most likely to say that they're managing their stress well. Health problems as well as money worries are cited as the biggest stressors for the over-65 age group, while job security and money problems are more worrying for the younger generation.

Making a note of what sparks your anxiety can help you identify the triggers.

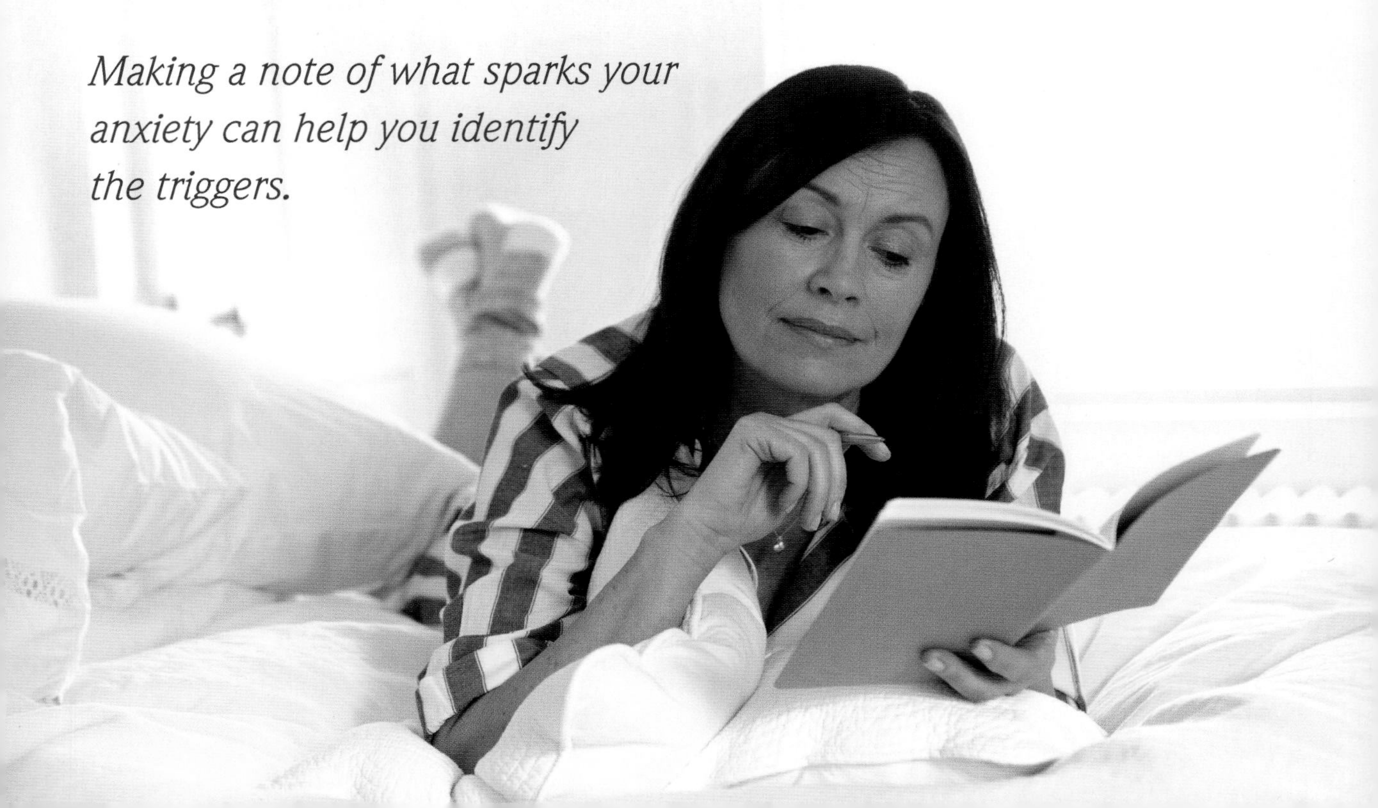

take CARE! When to seek **HELP** for **ANXIETY**

Generalised anxiety disorder (GAD) is the most common type of anxiety to affect us as we age. Symptoms include:

- Constant worrying or feeling nervous.
- Muscle tension or fatigue.
- Irritability or difficulty concentrating.
- Physical symptoms such as sweating, a racing heart, trembling, dizziness and feeling faint.

Impending retirement, a hospital stay, ill health or having to care for a loved one are common triggers. Another cause – easily confused with agoraphobia – is a fear of falling. This can make you avoid going out, which paradoxically increases your risk of falling as you then get less exercise.

If you have an anxiety problem, seek help as soon as you can. Left untreated it can exacerbate other problems such as migraine, arthritis and gastrointestinal upsets. Your doctor will be quite used to seeing patients with similar problems and can advise you on treatment. Depending on your specific symptoms, this could include medication and/or a talking treatment.

- **Be informed** Don't be afraid to ask questions about the problems you're experiencing, the treatments suggested, their side effects, any possible alternatives and how long it might be before you start to feel better.

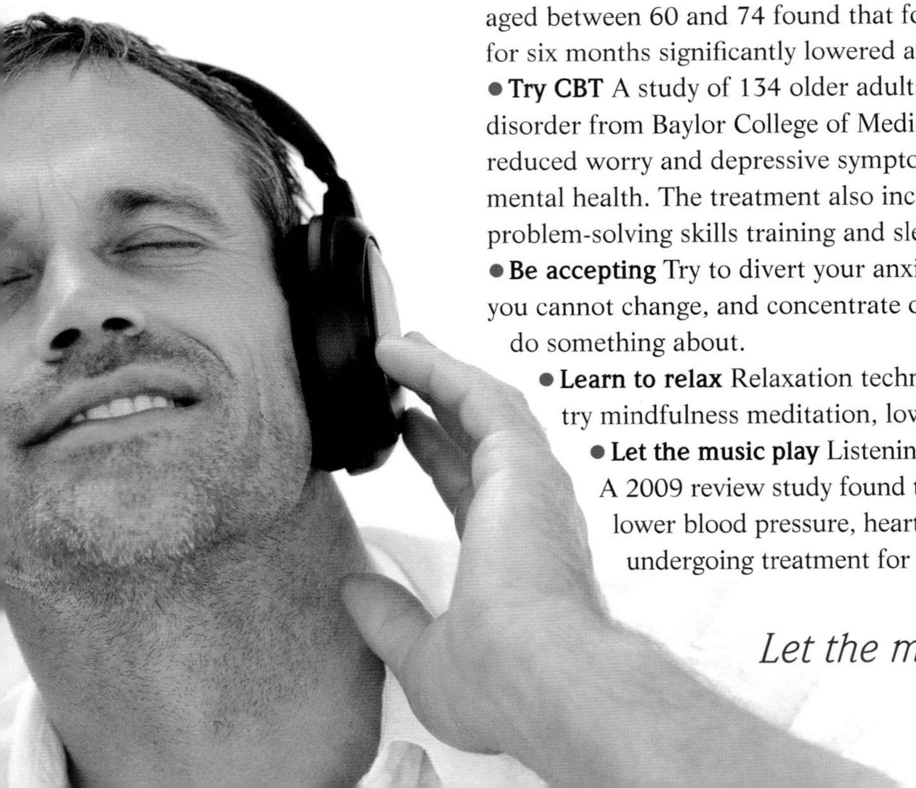

- **Get moving** It's hard to worry when you're doing something physical and you'll benefit from the release of calming endorphins, too. A study carried out at São Paulo University in Brazil of people aged between 60 and 74 found that following an aerobic program for six months significantly lowered anxiety and stress.
- **Try CBT** A study of 134 older adults with generalised anxiety disorder from Baylor College of Medicine, Houston, found that CBT reduced worry and depressive symptoms, while improving general mental health. The treatment also included relaxation training, problem-solving skills training and sleep management.
- **Be accepting** Try to divert your anxiety away from the things you cannot change, and concentrate on the things that you can do something about.
- **Learn to relax** Relaxation techniques can help with anxiety: try mindfulness meditation, low-impact yoga or tai chi.
- **Let the music play** Listening to music can help to calm you. A 2009 review study found that listening to music could lower blood pressure, heart rate and anxiety in patients undergoing treatment for coronary heart disease.

Let the music play.

FACING PROBLEMS
useful strategies

Some diseases, such as dementia and Parkinson's, become more common with age, although they are far from inevitable. Learning as much as you can about them will help you cope if you or a loved one are affected.

The latest Alzheimer's medications can benefit people at all stages of the disease.

It's normal to become more forgetful as you get older, but memory lapses are not necessarily a sign of dementia (*see* page 187 for the differences between forgetfulness and more serious problems). Memory overload, tiredness, illness or changes that occur in your brain as you age are common causes of forgetfulness.

But mild cognitive impairment (MCI) may also be to blame. This condition is more than just normal age-related forgetfulness, but less than full-blown dementia. According to a 2010 study carried out at Oxford University, one in six people over the age of 70 is thought to be affected, experiencing problems with memory, language or other mental functions, but not to a degree that interferes with daily life. Around half of those with mild cognitive impairment go on to develop dementia – mainly Alzheimer's disease – within five years of diagnosis. In others, dementia may set in if brain connections are lost through inflammation (*see* page 183), disease or injury, and the neurons start to die. It is true that the chances of developing dementia do increase with every birthday, but it is by no means inevitable. According to Alzheimer's Australia, less than one in 50 people between the ages of 65 and 70 has some form of dementia and this rises to about one in four after the age of 80.

ALZHEIMER'S DISEASE

There are many different types of dementia, with slightly different symptoms. The most common form is Alzheimer's disease. It develops when clumps of a starchy protein called beta-amyloid, known as 'plaques', form in the brain tissue. At the same time, 'tangles', made of another protein called tau, develop and wrap themselves around the synapses (the junctions between neurons).

take CARE! New HEADACHE SYMPTOMS

If you notice a new type of headache or an increase in frequency, see your doctor. Research from Canada's University of Toronto found headaches in older people can be a sign of underlying medical problems. They are an early symptom of temporal arteritis, for example, which often occurs in people over 55 and can lead to blindness if left untreated. If, on the other hand, you have suffered from migraines all your life, you'll be glad to know that they tend to get less severe – and happen less often – as you get older.

Other causes

Headaches may be a side effect of medication, and so can be relieved by changing the medication or dosage. They can also be caused by dentures that don't fit properly (which puts pressure on the teeth and gums). Tension headaches in later life may be linked to depression – especially if they occur for the first time after a major life change. So do talk to your doctor about your headaches rather than reaching for the pills.

Levels of certain nerve messenger chemicals also start to dwindle, in particular, acetylcholine, which is linked to memory and learning. Free radical damage and clogged and narrowed arteries in the brain are other contributing factors. Alzheimer's tends to creep up, so it may be some time before symptoms become obvious, but invisibly over time these plaques and tangles start to destroy more and more brain cells until eventually memory and other problems kick in.

DID **you** KNOW?

Scientists at Cape Western Reserve University in Ohio made an interesting discovery when they tested bexarotene, a cancer medication, on mice with an Alzheimer's-type disease. It reduced the number of plaques – the markers of Alzheimer's disease – at 'an unprecedented speed'. The mice's behaviour also indicated an improvement in brain function. Although the research is very new, there is some hope that it may provide a breakthrough that could be transferred to people.

Are you at risk?

The jury is still out over exactly what causes Alzheimer's, but genes and environmental and lifestyle factors all play a part. For instance, you are more likely to get Alzheimer's if you are older (the risk increases after 65), have a close relative with Alzheimer's or have inherited a certain genetic profile (in particular, the ApoE4 gene, found on chromosome 19). Other possible risk factors include prolonged high blood pressure, history of head trauma and obesity, but there's not such strong evidence for these. Gender also plays a part – women seem to be more at risk than men.

Seeing your doctor

If you suspect that you or a loved one may have dementia, it's vital to share your worries with your doctor as soon as you can, as early treatment may slow the disease's progression. It can help to make a note of symptoms beforehand, and to ask family members if they've noticed any changes in behaviour. Symptoms to look out for include:

- Confusion and forgetfulness.
- Mood swings.
- Difficulty recalling names of people or places.
- Frequently losing or misplacing things.
- Finding it hard to follow a conversation.

Getting a diagnosis

As yet, there's no definitive test for dementia. A skilled doctor may be able to assess whether you have the disease by asking about your family history, medical history and symptoms, examining you and carrying out checks on your thought processes and ability to perform daily tasks. You may also be tested to rule out conditions such as anaemia, chronic infection, severe depression, stroke, thyroid disease and/or vitamin deficiency. Further investigations such as an MRI scan or a more in-depth assessment of your memory, concentration and thinking skills may be needed. And researchers at the University of Edinburgh have developed new tests based on their earlier findings that people with Alzheimer's disease have a problem with doing two things at once (*see* page 203), which may help with better diagnosis in the future.

A diagnosis of Alzheimer's or any other type of dementia is bound to be shocking and may make you feel angry, confused, frightened and/or miserable. To help you to come to terms with it:

- **GO EASY ON YOURSELF** You're likely to experience many conflicting emotions. Give yourself time to adjust.

- **GET SUPPORT** You'll need all the help you can get from friends and family. Don't be afraid to reach out for support from groups and charities specialising in the condition (*see* Resources).

- **THINK AHEAD** This is the time to put your affairs in order – make a will (*see* Resources), get your finances sorted and think about your future healthcare needs and about who you trust to make

it's a **MYTH** ...

... that **ALUMINIUM** is a cause of Alzheimer's

Experts have been arguing for years over whether aluminium causes Alzheimer's. Why? Because some studies suggest that aluminium is associated with the plaques and tangles associated with the disease (*see* pages 199–200). According to Alzheimer's Australia, the balance of evidence suggests that aluminium doesn't play a specific role. A 2011 Japanese study of mice engineered to develop Alzheimer's is reassuring. It showed that even large amounts of aluminium over a long period did not accelerate progress of the disease.

what's NEW

DEEP BRAIN STIMULATION The surgical technique deep brain stimulation (*see* page 205) could one day reverse brain shrinkage caused by Alzheimer's, according to a 2011 study of just six patients from the University of Toronto in Canada. When DBS was applied to the fornix, an area of the brain involved in memory, two of the patients had significant increases in the size of the hippocampus after just 12 months. According to lead researcher Professor Andres Lozano, the hippocampus would normally have shrunk by around 5 per cent during this period. Not only that – these patients also experienced better than expected cognitive function.

decisions on your behalf when you're no longer able to do so. Think about setting up an advance directive or lasting power of attorney, so that someone else can handle your affairs.

Time for treatment

Although there is no cure for Alzheimer's, medications can improve symptoms and may slow progression in some people. There are two main types of medications: cholinesterase inhibitors, which work by preventing the breakdown of certain chemical messengers involved, and NMDA-receptor antagonists, which block substances released as Alzheimer's takes hold. Your doctor can also advise you and your family on useful lifestyle steps, such as increasing lighting and installing grab bars and handrails to make getting in and out of the bath easier.

VASCULAR DEMENTIA

There are other types of dementia besides Alzheimer's. The most common of these is vascular dementia, which is caused by furring and narrowing of the arteries in the brain. It is usually the result of a major stroke or a series of smaller strokes, which deplete oxygen flow to the brain. It is more of a risk in people who smoke, have high blood pressure, diabetes or high cholesterol.

The problems caused by vascular dementia depend on the part of the brain affected and the severity of the strokes. They can include memory loss, depression, poor concentration, confusion and mood swings. Some people have hallucinations and physical problems such as difficulty in walking and incontinence. Although there is no cure for vascular dementia, its progression can be slowed down by:

- Following a healthy lifestyle – exercise regularly and eat well.
- Taking medication for any underlying problems such as high blood pressure or diabetes.
- Getting a referral for physiotherapy, occupational therapy and speech therapy – ask your doctor about this.

BE **prepared** ... Living with **DEMENTIA**

Remaining independent is the goal of most people – and it is important that you maintain control of your life for as long as you are able. These tips will help:

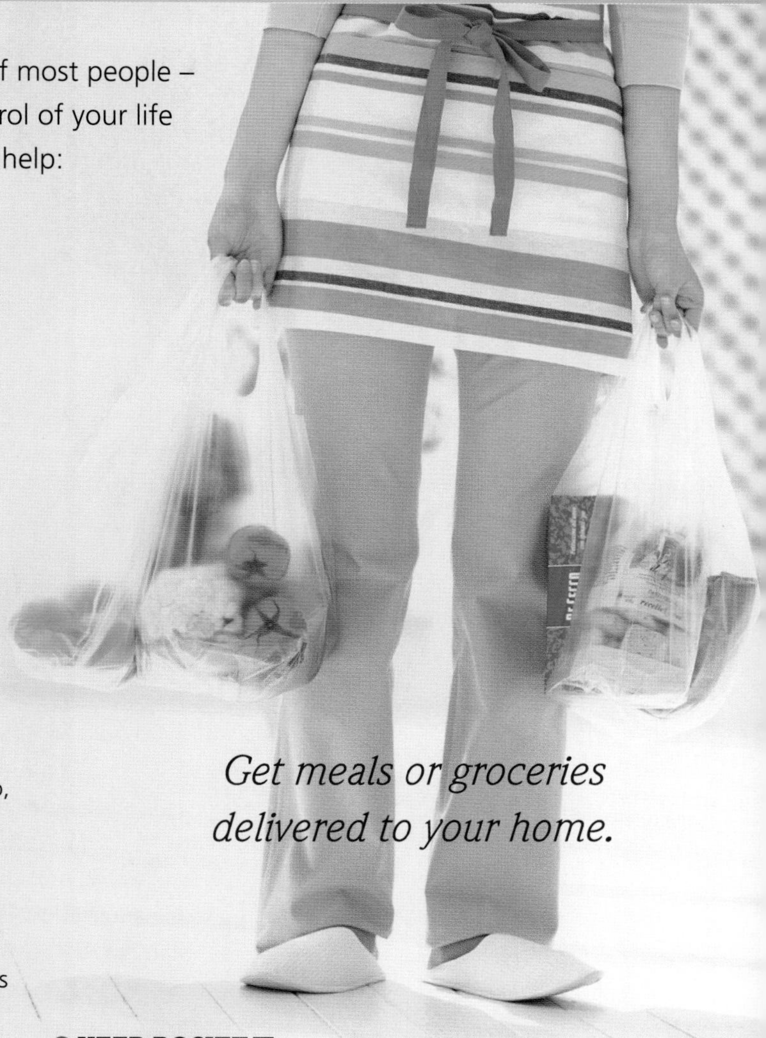

Get meals or groceries delivered to your home.

- **LOOK AFTER YOURSELF** Going for regular check-ups, taking prescribed medicines, eating well, exercising regularly, resting when tired and keeping an eye on your alcohol intake can improve your quality of life.
- **DEAL WITH CHANGE** Daily tasks may get harder. Try to do tricky tasks at the time of day you feel at your best, and allow yourself plenty of time. If something is hard, take a break or ask for help.
- **RESTRICT VISITORS** Group conversations may be hard to follow, according to researchers in Scotland. So ask friends and family to visit one or two at a time.
- **ONE THING AT A TIME** The same researchers have also shown that people with Alzheimer's find it hard to do two things at once. So, for example, don't try to walk and talk at the same time – stop walking or sit down if you want to talk.
- **HELP YOUR MEMORY** Keeping familiar pictures and objects around you can stimulate your memory. Label cupboards so you know where things are, and write notes to remind yourself to lock the door at night and when to put the rubbish out. Keep keys and glasses in a place you can remember.
- **ENJOY YOURSELF** Keep doing things that you enjoy such as listening to music, knitting, playing games, exercising or talking to a friend.
- **TAKE YOUR TIME** If it is hard to understand what someone is saying, ask the person to repeat what he or she has said or to write it down.
- **KEEP POSITIVE** Concentrate on what you can still do, rather than what you can't.
- **PAY BY DIRECT DEBIT** Ask your bank if they provide services to help pay bills and keep track of your accounts. Or set up direct debits for paying bills.
- **USE HOME DELIVERY** Get meals or groceries delivered to your home. Also consider stocking your freezer with microwave meals.

PARKINSON'S DISEASE

One in 100 people over 60 are thought to have Parkinson's disease. It develops when brain cells in part of the brain stem die, leading to low levels of dopamine. One of this brain chemical's many functions is to drive movement. Symptoms of Parkinson's vary but often include tremor (shaking) – which may start in the hand and spread up the arm then to the foot on the same side – as well as slowness of movement and rigidity. These can, in turn, cause difficulty walking, stiff muscles and poor balance. Some people also have problems with eating and swallowing, digestion and speech. It's quite common to develop anxiety and depression with Parkinson's, and some people have difficulties with memory or thinking.

Parkinson's symptoms can change from day to day, and the rate at which the disease progresses also varies from person to person. The symptoms usually appear slowly and develop gradually. Some people live with the disease for years with only mild symptoms, so don't assume the worst if a diagnosis confirms you have the disease.

Scientists don't know why people get Parkinson's, but there's evidence that it is due to a combination of genetic, environmental and lifestyle factors. You are more likely to develop Parkinson's if you're over the age of 55 or a man, or if you have a close relative who had it at a young age. People of African and Asian origin appear to have a lower risk than Caucasians.

Getting help

Parkinson's can be hard to diagnose because the symptoms may not be marked and there are no definitive tests. The first sign for some is difficulty manipulating a pen (and handwriting often gets smaller) because of the disease's effects on the fine motor skills.

Your doctor will take a medical history and carry out a neurological examination, which may include observing you as you sit, stand, walk and extend your arms, as well as checking your balance and coordination. You

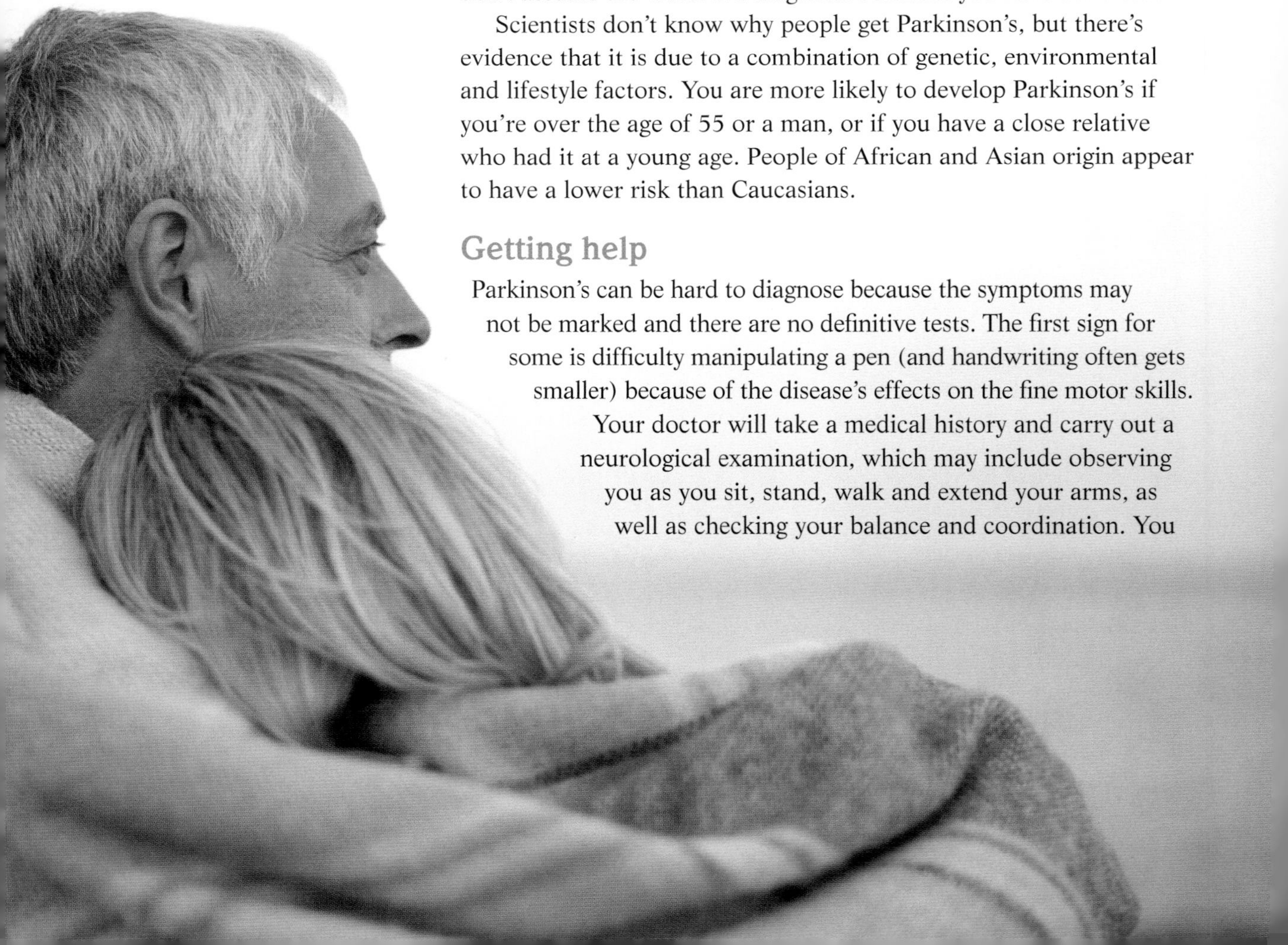

may be sent for tests, including a SPECT brain scan, which can detect dopamine deficiency, or an MRI scan to rule out other conditions.

Parkinson's is usually treated with medication, such as levodopa, which is converted to dopamine in the brain. Different medications are used, and you may need a combination. Many people find that a particular medicine is effective at first, but as time goes by it may become less so. You will see your doctor regularly to review medication, and should let him or her know about any side effects you experience – your medication may need to be changed or additional medications given to control the problem. Be sure to take your medication regularly, and at the same time of day (*see* pages 43–44 for tips to help you remember).

Surgical techniques can also help; the most common is deep brain stimulation (DBS), which can help to alleviate symptoms such as slowed movement and tremor. It involves placing a wire into the brain that is attached to a device similar to a pacemaker. The device is implanted into your chest wall and generates a small electrical current, which stimulates the affected part of your brain.

what's NEW

TAKE TIME TO TANGO A study carried out at Washington University School of Medicine in the USA showed that a group of people with Parkinson's disease had less severe symptoms after attending twice-weekly Argentine tango classes for 12 months. The control group – who didn't take the classes – showed no improvements. This led researchers to the exciting conclusion that taking part in tango classes in the long term may help slow the progression of the disease.

Living with Parkinson's

Here are some helpful tips to help you keep on top of your condition:

- **Move it** Research shows that people with Parkinson's who exercise regularly do better than those who are inactive. Walk as much as you can to help improve your balance, even if it means you have to hold on to something. Practise bending, stretching and breathing exercises to keep muscles flexible. It may be easier to do some exercises in bed (*see* pages 159–161, though check with your doctor first).
- **Watch your moods** Depression and anxiety are common in people with Parkinson's. Sharing problems with other people who are also affected can be a great help.
- **Stay safe** Ask your doctor to refer you to an occupational therapist, who can visit you at home to give you advice on how to manage everyday tasks – and to do a safety check.
- **Watch how you eat** Cut your food into smaller portions to aid digestion and stay upright for half an hour after eating. Good nutrition is essential – so ask your doctor to refer you to a dietitian.

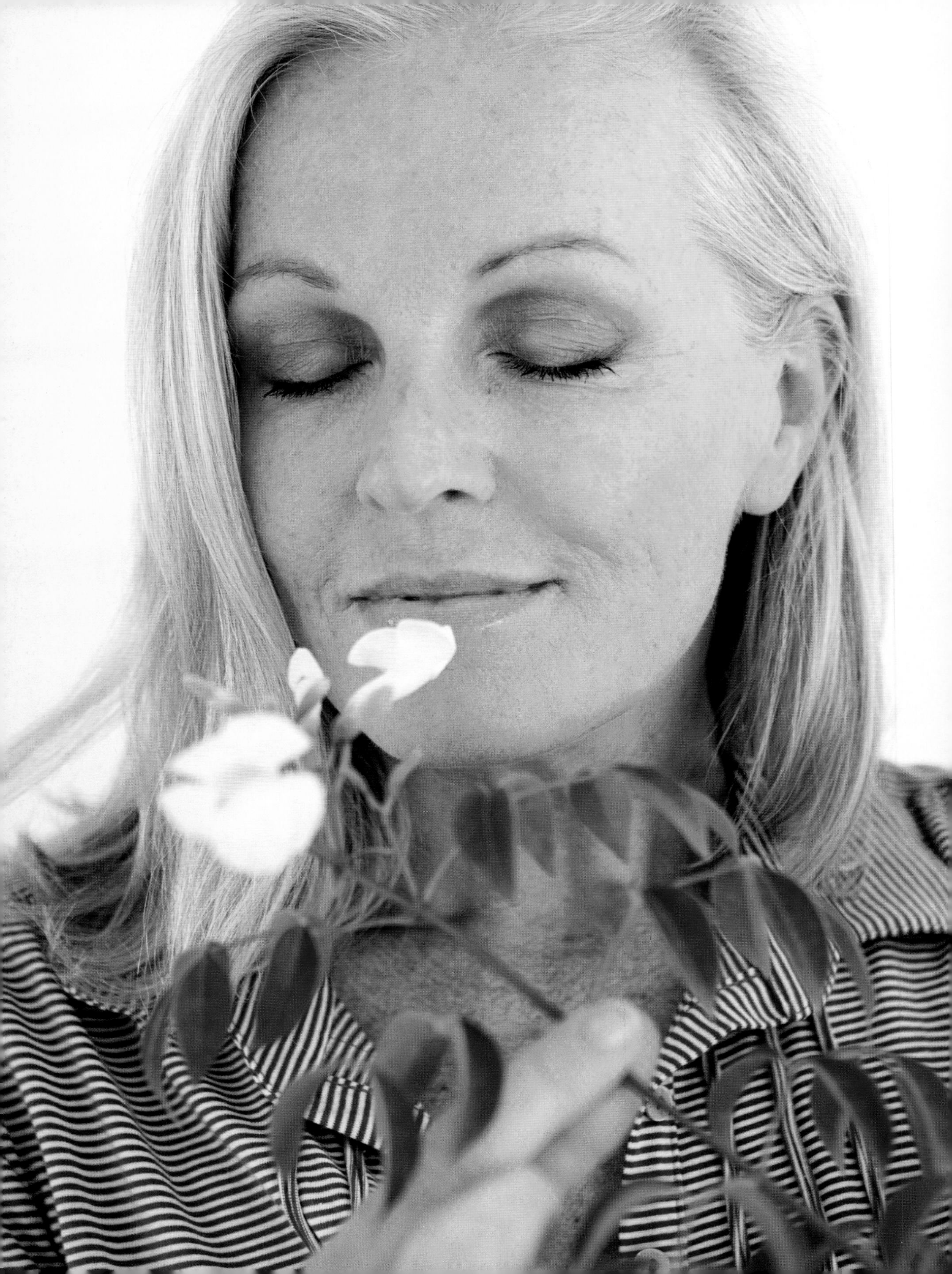

8

Super SENSES

Your five senses are the network that connects you with the world, and the conduit through which you receive many of its pleasures and benefits. All the senses tend to dull somewhat with age – few people, for example, get through life without needing glasses. But there are many ways of treating or correcting sensory problems, and there are many steps you can take to ensure that you never lose the enjoyment of a beautiful landscape, great music or fine food.

Daily exercise can cut your risk of cataracts by a third, according to US research.

YOUR EYESIGHT
seeing into the future

Eye problems tend to become more common with age, but recognising them is half the battle, because there are so many ways to compensate for visual changes.

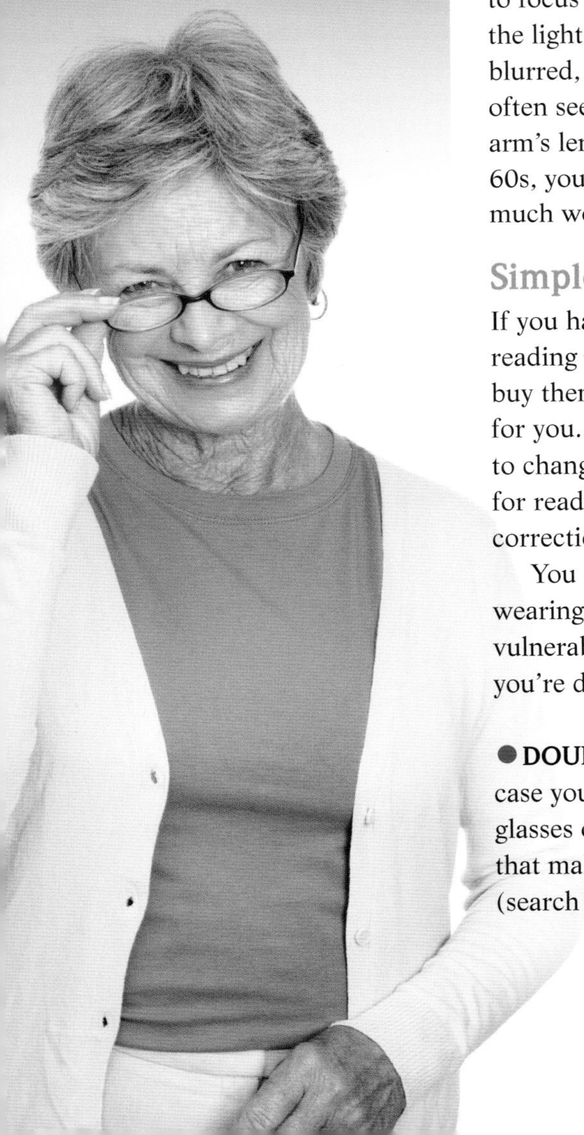

You almost certainly find it harder to focus close up than you did when you were young. This natural change to the eyesight – presbyopia – starts during the 40s. It occurs because the lens of your eye becomes less flexible, so it can't change shape as easily to focus on nearby objects and create a sharp image on the retina, the light-sensitive layer at the back of your eye. Near objects become blurred, making it more difficult to read fine print – this is why you often see people of a certain age holding a newspaper or menu at arm's length. The good news is that by the time you're in your mid-60s, your focus has usually stabilised and the problem doesn't get much worse.

Simple solutions

If you had normal vision before, presbyopia is easily corrected by reading glasses, which magnify text or other near objects. You can buy them over the counter, or your optometrist can prescribe them for you. If you were already short- or long-sighted, you may need to change your prescription, have an additional pair of glasses for reading, or consider bifocals or varifocals, which incorporate corrections for near and far vision into the same lens.

You can't damage your eyes by not wearing your glasses, or by wearing the wrong corrective lenses, but you do make yourself more vulnerable to headaches, and you'll be less efficient at whatever you're doing.

- **DOUBLE UP** Once you need glasses, always have a spare pair – in case you lose or break them. If you tend to mislay them, hang your glasses on a chain round your neck or attach them to a key finder that makes a sound when you whistle or clap in close proximity (search online for 'key locator' or 'key finder').

Quiz Check your **eye health**

The good thing about eye symptoms is that they're often obvious. So it's usually possible to catch problems early, when they can be treated and cured, or at least further deterioration can be prevented. Do the quiz to see if you need to take action.

Yes	No	DO YOU:
☐	☐	1 **Need glasses for reading or computer work?**
☐	☐	2 **Have a blurry or dim patch in the centre of your vision?**
☐	☐	3 **Find bright lights (such as headlights at night) dazzling?**
☐	☐	4 **Get tired or experience headaches or eyestrain after prolonged reading or computer work?**
☐	☐	5 **Eat oily fish once or twice a week?**
☐	☐	6 **Have diabetes?**
☐	☐	7 **Smoke?**
☐	☐	8 **Find it difficult to drive at night?**
☐	☐	9 **See floaters regularly?**
☐	☐	10 **Have a family history of glaucoma?**
☐	☐	11 **Have regular eye checks (at least every two years, or more often if recommended by your optometrist)?**
☐	☐	12 **Have high blood pressure?**

Yes	No	
☐	☐	13 **Have difficulty reading small print on labels, such as medicine bottles?**
☐	☐	14 **Eat seven or more portions of fruit and vegetables most days?**
☐	☐	15 **Find it takes longer for your eyes to adapt when you come indoors after being in bright sunlight?**
☐	☐	16 **Sometimes find that straight edges, such as door or window frames, appear wavy or distorted?**
☐	☐	17 **Know you have high cholesterol?**
☐	☐	18 **Have dry, itchy or irritated eyes?**
☐	☐	19 **Feel that colours are not as vivid as they once were?**
☐	☐	20 **Have red or inflamed eyes with no obvious cause?**
☐	☐	21 **Feel as if your visual field is narrowing or that you're looking down a tunnel?**
☐	☐	22 **Find your eyes are irritated by strong sunlight or wind?**

YOUR ANSWERS

Yes to Qs 1, 3, 8, 13, 15 or 19: You may have presbyopia, cataracts or other age-related eye changes. Be sure to see your optometrist regularly to have your eyes tested.

Yes to Qs 2, 16 or 21: These are potentially worrying symptoms. See your optometrist or doctor to make sure your vision is not compromised by serious eye disease.

Yes to Qs 4, 9, 18 or 22: These problems are usually not serious and have simple solutions that can ease symptoms.

Yes to Qs 5, 11 or 14: Well done. All of these help to protect your eyes from serious problems.

Yes to Qs 6, 7, 10, 12, 17 or 20: You may be at risk of eye disease. Have regular eye tests and report changes to an optometrist or doctor promptly.

what's NEW

EYE SURGERY One possible alternative to reading glasses in the near future is a lens implant, in which the natural lens is replaced with a synthetic one that gives the correct focus. This simple operation is similar to cataract surgery (*see* page 217), but side effects such as blurring and glare may occur. A very recent development is the corneal inlay: a tiny and virtually invisible device inserted on the cornea, the clear surface at the front of the eye. The surgery may have fewer risks since only the surface of the eye is affected. An inlay works much like a contact lens, by altering the way light rays enter the eye, but it is permanently implanted. Early trials have yielded promising results.

To avoid the need to keep switching between different corrective glasses, a new approach – monovision – corrects just one eye for close work, enabling the other to be used for distant vision, for example, when driving. Monovision may be achieved with a contact lens or with laser surgery in just one eye. Having the two eyes focusing at different distances is disorienting at first, but within a short time your brain learns which eye to favour in which situation.

Getting checked

Having regular eye tests is essential to keep your prescription up to date and to detect any other eye conditions as early as possible. Many eye diseases become more common in the over-60s. All can be readily detected during a routine eye examination, so it's important to have your eyes checked at least every two years, and more often if your optometrist recommends this or if you have conditions that can lead to eye problems, such as diabetes or high blood pressure.

● **DON'T MISS AN EYE TEST** The health of your eyes can tell your optometrist a lot about your overall health. High blood pressure, for instance, causes few symptoms, so the problem may be detected for the first time by a routine eye test. Your optometrist can also spot signs of other diseases in your eyes – including thyroid disorders, high cholesterol, liver disease and even brain tumours. In one US study, eye tests detected signs of chronic diseases before any other medical examinations – 65 per cent of the time for high cholesterol, 20 per cent for diabetes and 30 per cent for hypertension.

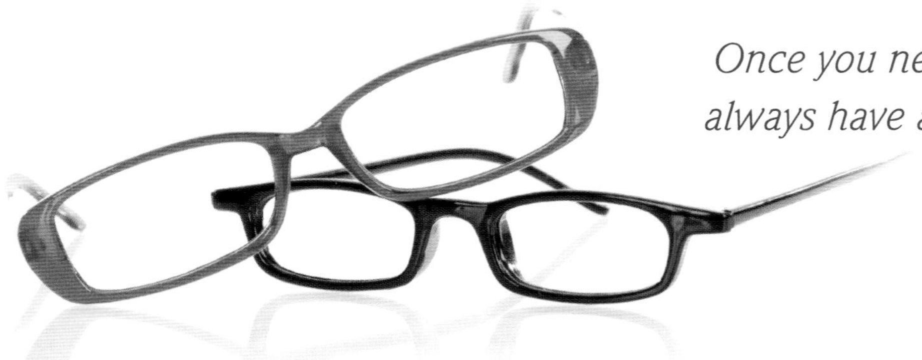

Once you need glasses, always have a spare pair.

take CARE! Spot the EMERGENCY SIGNS

If you develop any of these problems, seek help immediately, if necessary by going to the Emergency department of a hospital or calling an ambulance.

- Sudden loss of vision, or everything becoming suddenly dim or hazy.
- Abrupt loss of vision on one side.
- Vision loss like a curtain coming down in front of one eye.
- Intermittent visual loss in one or both eyes.
- Sudden distortion of your central vision (the middle part of your visual field).
- Eye symptoms accompanied by feeling generally unwell, especially if you also have a headache or tenderness in the temples.
- A sudden shower of floaters and/or flashing lights.
- Persistent severe pain in your eye.
- Sudden blurred or double vision.
- Swelling of the eye.
- Irregular pupils.

OTHER CHANGES

As well as becoming less flexible, your lenses become yellower and more opaque as you get older. Clouding of the lens may develop into a cataract (*see* page 217). At the same time, your pupils gradually shrink, so less light can get into your eye, and light tends to scatter more, increasing the effect of glare. What does this mean? Well, generally speaking, you need a lot more light to see clearly than you did when you were younger – and it needs to be uniform lighting rather than sharp pools of light contrasting with deep shadows, such as from a spotlight (this is fine for doing tasks but shouldn't be your only light source).

Changes to the eye also reduce your peripheral vision, perception of colour and depth, and your ability to tell where one surface ends and another begins (contrast discrimination). It's harder to see in dim light and to adapt to sudden changes in light levels. And if you are finding it harder to drive in the dark, you are not alone: night vision gets poorer with age. Here are some other changes to expect:

- **FLOATERS** become more common. These are specks, cobwebby strings or shadows that drift across your field of vision, especially when you're looking at a light, uniform background such as the sky.

DID **you** KNOW?

Smoking increases the likelihood of many eye-related diseases. It may treble your risk of macular degeneration – a painless condition that eventually leads to loss of vision in the centre of the visual field – according to scientists at the University of Manchester. Meanwhile, researchers at the University of California found that smoking doubles the risk of uveitis (eye inflammation). Quitting can halt or even reverse the damage.

Floaters are due to bits of debris from the gel inside your eyeball, and they move when you move your eyes. They can be annoying but are usually quite harmless. However, if you get a sudden shower of floaters accompanied by flashes of light, seek medical attention urgently (it may be a symptom of retinal detachment – *see* page 217).

DID **you** KNOW?

Tears of emotion are chemically different from those produced when you get a speck of dust in your eye or if you peel an onion. Experts think emotional tears help to rid the body of stress chemicals.

● **DRY EYES** become more common. The flow of tear fluid – the film across the front of the eye that keeps it moist – reduces; there is also less oil in the fluid, so the film breaks up more easily. Women usually suffer more than men as the condition is linked to fluctuating hormone levels. It may cause irritation and itching, but can be readily relieved by using lubricating eyedrops ('artificial tears') or ointments.

● **INCREASED TEAR FLOW,** the opposite problem to dry eyes, can also be an issue, and your eyes may be more sensitive to wind, light or sudden temperature changes. Increased eye watering can signal a problem that needs treatment, such as conjunctivitis or a blocked tear duct, so get your eyes checked if it persists.

● **IRRITATION OF THE EYELIDS** Your eyelids may become extra sensitive and more prone to crusting, redness and inflammation (blepharitis). This is due to blockages in the tiny glands in your eyelid that help the tear film to spread across your eye, and can make your eyes feel sore and gritty. Sometimes a stye – a red, swollen pimple – appears at the lid margins. Strong sunlight or a smoky atmosphere may also increase irritation. Gently cleaning your lids with cotton wool soaked in warm water usually helps, and eye lubricants can ease irritation. In severe cases, or if the irritation doesn't get better within two weeks, seek medical advice. You may need an antibiotic cream.

AMD – AND HOW TO TACKLE IT

Age-related macular degeneration (AMD) is a leading cause of sight problems as you get older. The Macular Degeneration Foundation estimates that one in seven people over 50 is affected.

AMD occurs when the macula, the central area of your retina responsible for detailed vision, is damaged, causing blurring in the centre of your visual field and eventually a central blind spot. There are two forms. In dry AMD, yellow deposits called drusen build up

6 simple ways to go **EASY ON YOUR EYES**

Human eyes aren't designed for prolonged close work. Reading, normal computer use or eye-intensive hobbies such as needlework or model-making won't permanently harm your eyes, but they may cause tiredness, headaches and temporary blurred vision. Fortunately, there are many simple measures you can take to avoid eyestrain when doing close work.

1 SIT RIGHT Make sure your computer screen is set at the right angle – below eye level and slightly tilted backwards – and sit the correct distance away, with your eyes at least 60 cm from the screen.

2 DON'T SQUINT Always wear the right prescription glasses or lenses if you need them. If you're still straining to see your computer screen, increase the font size rather than squinting or leaning forward.

3 BLINK A LOT Intense focusing on a printed page or especially a computer screen tends to reduce your blink rate. As blinking keeps the front of your eyes moist, a fixed gaze makes your eyes more prone to irritation. You may have to concentrate on deliberately blinking more, ideally every 4 or 5 seconds.

4 REST YOUR EYES Try not to do close work when you're already tired.

5 GLANCE UP REGULARLY Do it for just a second or so every few minutes – preferably look into the far distance – and take a complete break for a few minutes every half to three-quarters of an hour: make a cup of tea, do some brief exercise, go for a quick stroll in the garden.

6 BRIGHTEN UP Ensure you have good lighting at your working area, positioned above or to your side, not directly in front or behind it.

in the retina and blood vessels become brittle, damaging the macula. In wet AMD, new blood vessels grow and leak beneath the macula, causing scar tissue. Wet AMD – which accounts for about 10 per cent of cases – is more serious and progresses more quickly.

Once vision is lost in AMD, it cannot be regained, but as it affects only the central vision it never causes complete sight loss. People with AMD may have difficulty reading, driving or recognising faces, but can carry on with many day-to-day activities.

You're more likely to get AMD if you smoke, are long-sighted or have a family history of it, but there's much that you can do to reduce your risk:

- If you smoke, stop.
- Wear sunglasses that block ultraviolet A and B rays in strong light. Or have photochromic lenses fitted to your ordinary glasses, which darken in sunlight (check they have UVA and UVB protection).
- Keep your BMI within the healthy range (*see* page 96).
- Eat less saturated fat.
- Have an eye-healthy diet: eat plenty of fruit and vegetables (for anti-oxidant vitamins) and oily fish (for omega-3 fatty acids).
- Exercise. Vigorous exercise cut the risk of AMD by up to 54 per cent in a US study of 1313 women aged 55 to 74; also eating healthily and not smoking reduced the risk by 71 per cent.

Act quickly

If you spot the symptoms of AMD early, prompt action – mainly through dietary changes and stopping smoking – can help to slow any loss of vision. These are the most common signs:

- Straight lines appear wavy.
- Your central vision is blurred, causing difficulty reading fine print. The affected area slowly expands; a central dark spot may appear.
- Colours may seem faded and increased light is needed to see.

● **TALK SUPPLEMENTS** Ask your ophthalmologist about the Age-Related Eye Disease Study (AREDS) at the US National Eye Institute in Maryland. It found that a combination of vitamin and mineral supplements led to a 25 per cent reduction over six years in the risk of dry AMD progressing to an advanced stage. Some ophthalmologists may now recommend supplements to match the AREDS formula. The components are – vitamin C: 500 mg; beta-carotene: 15 mg; zinc: 80 mg; copper: 2 mg (added to prevent

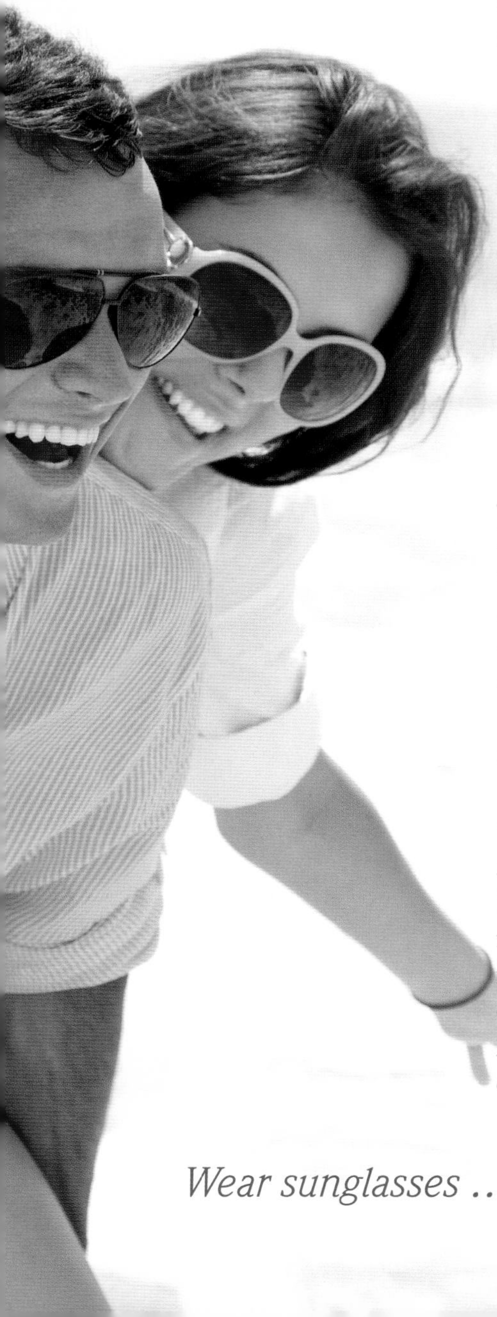

Wear sunglasses ...

6 TOP FOODS for an EYE-FRIENDLY diet

The macula, or 'yellow spot', contains exceptionally high levels of two anti-oxidant plant pigments, lutein and zeaxanthin (lutein is also found in the lens and other tissues of the eye). Both lutein and zeaxanthin are found in dark green and orange-yellow fruit and vegetables. These foods seems to protect against AMD and cataracts.

1 KALE This dark green leafy vegetable has exceptionally high concentrations of lutein and zeaxanthin, which reduce the risk of AMD.

2 WINE Among 3072 people aged 45 to 74 participating in a major US study of diet and health, 9 per cent of non-drinkers developed AMD compared with only 4 per cent of wine drinkers. Researchers found that wine was associated with a one-fifth lower risk of AMD after other risk factors were taken into account. It may be because red wine contains anti-oxidant chemicals called polyphenols.

3 LOW-GI FOODS In a subset of 4003 participants in the Age-Related Eye Disease Study (AREDS) at Tufts University in Boston, low-GI (glycaemic index) diets, and diets with higher lutein, zeaxanthin, omega-3s, zinc and vitamins C and E reduced the risk of AMD.

4 ORANGES Make citrus fruits an essential part of your diet. In a study of 677 people by the London School of Hygiene and Tropical Medicine, higher blood levels of vitamin C were associated with a 64 per cent reduced risk of cataracts. And a University of Eastern Finland study found that people with the highest blood levels of lutein and zeaxanthin (both found in oranges) were over 40 per cent less likely to have a cataract than those with the lowest levels.

5 OILY FISH Omega-3 fatty acids in oily fish protect against eye disease even among people already at risk. In a group of 1837 people in the AREDS study (*see* opposite) at moderate-to-high risk of AMD, those with the highest omega-3 intake were over 30 per cent less likely to develop AMD over the next 12 years.

6 GREEN TEA Rich in anti-oxidants, green tea reduces lens clouding in animal experiments and may help to protect against cataracts.

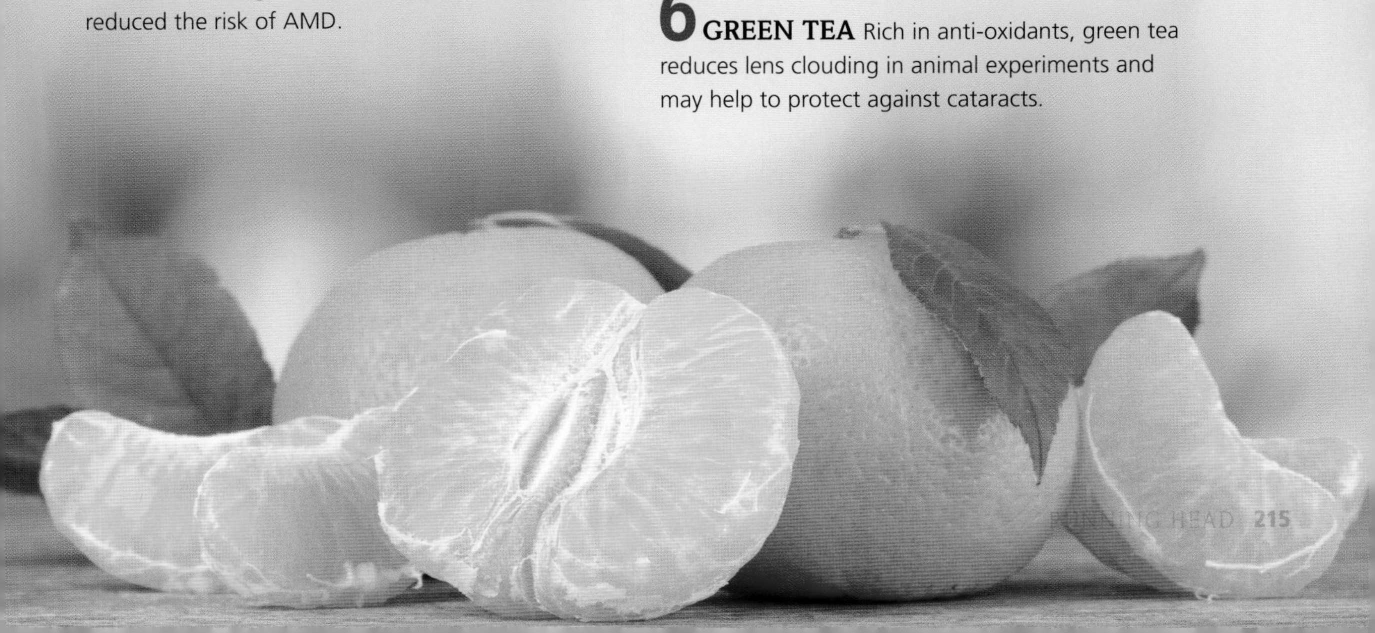

what's **NEW**

ECCENTRIC VIEWING FOR AMD

Losing your central vision due to macular damage forces you to use your peripheral vision. Eccentric vision is a technique that teaches you to use this residual vision more effectively to make everyday activities easier, including walking, reading, recognising faces and watching television. It is often combined with another technique called 'steady eye' for reading, in which you learn to keep your head and eyes still but move the page through the areas where your sight is clearest.

deficiency caused by zinc); and vitamin E: 400 IU. They should be taken only under medical supervision (vitamin E and zinc may have side effects), and should not be taken if you smoke (beta-carotene as a supplement is associated with an increased risk of lung cancer in smokers).

Treatment of wet AMD may involve medications such as ranibizumab to prevent new vessels forming or photodynamic therapy, in which a light-activated medication is injected to destroy the vessels.

OTHER SIGHT RISKS

Your risk of serious eye conditions increases as you age. But the damage is often limited by early treatment – always seek medical attention for eye symptoms (*see also* page 211).

● **GLAUCOMA** Once you reach 40 (or earlier if you're African or of African descent), your risk of glaucoma, a potentially sight-robbing condition, rises. High pressure in the eye is an important risk factor – this is what is treated because lowering eye pressure enough will help preserve the vision the patient has left. Glaucoma can run in families and causes few or no symptoms early on, but it's readily detected during an eye test. Otherwise, you may be unaware of a problem until you start to lose your side vision. Your central vision is affected only in the advanced stages.

● **RETINOPATHY** This refers to damage to the retina. In people with diabetes, high blood-glucose levels affect blood vessels in the retina, which become swollen and leaky, leading to diabetic retinopathy. Sometimes new, fragile blood vessels proliferate. Eventually this causes patchy vision loss, blurring, dark spots or shadows and sometimes pain, but symptoms may not be noticeable at first. The retinal changes can be seen during an eye examination, and laser treatment can often stop any damage or slow its progress. If you have diabetes, you're also at increased risk of cataracts and glaucoma, so it's especially important to have regular eye tests.

BE prepared ... CATARACTS and modern surgery

By the age of 80 around half of us will develop a cataract – a cloudy patch in the lens of the eye. This is the leading cause of impaired vision throughout the world, but a surgical procedure can cure the problem in 95 per cent of cases.

With age, protein deposits may build up in the lens of the eye, causing blurred, hazy or cloudy vision, muted or yellowed colouring, glare and difficulty seeing in low light. This clouding of the lens is a cataract, and it may affect one or both eyes.

Women and people with light-coloured eyes or a family history of cataracts are more at risk, as are those with diabetes or high blood pressure. Exposure to sunlight or radiation, eye injury or surgery, excess alcohol, steroid use and obesity are also risk factors; smoking can increase your chances of cataracts by 48 per cent, according to a study in Singapore.

At first a change of prescription in glasses or contact lenses may help. But cataracts usually worsen over time, so surgery is generally needed.

What's involved

Modern treatment is speedy and safe, with an operation usually carried out under local anaesthetic to replace the cloudy lens with a clear artificial one. One eye is usually done at a time and vision improves almost immediately, though it may be blurry at first. If you also have refractive errors, such as short-sightedness, replacement lenses can correct this.

Managing your diabetes well and keeping blood-glucose levels stable help to prevent diabetic retinopathy. Hypertensive retinopathy is a similar form of retinal damage that occurs in people with high blood pressure. Changes can be detected during an eye test. Later on, double or dimmed vision, headaches and sometimes vision loss can occur. The retina may recover when blood pressure is controlled.

● **RETINAL DETACHMENT** This is more common with age, especially in people who are short-sighted, have a family history of the condition, or have had an eye injury or cataract surgery. It happens when the retina peels away from the layer of supporting cells at the back of the eye. A common warning signal is a sudden intense burst of floaters and/or flashing lights. As detachment occurs, the effect is of a curtain dropping over the field of vision. This is a medical emergency, and if you suspect it, seek help straight away: surgery or laser treatment can prevent sight loss in over 90 per cent of cases.

Get a hearing aid if you need one. A US study found that four out of five people don't bother.

YOUR HEARING
how to safeguard it

From your 50s and 60s onwards, you are likely to suffer a degree of hearing loss. It may be more difficult to hear conversations at a party, or in a busy restaurant. But becoming deaf is far from inevitable – especially if you safeguard your ears throughout your life. Diet, too, has a role to play.

Children generally have much better and more acute hearing than adults. They can hear higher frequencies, which is why sonic deterrents – devices that emit shrill ultrasonic tones that older people usually can't detect – have been successful in dispelling gangs of loitering teenagers. But in our noisy society, young people are starting to suffer the effects of cumulative exposure to loud noise, resulting in noise-induced hearing loss (NIHL). Excessive noise can damage the tiny sensory cells (also known as hair cells) in your inner ear, which detect and convert sound to nerve impulses.

Hearing loss may also be described as conductive (when something, often earwax, blocks the transmission of sound waves to the inner ear), sensorineural (damage to the hair cells or to the auditory nerve), congenital (present from birth) or central (a rare condition caused by damage to the auditory pathways or centres in the brain).

Age-related hearing loss

With age, your eardrum thickens and the tiny bones of your middle ear (the ossicles), which convey sound vibrations to the inner ear, stiffen. Inner ear damage, together with slowed nerve and brain function, may further reduce your hearing capacity. Age-related hearing loss – called presbycusis – occurs naturally as part of the ageing process. It affects a third of people over 65 and up to half of those over 75.

There are other factors that contribute to hearing loss, such as noise exposure, genetic factors, disease and individual susceptibility. Cardiovascular disease, diabetes and hypertension – all common over the age of 60 – can worsen hearing loss, and it can also

6 ways to be **KIND TO EARS**

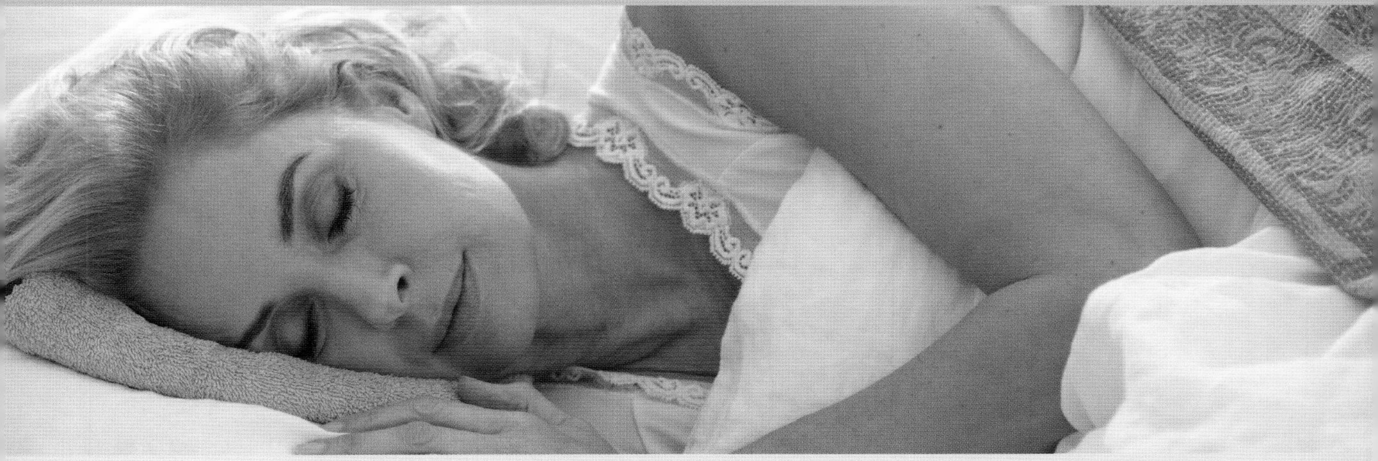

1 TACKLE EARWAX You produce more earwax as you get older – and too much can muffle sounds (a common cause of hearing loss). Ears are self-cleaning as long as the wax doesn't harden. So put a drop or two of olive oil in your ear overnight to soften the wax (protect your pillow with a towel).

2 TREAT SNORING If you or your partner snores, take action to resolve the problem (*see* pages 249–250). Meanwhile, wear earplugs to bed. At close range, snoring can reach levels of 90 dB – louder than a road drill. In one small study at Queen's University in Ontario, Canada, all four bed partners of chronic snorers had noise-induced hearing loss in one ear – the one nearest the snorer.

3 CUT DOWN ON SATURATED FAT It raises cholesterol levels (*see* page 86), which can worsen atherosclerosis and accelerate hearing loss due to reduced blood flow to the inner ear. When doctors at the Hospital El Bierzo in León, Spain, tested 180 people aged over 65 with hearing impairment, they found that those with high cholesterol had significantly worse hearing loss.

4 GET ENOUGH EXERCISE Scientists at Miami University in Ohio, USA, have shown that two months of aerobic exercise training in relatively unfit volunteers increased hearing sensitivity as well as cardiovascular fitness. Don't exercise while listening to loud music – apart from the noise level itself, Swedish scientists have shown that combining loud music with exercise may increase hearing damage.

5 EAT A HEALTHY, BALANCED DIET A study of 2111 people aged 49 to 99 at Vanderbilt University in Tennessee showed that those whose diets included more foods providing vitamin C, vitamin E, riboflavin (a B vitamin), magnesium and lycopene (a plant chemical found in high concentration in tomatoes) had better hearing.

6 EAT OILY FISH A study at the University of Sydney of 2956 participants aged 50-plus showed that the higher the dietary intake of omega-3 fatty acids, found in oily fish and some plant foods, the lower the risk of developing age-related hearing loss; higher omega-3 consumption reduced the risk of established hearing loss becoming worse, too.

be associated with stroke and various neurological conditions. Atherosclerosis both contributes to hearing loss and exacerbates noise damage. But forewarned is forearmed, because it is possible to fight back, both against the diseases that can rob you of your hearing and against noise pollution.

Noise reduction

In the 1960s, ear specialist Dr Samuel Rosen conducted hearing tests on the Mabaan people, whom he described as living in Stone Age conditions in a remote area of Sudan. Even those in their 70s had excellent hearing, comparable with that of 20- to 30-year-olds in Western civilisations. How come? The answer is that these people quite literally lived a quiet life – other than transient animal noises, few environmental sounds were intense enough even to register on a sound meter.

Follow-up studies showed that when Mabaan people moved to urban areas, hearing loss became more common, along with high blood pressure and cardiovascular disease.

Here are three simple ways to reduce unnecessary noise:

- **Turn it down** Keep the volume low on your radio, television and sound system (in the car and at home).
- **Get earplugs** Wear them when you can't avoid loud noise: using power tools, mowing the lawn, at the cinema, riding a motorbike.
- **Stand back** At any event with amplified sound, position yourself as far away from the speakers as possible.

'We have two ears and one mouth in order that we may hear more and speak less.'

Diogenes, Greek philosopher

HOW SHARP IS YOUR HEARING?

While it's easy to shut your eyes and imagine how it feels to lose your sight, it's much harder to envisage hearing loss. It tends to creep up on you, isn't readily noticeable and often causes no other symptoms, so people with early hearing loss are often the last to know about it. What's more, it can be hard to admit that there's anything wrong – hearing loss is one of those things that makes you feel old. Yet experts stress that hearing loss itself is much more noticeable to others than a modern hearing aid.

- Early hearing loss typically begins with difficulty in hearing high-frequency (pitch) sounds – women's voices, telephones ringing, birdsong.

take CARE! MEDICATIONS and HEARING

Numerous medications can damage your inner ear – a phenomenon known as ototoxicity – causing hearing impairment, tinnitus or balance problems. Difficulties may begin after just one dose, or may appear after weeks or even months, and may be temporary or permanent.

The main culprits include aspirin, quinine and certain antibiotics, as well as diuretics and chemotherapy medications. Aspirin ototoxicity is particularly common, occurring in up to one in 100 people, and older people are more at risk. It most often causes tinnitus, sometimes with mild hearing loss. Fortunately, recovery usually occurs within three days of you stopping taking it.

● **SEEK HELP** If you notice any new ear symptoms, speak to your doctor about whether your medications could be responsible.

- Soft consonants – f, g, s, t and z – may be harder to hear or to distinguish in words that sound alike, such as 'sat' and 'fat'.
- It's harder to follow conversations against background noise or to understand rapid speech, unfamiliar words or complicated language.
- It's more difficult to pinpoint where a sound is coming from.

Don't ignore it

If you've noticed that your hearing has deteriorated, or if others have commented on it, ask your doctor for an assessment. Hearing loss can affect many aspects of daily life – you may be missing important conversations, for example. Continually straining to hear is also draining, and hinders your communication with loved ones. It may lead you to withdraw from social situations, causing isolation and possibly leading to depression. Hearing loss may even promote cognitive decline, since social interactions protect against it.

In one study at Johns Hopkins University in Baltimore, older people with hearing loss were more likely to develop dementia, and the risk rose with increasing severity of hearing loss. The same researchers found that only a fifth of people with poor hearing used hearing aids. And scientists at the University of Pennsylvania have shown that reduced hearing in older adults accelerates loss of brain density in areas linked to speech processing. 'Preserving your hearing doesn't only protect your ears, but also helps your brain perform at its best,' comments lead researcher Dr Jonathan Peelle.

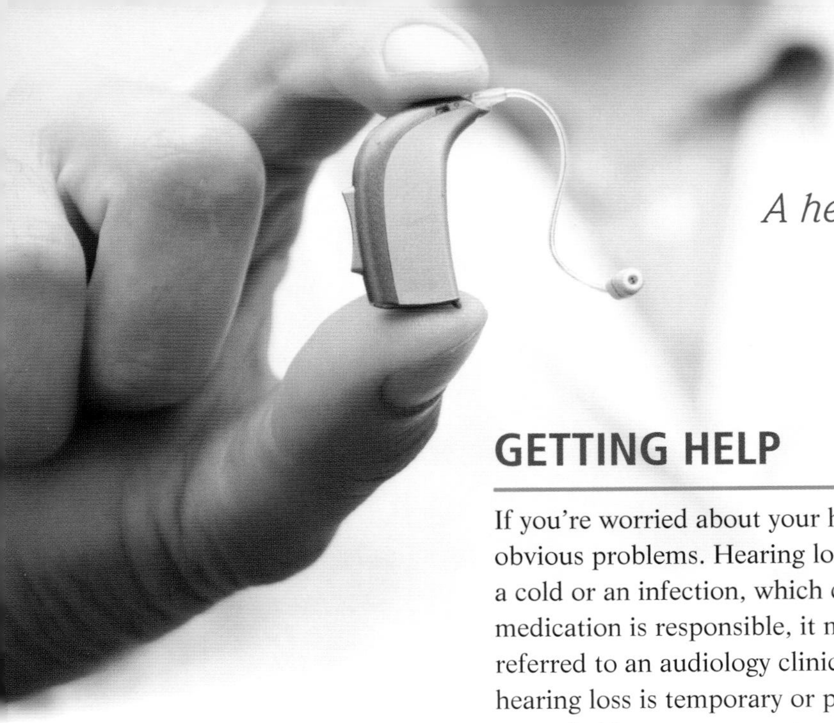

A hearing aid should improve hearing loss by about 50 per cent.

GETTING HELP

If you're worried about your hearing, ask your doctor to check for obvious problems. Hearing loss may be due to a build-up of earwax, a cold or an infection, which can all be treated, or if a particular medication is responsible, it may be changed. Otherwise, you'll be referred to an audiology clinic for tests and to assess whether your hearing loss is temporary or permanent. You'll be advised about any suitable treatment and may be referred to an ENT specialist to investigate the underlying cause.

Your hearing specialist may suggest that you would benefit from a hearing aid. There are different types, but in most cases a modern (digital) hearing aid would be recommended. In severe cases, a cochlear implant or a hearing dog may help. Your specialist can also provide information on devices to help around the house, such as telephone amplifiers or a loop system. This is a wire loop installed permanently or temporarily around an area to amplify sound for anyone within the loop wearing a hearing aid with a telecoil (a t-switch or t-coil). The following can also help:

- Position yourself in front of people when chatting and ensure that you have good home lighting to help you see faces – most people with hearing problems speech read (lip read) to some extent.
- Move closer. A voice on the other side of a typical living room can be up to 150 times quieter than one by your ear.
- Minimise background noise when talking – turn off radios and TVs.

Using a hearing aid

Hearing aids have come a long way. Modern (digital) hearing aids can be specifically programmed to your hearing loss. For example, in most age-related hearing loss, it is higher frequencies that people struggle to hear, which affects the clarity of speech. A digital hearing aid can be programmed to give more high-frequency sound, thus improving speech clarity. Feedback (whistling) from the hearing aid

focus ON ... TINNITUS

Noises in the ears with no external source – tinnitus – affect about one in five people, and become increasingly common after the age of 60.

The sounds of tinnitus – ringing, whistling, buzzing, clicking or hissing – are usually intermittent, mild and noticed mainly in quiet conditions, such as in bed. Occasionally tinnitus is constant, and may be severe enough to disrupt sleep and concentration.

Tinnitus can occur on its own, following exposure to loud noise, or it may accompany hearing loss, the inner ear disorder Ménière's disease, ear infection, earwax or circulatory disorders. It may be a side effect of medications, particularly aspirin (*see* page 221). Your doctor can check for an underlying cause.

If tinnitus bothers you, it may be improved by:

- Reducing stress.
- Avoiding alcohol and caffeine.
- Following a low-salt diet.
- Using external sound – music, or 'white noise' devices – to mask the noise. This can aid sleep.
- A hearing aid (in tinnitus with hearing loss).

Your doctor may also give you antidepressant or anti-anxiety medications. In severe cases, you may be offered tinnitus re-training: this involves having programmed sound to mask individual tinnitus frequencies, and counselling to help you switch focus.

is more controllable. The aids are often fully automatic and adjust themselves according to the situation you are in, which can help with background noise. As well as more effective versions of traditional behind-the-ear devices, hearing aids can now sit completely inside your ear canal, virtually invisible from the outside. (You can now also buy 'Hearrings', cleverly designed pieces of jewellery that attach to specially developed ear moulds of behind-the-ear hearing aids.) Wireless technology even enables aids to pick up signals directly from TVs, mobile phones and MP3 players, providing consistency and clarity of sound, so you can enjoy your favourite music again, talk to your grandchildren on the phone, and watch television at a volume to suit everyone.

- **BE REALISTIC** Hearing aids won't give you perfect hearing, but should help you hear everyday sounds. Allow yourself time to adapt – it can take up to three months for your brain to relearn how to process altered sound. Always have spare batteries, especially if you go into hospital, so that you don't have problems communicating with staff.

With age you become less sensitive to itching and pain – which can be a mixed blessing.

FEELING GOOD
touch and sensitivity

It's not just the more obvious senses of vision and hearing that change with age; your whole range of sensations – from touch to your sensation of heat and cold – alters, too. Awareness is key to helping you overcome any problems.

With age comes a natural reduction in your sensitivity to touch, pressure and temperature – in other words, you need more input before you feel the sensation. What this means in practical terms is that you'll now benefit from paying extra attention to touch. Take time to notice and enjoy the sensation of touching and interacting with the world around you. The more you do so, the more you will appreciate what makes you feel good.

The impact

Changes in these hidden senses can have a knock-on effect:

- Reduced temperature sensitivity may make you more at risk of hypothermia (dangerously low body temperature) or cold injuries such as frostbite, especially if your circulation is reduced by atherosclerosis or your nerves are affected by diabetes.
- Becoming less aware of body position and poorer balance mean you are more at risk of falls.
- Lower pain sensitivity puts you at increased risk of injury or burns, and this becomes more likely if you have experienced other age-related problems such as stroke, or if you suffer from arthritis.
- Being less able to sense touch, pressure and pain increases your risk of pressure sores if you're immobilised.

Even if your ability to sense pain is unimpaired as you get older, both your reflexes and reaction time may well slow with age – meaning you may be less quick to withdraw from painful stimuli and more likely to suffer injuries such as burns. You may also be less able to sense or react to danger, so it's important to make use of all the senses you have, for example, listen as well as look while crossing the road.

7 steps to STIMULATING SENSATION

Lowered touch sensation can mean you miss out on sensual pleasures, physical communication and intimacy. Touch can release endorphins, the body's pleasure chemicals, and is good for your overall wellbeing. It lowers anxiety, improves mood, relieves pain, boosts healing and even calms erratic heartbeats. Using your senses helps to maintain them – here are some enjoyable ways to keep on touching.

1 BE KIND TO YOUR SKIN Older skin is more frail and has less protective oil, so use a soap-free wash and moisturise well, all over.

2 STIMULATE YOUR SKIN This helps to retain touch sensitivity. The most sensitive areas, with more nerve endings than elsewhere else, are your face (especially your lips), hands (especially your fingertips), feet and neck.

3 ENJOY A HEALING MASSAGE It's been shown to relieve stress, anxiety and depression and helps with pain, stiffness and blood pressure control. Older people who have massages have better emotional wellbeing and fewer limitations due to physical or emotional issues than those who don't, according to a study of 144 people aged 60 or over at the University of Kentucky.

4 INCREASE CONTACT If you have a partner, look at ways to boost sexuality and improve your sex life (*see* pages 282–285). According to a 30-year study at Gothenburg University in Sweden, men and women reaching their 70s today have more sex than previous generations and report higher satisfaction with their sexuality than those 30 years ago.

5 SHARE THE LOVE Compensate for reduced sensations by encouraging more cuddling.

6 GET A FURRY FRIEND If you live alone, think about getting a pet to cuddle so that you have some daily physical contact.

7 CHALLENGE YOUR BRAIN Exercises that stimulate your sensory inputs, called neurobics (brain aerobics), can activate underused sense pathways, boosting both sensation and brain connections. The idea is to switch routines, use different senses or combine sensations – for example, use your opposite hand to brush your teeth, get dressed with your eyes closed or listen to music while stroking something soft and silky.

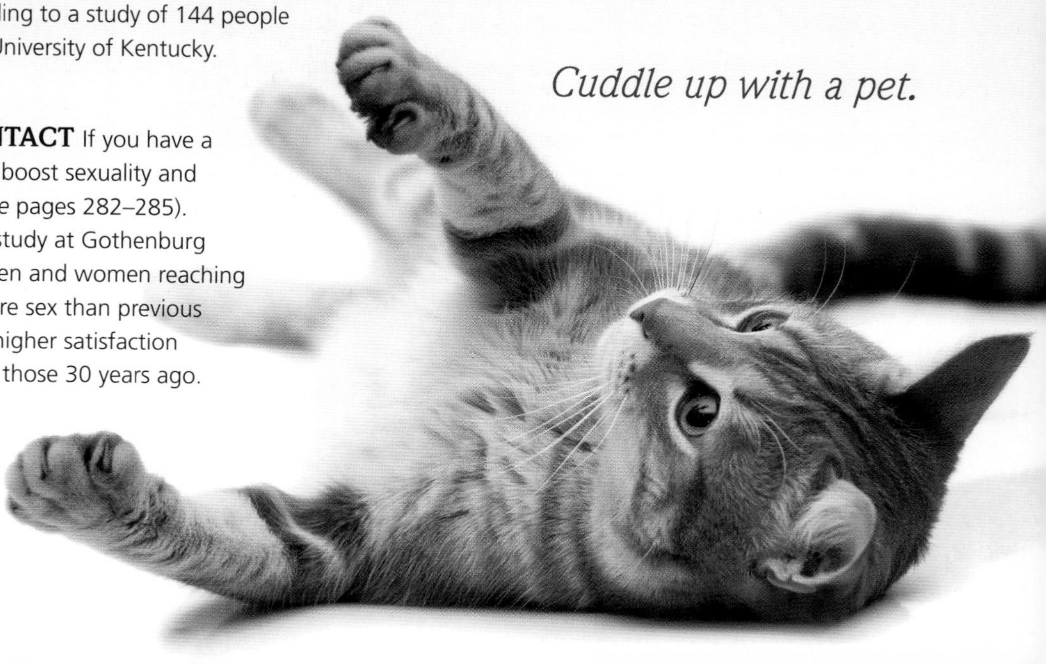

Cuddle up with a pet.

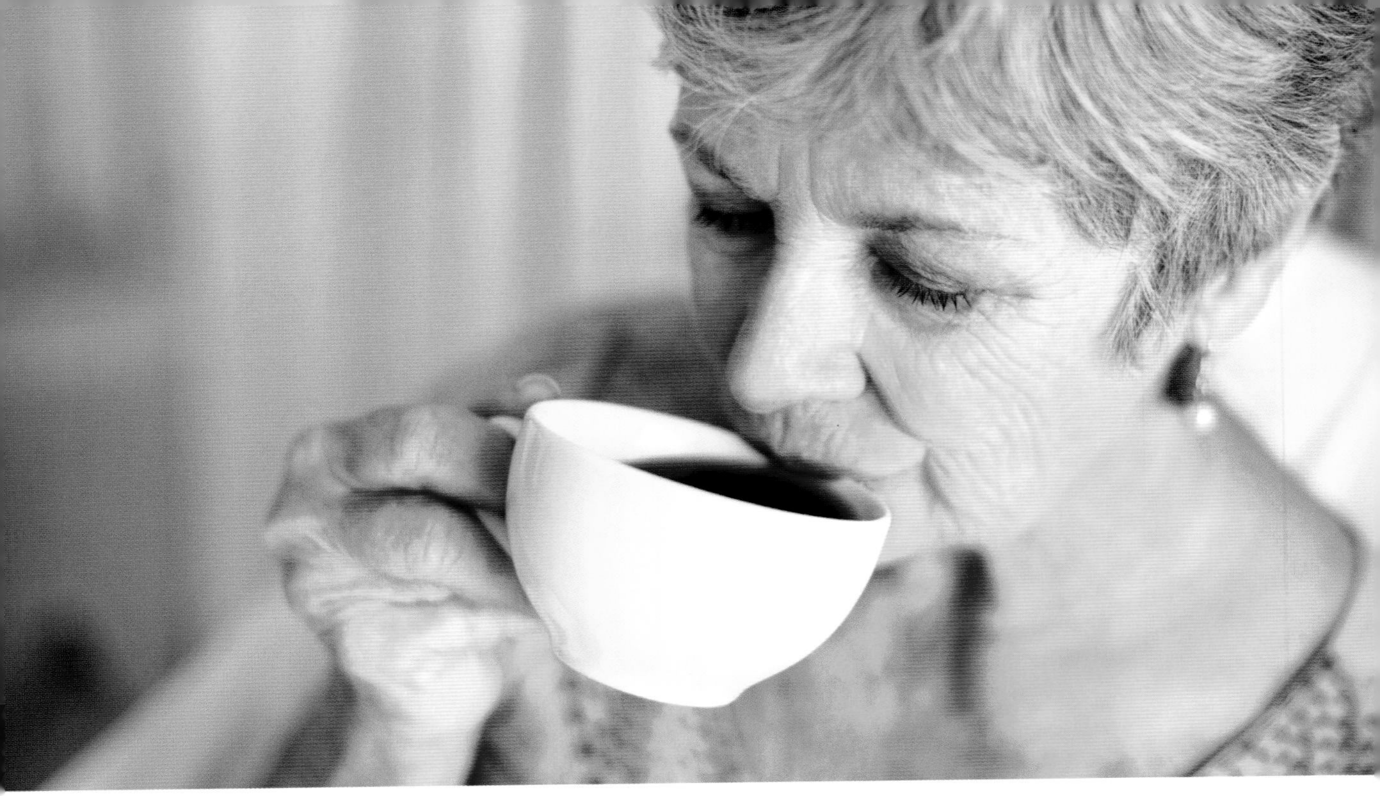

Don't get distracted. A hot drink can still scald you 10 minutes after it's been poured.

Here are four handy ways to compensate for reduced sensations (*see* opposite for ways to avoid falls):

- **Take extra care** Don't get distracted when using pans or kettles. Even a hot drink can still scald 10 minutes after it's been poured.
- **Check yourself out** Inspect your skin for injuries, particularly on your feet and especially if you have a condition such as diabetes that compromises your circulation or nerve function. Look carefully and don't rely on pain sensations to decide whether an injury is serious.
- **Get a thermometer** Use it to check the temperature to help you decide what to wear, indoors or outdoors, rather than relying on sensing whether it's hot or cold.
- **Turn the thermostat down.** Scalds from tap water are not that common, but when they occur they can be serious, and older people are more vulnerable. Setting the hot-water tank thermostat to a maximum temperature of 49°C minimises the risk.

A NEW RISK OF FALLING

You are more likely to fall as you get older. This is partly because of changes to your sense of balance, touch and sight, and partly because your muscles get weaker. Each year, around one in three people over 65 has a fall, 5 to 10 per cent of which result in injury. And falls become increasingly dangerous as you get older, because your bones become more brittle (*see* pages 164–165) and more likely to break.

There are many reasons why this happens. Your sense of balance may be disturbed and your ability to sense where the parts of your body are in space diminishes, reducing your coordination and ability to tell where your feet are on the floor, or to move around with agility or confidence. Loss of touch and pressure sensation, especially in your feet, can add to the problem.

As well as diminished balance and sense of position, various inner ear disorders such as Ménière's disease can cause vertigo, dizziness or giddiness, as can stroke, low blood glucose and heart rhythm disorders. Arthritis and neurological conditions such as Parkinson's disease can also make it considerably harder to stand steadily or walk. And so, too, can side effects of medications for conditions such as cardiovascular disease or high blood pressure. Medications that increase drowsiness – including sleeping tablets and alcohol – can increase the hazards.

'Life is like riding a bicycle. To keep your balance, you must keep moving.'

Albert Einstein,
German-born physicist

Help yourself

But there's plenty you can do to cut the risk, such as safety-proofing your home to avoid tripping hazards (*see* pages 232–234). But the number-one solution is exercise – exercise programs to improve strength and balance reduce falls in older people by up to 55 per cent according to Age UK.

You can compensate for reduced strength or lowered sensation by:

- Building muscle mass with resistance exercises (*see* pages 142–145).
- Strengthening your bones by doing weight-bearing exercises (*see* page 162).
- Improving balance with balance training (*see* pages 154–155).
- Improving flexibility and mobility (*see* pages 147–151).
- Eating a bone-friendly diet with plenty of calcium and vitamin D, or supplements if necessary (*see* pages 85–87 and 163).
- Taking care of your vision and hearing and ensuring any untoward symptoms are checked and treated promptly.
- Having treatment for conditions that can impact on your senses, such as diabetes, high blood pressure and cardiovascular disease.
- Reviewing your medications to avoid medication side effects.
- Asking your doctor about hip protectors if you are at high risk, to guard against fracture if you do fall.

Sensitivity to taste is strongest in the morning, so be sure to enjoy a good breakfast.

TASTE AND SMELL
appetite for life

Don't underestimate the importance of your senses of taste and smell – both play key roles in your wellbeing and enjoyment of life, and not just because they contribute to your appreciation of flavour.

Your sense of taste changes throughout life. As a child, you tend to crave sugary tastes, then, in adulthood, you start to appreciate more sophisticated and bitter flavours, such as olives, dark chocolate and spinach, and develop a more refined palate, so that you enjoy fine wine or mature cheese. But as you get older still – and especially if you develop certain diseases or take more medicines – your sense of taste and smell can become blunted or distorted (the most common distortion being a metallic taste). Your sense of smell – which plays a huge part in your sense of taste (*see* page 230) – is most accurate between the ages of 30 and 60, and it generally declines thereafter, as does taste sensation, especially for salty and sweet tastes.

Why does this happen? The specialised cells that allow us to detect smells and tastes are unique in the nervous system because they are replaced when they get old or damaged. But eventually the number of cells that die off exceeds the number replacing them, and sensation declines. In addition, the sensitivity of nerve endings in your mouth, nose, throat and the moist surfaces of your eyes – which help you identify certain chemical sensations such as the heat of chillies or the coolness of menthol – also declines with age. Temperature and texture also contribute to the experience of eating through other receptors in the mouth, and these, too, can be affected by ageing.

What you can do

Don't dismiss any blunting of taste or smell sensations as merely a consequence of ageing. Sometimes illness or other factors can play a part – respiratory infections, allergies, nasal polyps, sinus disease, dental problems, head injury, neurological disorders (including stroke and Alzheimer's disease), cancer, hormonal disturbances, zinc deficiency, exposure to chemicals or radiation, smoking and

focus ON ... DRY MOUTH

As you get older, you're at increased risk of a condition called xerostomia, or dry mouth, which is caused by a reduction in saliva secretion. It can make eating and swallowing difficult and also reduces your ability to taste (for which saliva is essential).

As well as impairing taste and swallowing, having a dry mouth can lead to bad breath, sore throat, tooth decay and gum disease. It is often a side effect of prescribed and over-the-counter medications, which are more likely to be taken by older people: medication for high blood pressure, urinary incontinence, Parkinson's disease, diabetes and snoring as well as chemotherapy medications or radiation treatment, for example.

See your doctor for a medication review, and ask about treatment to increase saliva production.

The following measures can all help:

- Sip water frequently throughout the day.
- Chew sugar-free gum.
- Brush your teeth regularly.
- Stop smoking and limit caffeine and alcohol – all can make dry mouth worse.
- Avoid alcohol-containing mouthwashes, antihistamines and decongestants.
- Breathe through your nose if you can, not your mouth.
- Try over-the-counter remedies to increase saliva flow – ask your pharmacist.
- Humidify indoor air, especially overnight – bowls of water on top of radiators can help.
- Visit your dentist to check for dental problems.

many medications can all contribute to loss or distortion of smell or taste sensations. And many of these problems are treatable.

That's important because the consequences of taste or smell disturbances are more wide-ranging than you might think. Reduced flavour perception lessens your enjoyment of food and may lead to reduced appetite and weight loss. Your social life may also suffer if you can't detect, for example, that your home smells unpleasant (from lingering pet or food odours) – or, worse, that you do.

Not only that – it's tempting to compensate for loss of flavour by eating more fatty and sugary foods, promoting weight gain, or by adding extra salt, which may exacerbate high blood pressure and promote cardiovascular disease. In one small study in Germany, people who had lost their sense of smell needed up to eight times as much tastebud stimulation to recognise flavours.

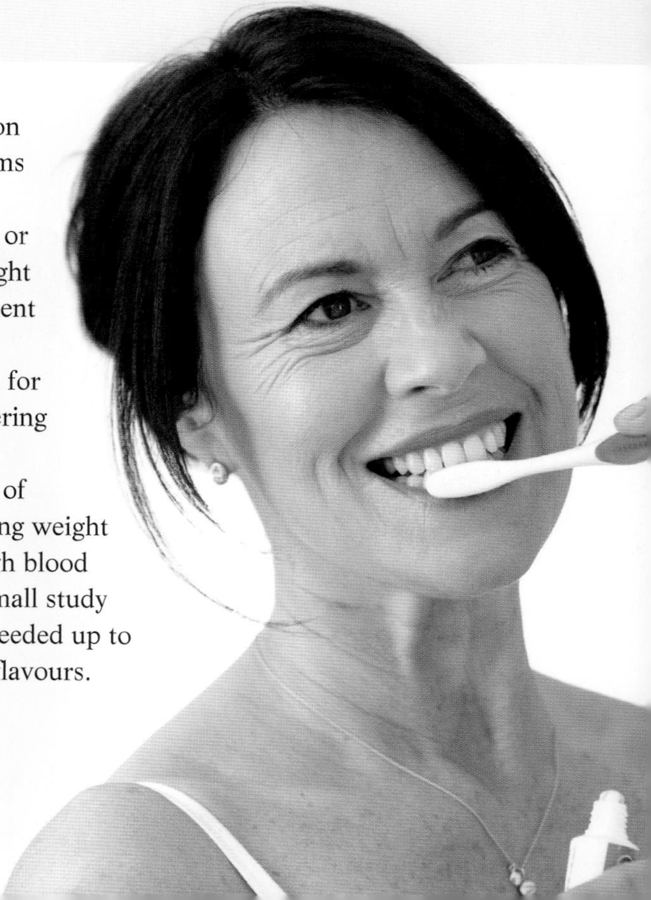

Brush your teeth regularly.

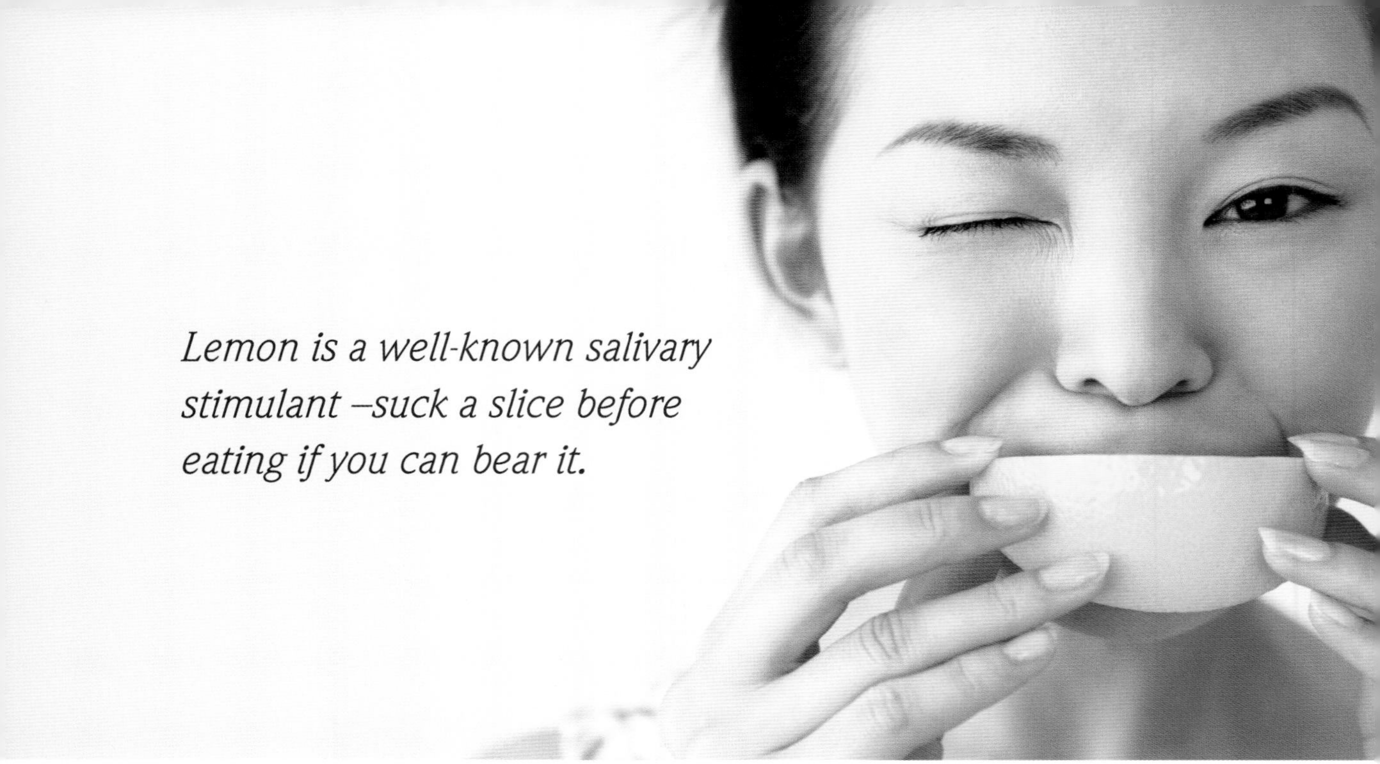

Lemon is a well-known salivary stimulant –suck a slice before eating if you can bear it.

Impaired taste and smell can therefore lead you to eat a nutritionally unbalanced diet – and this can affect your health. In what can become a vicious cycle, nutritional deficiencies sometimes further impair your taste/smell sensations. High blood pressure and diabetes, which may be a consequence of weight gain, can also impact on your taste and smell. That's not all: nutritional imbalances may also lead to other problems such as cardiovascular disease, and hinder your body's ability to recover from illness or surgery.

Seek medical advice if you suspect you have a problem. Your doctor can test you for smell and taste impairment using a special 'scratch and sniff' card and various solutions that you sip or which are applied directly to your tongue. Often, smell and taste sensations can be returned, or at least further loss be prevented, when an underlying disorder is treated or a medication stopped or changed.

We don't tend to think of taste and smell as contributing to our safety in the same way as vision and hearing, but these senses are nevertheless vital in helping us detect danger. That's why we find the smell and taste of rotten food revolting, and why smoke, toxic gases and poisonous fumes often smell noxious. If you have reduced taste or smell sensation, it's important to take extra care. People with total or partial loss of smell are almost twice as likely to have accidents when cooking, to eat or drink spoiled foods or toxic substances, or to fail to detect gas leaks or fires (*see* page 234 for safety tips).

DID **you** KNOW?

About three-quarters of the sensation of taste comes from smell, which contributes to the perception of flavour, especially with highly aromatic foods such as chocolate or coffee. That's why you can't taste properly when you have a cold with a blocked nose. Many people who think they've lost their taste sensation in fact have a problem with smell.

TASTE BOOSTERS

Even if you can't get back the refined palate you had in your middle years, there's plenty you can do to ensure that food is as enjoyable as ever. Try these clever ways to trick your senses into working harder:

- **Get your juices flowing** Increase your saliva flow, which is vital for taste sensations. Lemon is a well-known salivary stimulant, if you can bear to suck a slice before eating; a lemon-flavoured boiled sweet can have the same effect.
- **Start early** Be sure to eat breakfast – taste sensitivity is strongest in the morning.
- **Be inventive with your flavourings** Avoid piling on salt, which can have detrimental health effects that may worsen taste loss. Instead use aromatic herbs and spices to flavour your food. Consciously savour the smell of food both when it is cooking and when you eat it.
- **Add umami** As well as sweet, sour, salty and bitter, there is a fifth taste receptor that responds to a flavour called umami, roughly translated as 'savoury deliciousness'. It's due to glutamate, found naturally in foods such as Parmesan, mushrooms, ripe tomatoes and meat stock. Use these foods to enhance the overall flavour of a dish (rather than adding other flavours as with herbs and spices). Or simply sprinkle the glutamate-salt food flavouring MSG. Despite much media concern, MSG is in the safest category of food additives and is used routinely instead of ordinary salt in much Asian cuisine.
- **Aim for texture** Eating foods with a crunch, or varying textures, can boost appetite.
- **Take care with temperature** Very hot or cold foods and drinks can injure your tastebuds, which may take time to recover – after the age of 50 your tastebuds regenerate more slowly. This also applies to 'hot' spices: when you 'get used' to them and can eat hotter and hotter curries, it's actually because you're knocking off your tastebuds. This is fine if you're 20 because you replace them pretty quickly, but not so good for the over-60s.
- **Do what top chefs do** Exhale through your nose after swallowing, to help you appreciate the flavours by stimulating smell receptors.

what's NEW

ALL THE SENSES There's evidence that the senses are cross-wired to an extent, so concentrating on all aspects of the food you are eating – appearance, smell, taste, texture and even sound (such as crunching) will boost appreciation of flavour. An experiment involving top UK chef Heston Blumenthal found that diners perceived chips as being crisper if they ate them while wearing headphones that amplified the sound of their crunching. And in 2012, researchers in Montreal and Philadelphia discovered that they could enhance volunteers' sense of smell simply by electrically stimulating the brain's visual cortex.

Safety-proof your living space; 60 per cent of fatal falls happen at home.

KEEPING SAFE by thinking ahead

Your senses are your body's early alert system for detecting danger, so any changes here obviously make you more susceptible to hazards. Taking steps to safety-proof your environment, as well as being extra careful when you're driving or out and about are the sensible way to compensate.

You can relax and enjoy life more if you feel safe. Carrying a personal alarm, which you can get separately or have incorporated with a home alarm system, gives you peace of mind in case you fall or become incapacitated. You wear the alarm, for example, round your neck or as a wrist band. It connects to a 24-hour call centre, enabling you to press a button to call for help quickly if you need it (*see* Resources).

SAFETY AT HOME AND OUTDOORS

Falls are a major cause of injury and death among older people, and around 60 per cent of all fatal falls occur at home. Here are some essential ways to keep yourself safe.

At home

To reduce your risk of a nasty fall, be alert to possible hazards around the home, and do something about them. Fix tripping hazards such as loose carpets, rugs or uneven flooring, avoid slippery floor coverings and stay off wet floors. Make sure floors, stairs, halls and corridors are kept clear of clutter and avoid trailing wires. Also:

- Move low furniture away from main routes across rooms.
- Make any pets that could cross your path more noticeable, for example, with a bell or a fluorescent collar.
- Fit grab handles to the bath and use non-slip mats and floor rugs.
- Increase contrast to see important items – install dark-coloured light switches on pale walls, or put bright tape around them. Avoid heavily patterned carpets on or near staircases as these can obscure the treads. Fix a strip of contrasting tape to stair edges.

Dress appropriately for the weather, and stay at home in extreme weather conditions.

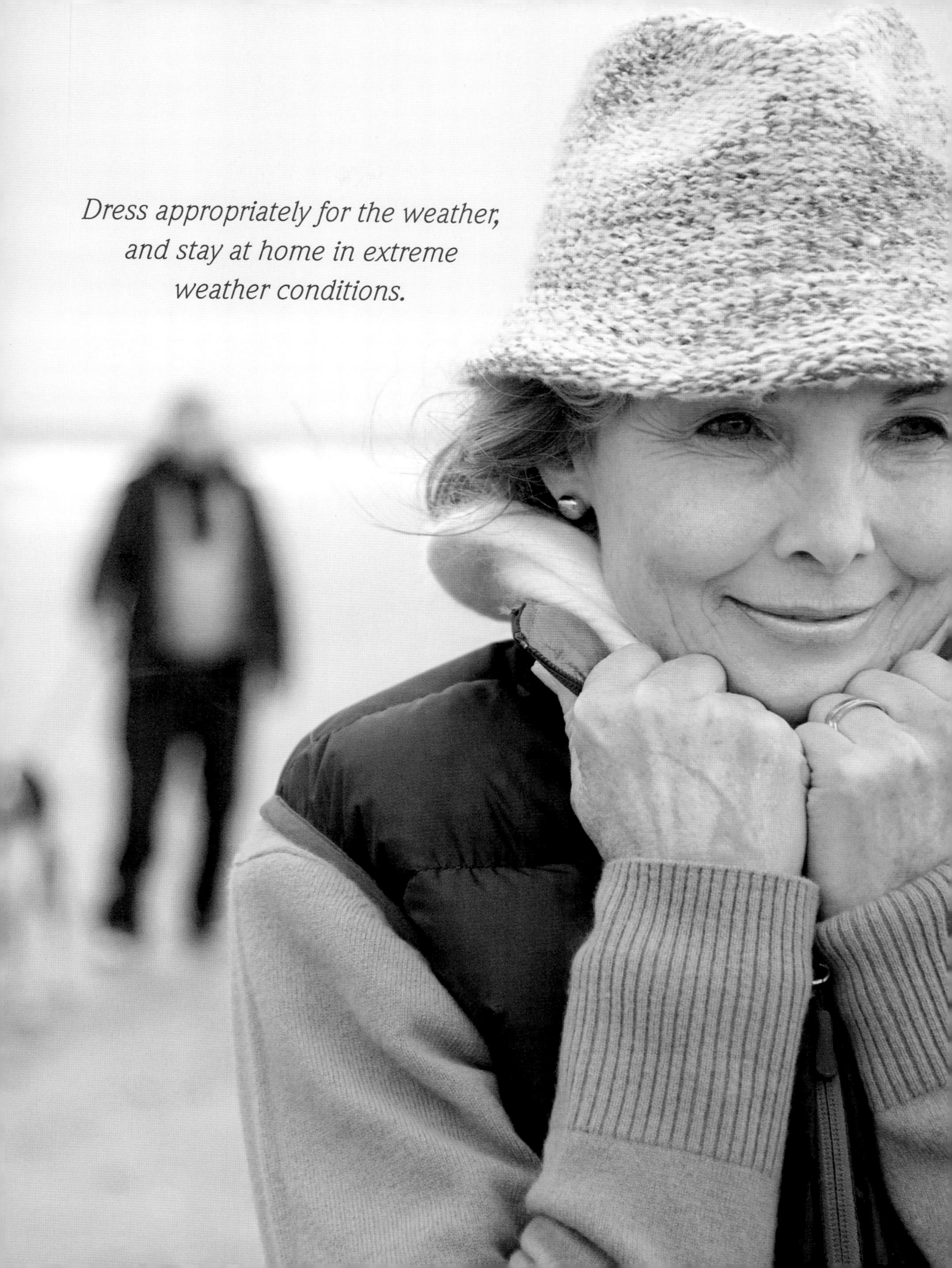

take CARE! Detecting DANGER

If your senses are compromised, you may be less alert to danger signals. You may not spot a burning ember on a carpet, hear a fire alarm or smell a gas leak. Even loss of taste can be hazardous if you don't notice that an item of food tastes rotten. Sometimes you can use your other senses to compensate, or ask other people to help.

Even so, safety gadgets are vital – though don't forget that you can't rely on them when you're away from home. If you're hard of hearing, for example, make sure hotel staff or friends know that you may not hear a fire alarm overnight, so they need to alert you. If your night vision is poor, ask your hosts to clear the route to the bathroom of tripping hazards (and remember to pack a torch). A little forward planning can usually help to ensure your safety.

Here are other ways to support your senses when it comes to recognising hazards.

- Fit at least one working smoke alarm on each floor, and test them regularly.
- Keep a fire extinguisher or fire blanket by your stove.
- If you use gas or solid fuels, have a carbon monoxide detector and install a sensor to check for gas leaks that you might not smell.
- Take care when using household products intended for well-ventilated areas: always read labels.
- Store and prepare food correctly (*see* page 93). Never eat anything past its use-by date and take care with leftovers.
- If you have a health problem that could leave you suddenly incapacitated, carry a personal alarm linked to a monitoring station.

- Install bright home lighting, especially in the kitchen and stairway. Use halogen or fluorescent lights; avoid energy-saving bulbs, which take time to warm up.
- Place task lighting for detailed work 0.5 m to 1 m away – this gives 25 times more light than a ceiling lamp 3 m away.
- Fit red night lights in hallways and bathrooms to give a dim light.
- Install motion-sensitive lights that activate as you approach.

When you are out

- **Look after your head** Head injury is a common cause of sensory loss. Always wear your seatbelt in the car and a helmet if riding a bicycle or motorbike, or when skiing, skating or horse riding.
- **Cross safely** If your senses are compromised, it's especially important to use road crossings properly.
- **Watch the weather** Dress for the weather, and stay at home in extreme weather conditions, such as heatwaves. Keep your cupboard well stocked with tinned and packaged food.

DRIVING

Driving is an important part of independent life for most people. But many issues can make it harder as you get older. Even if you retain generally good eyesight, the vision changes that come with age can alter your depth and motion perception, peripheral vision, contrast discrimination (*see* page 211) and your ability to see in reduced light.

On top of this, hearing loss may make you less aware of potential hazards such as screeching brakes. And your coordination and reaction times may not be all that they once were, so you're less able to react quickly to unexpected eventualities. Symptoms such as restricted movement, dizziness, pain and stiffness can all hamper driving ability. And you may be more easily distracted, especially in unfamiliar locations. The effects of medications, too, can make you less competent or less alert. These don't mean you necessarily have to stop driving, but you may have to make adaptations (*see* below).

Particular danger zones for older drivers include:

- Night driving, especially in areas with poor illumination or on unlit roads.
- Turning right, across the path of oncoming traffic.
- Seeing pedestrians or vehicles turning into your path.
- Noticing red lights.
- Merging with other traffic.
- Reversing and manoeuvring near kerbs.

If you're having difficulty, talk to your doctor – asking for help doesn't mean that you have to give up driving. Hearing and vision checks may detect easily solvable problems, and you may be able to stop taking or change a medication that's causing particular side effects. Car modifications can make it easier to drive if you have impaired mobility (*see* Resources). An occupational therapist with special training can give you tips and strategies, after a full assessment. The following tips may also help to make driving easier:

- Plan your route if you have a long journey, and allow extra time.
- Where possible, stick to well-lit and familiar roads at night.
- If you know you have to drive at night, avoid sunlight or bright lights during the afternoon to enable faster dark adaptation.
- Anticipate reduced vision when moving from a brightly lit to a shady area, such as entering a tunnel or passing under a bridge.
- Older people are more susceptible to fatigue. If you can, break up long journeys or allow yourself enough time for rest stops.

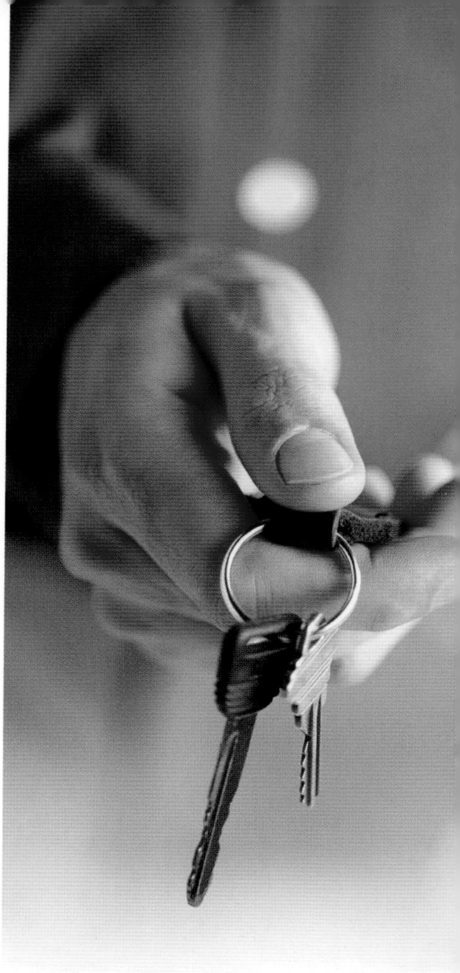

Driving is an important part of independent life for most older people.

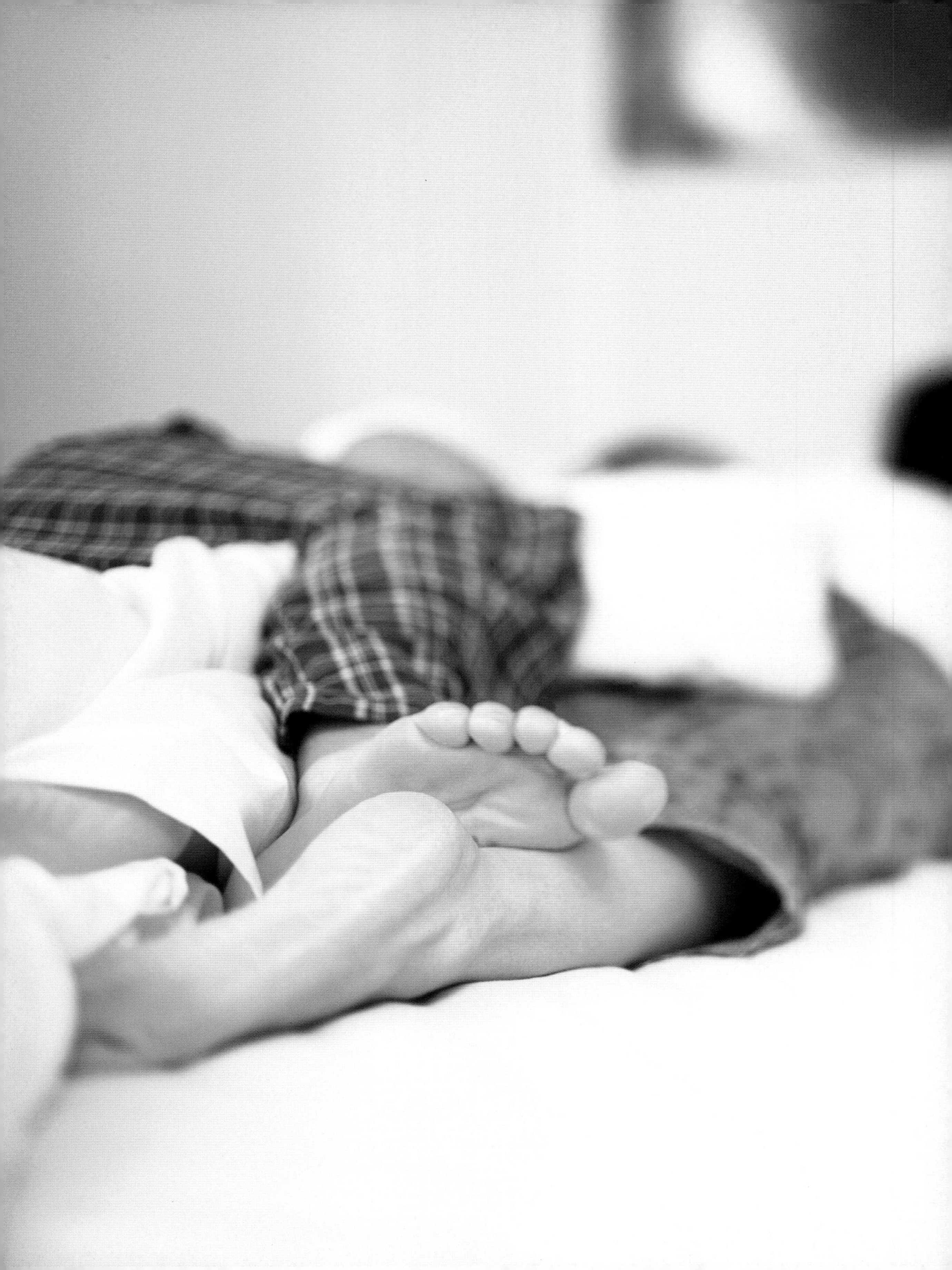

9

Sleep easy, SLEEP WELL

A good night's sleep makes a world of difference to how you feel. So if you find that you can't sleep as well as you did when you were 20, don't simply accept it as one of the annoyances of getting older. There are all sorts of beneficial strategies that you can try. These can improve your sleep pattern, which will make a significant and long-lasting difference. Help is available for more serious problems, too. And they are worth resolving as new research shows a clear link between sleep deprivation and illness. Happily, the reverse is also true: a good night's sleep promotes better health.

Adults typically need 7 to 8.4 hours' sleep a night. Fewer than 6 hours can raise heart attack risk.

NOURISHING SLEEP for body and mind

Sleep is much more than the shut-down scientists once thought it to be. Some parts of your brain remain highly active at night, helping to resolve mental and physical problems. Improving your sleep pattern boosts this healing process, bringing great dividends in later life.

The way you sleep is likely to alter as you get older. For a start, your sleep may be more fragmented and lighter, and you may take longer to nod off. Your sleep may become less 'efficient' – that is, you take longer to get the amount of sleep you need, and so you may start to supplement your night-time sleep with a daytime nap. For women, sleep disturbances that occur during the menopause because of hot flushes and night-time sweating may persist into later life.

Changing sleep patterns

The changes that occur with age may be linked to our levels of two sleep-promoting hormones. One is human growth hormone (HGH), which is associated with deep sleep: it is known that we produce less HGH as we grow older. The other sleep-related hormone is melatonin, which regulates our body clock. It helps to promote sleep by acting on receptors in the brain that control the sleep cycle. Its production is stimulated by darkness, and usually peaks between 2 am and 4 am. One German study suggests that the disturbances that some

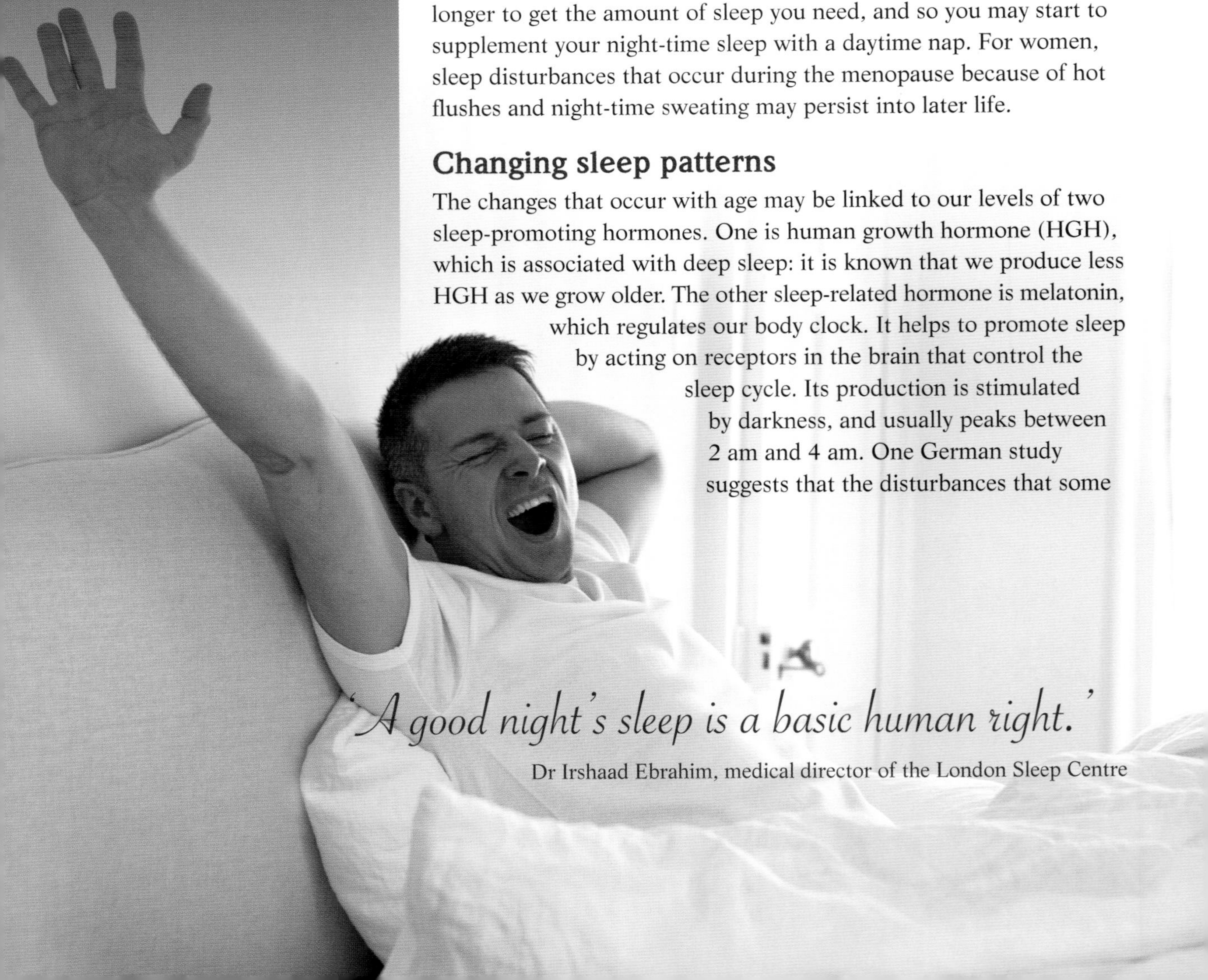

'A good night's sleep is a basic human right.'

Dr Irshaad Ebrahim, medical director of the London Sleep Centre older people experience – feeling sleepy early in the evening, waking up too soon, having trouble dropping off – could be caused by melatonin being released at the wrong time of day. This kind of research offers hope that new solutions may be found to the sleep problems of later life.

How much is enough?

Adults of all ages typically need between 7 and 8.4 hours' sleep a night, but individual requirements vary. What constitutes lack of sleep for one person may be plenty for another. Some people thrive on very little sleep; Margaret Thatcher reputedly got by on 4 hours a night. But too little sleep can make you unwell. Lack of sleep damages your immune system and is associated with conditions such as heart disease and hypertension. One German study suggests that lack of sleep can even lower your pain threshold, and other consequences include irritability, depression, poor memory, increased daytime sleepiness and raised accident risk. An Australian study found that older people rate their health and quality of life by how much sleep they get.

it's a **MYTH** ...

... that **OLDER PEOPLE** need much **LESS SLEEP**

It used to be thought that by their late 70s, people typically needed about 30 to 60 minutes a night less than they did as young adults. But older people may be better off trying to get the same amount as they needed in their 30s. A study of older adults reported at the American Association for the Advancement of Science in February 2010 showed that getting enough sleep may help ward off cognitive decline.

The cortisol effect

Research suggests that the amount of sleep you get may also impinge on the production of cortisol – a stress hormone linked to health problems. Cortisol levels peak early in the morning, and contribute to higher cardiovascular risk at that time. (This is why older people are advised not to exercise or shovel snow first thing in the morning as sudden activity or exposure to cold increases the risk.) A US study of people with an average age of 60 found that sleeping fewer than 6 hours a night increased cardiovascular risk. Similarly, a 2011 Canadian study suggested that sleeping for longer protects older people from developing higher levels of cortisol over time.

So, if you find yourself getting up later these days, this could be your body's way of making sure you're getting enough sleep for optimum health. The acid test is how you feel: when you wake, are you less than refreshed? Do you get sleepy in the daytime? If a lack of sleep is making you unhappy, you should do something about it.

Quiz How do you SLEEP?

Have you noticed that your sleep patterns have changed since you were younger, or have you always been a sound and solid sleeper? Answer the questions below to get some clues about the nature of your sleep, and to find out what to do about any problems. Choose the answer that best suits your experience.

	Always/Often	Sometimes	Rarely
1 I wake feeling refreshed and well rested.	☐	☐	☐
2 I have trouble sleeping.	☐	☐	☐
3 I have trouble getting off to sleep.	☐	☐	☐
4 I get to sleep fine, but wake up in the night.	☐	☐	☐
5 I worry about not sleeping.	☐	☐	☐
6 I try to make up for lost sleep by having a lie-in.	☐	☐	☐
7 I keep to a set bedtime.	☐	☐	☐
8 I have coffee or alcohol less than 2 hours before bedtime.	☐	☐	☐
9 I snore (or have been told I do so).	☐	☐	☐
10 I use over-the-counter sleeping aids.	☐	☐	☐

Score

Always/Often: If you ticked this box for questions 2, 3, 4, 5 or 10, then you have a chronic (ongoing) sleep problem. If you never feel refreshed or have frequent trouble sleeping (question 2), you are not getting the rest you need. You may have sleep-onset difficulty (3), which alcohol or caffeine (8) can exacerbate, or a sleep-maintenance problem (4) due to alcohol, depression, environmental disturbances or snoring (9). If you're perpetually anxious about your sleep (5), you may have depression. Not having a routine bedtime (7) and attempting to make up for lost sleep (6) may be causing a body-clock problem. Using non-prescription sleeping aids (10) is not advisable without medical supervision. Ask your doctor for advice; lifestyle changes could help or you may need to consult a sleep specialist.

Sometimes: Ticking this box to questions 2, 3, 4, 5 or 10 indicates that you have a short-term or intermittent sleep problem. Talk to your doctor – and look at the Good Sleep Plan opposite.

Rarely: Top marks for sleeping. But have a look through the Good Sleep Plan to see if there are tips that could help you get an even better night's rest.

THE GOOD SLEEP PLAN
easy if you know how

Get to bed early, live longer? An Italian study of over-80s found a link between the two.

You can enhance your sleep by rethinking old established bedtime habits and by making some simple and rewarding changes to your lifestyle. Here's how.

You may have heard people talking about 'sleep hygiene'. What this means is the combination of habits and factors that affect how you sleep, determining the quantity and quality of the hours you spend in bed. Here's how to make it work for you.

Before you lie down

The time you go to bed, and the way you spend the evening, can make the world of difference to how you sleep:

1 **Keep to a schedule** Go to bed and get up at the same time each day to keep your circadian rhythms – your personal 'body clock'– in kilter. It's important to stick to a schedule as you get older because, if you no longer have to get up and go to work, you can easily adopt an any-old-time approach to sleep/wake times. Make sure the time you set for going to bed is when you feel sleepy.

2 **Wind down** Relax before going to bed by having a warm bath or listening to soothing music.

3 **Avoid stress** Upsetting TV shows or reading matter, and heavy conversations or arguments can set your mind buzzing, interfering with sleep. Make the evenings a time for pleasant activities. And if you have concerns preying on your mind, make a list of them and put it outside the bedroom – to be dealt with calmly tomorrow.

4 **Switch off** Make the half-hour before bedtime technology-free – light emitted by televisions, computers and iPads inhibits production of the sleep-inducing hormone melatonin, by making the brain think it's still daytime. Moreover, Australian researchers found that exposure to electromagnetic radiation from mobile phones interferes with sleep by stimulating brain activity. It's fine to use an e-reader so long as it's not backlit.

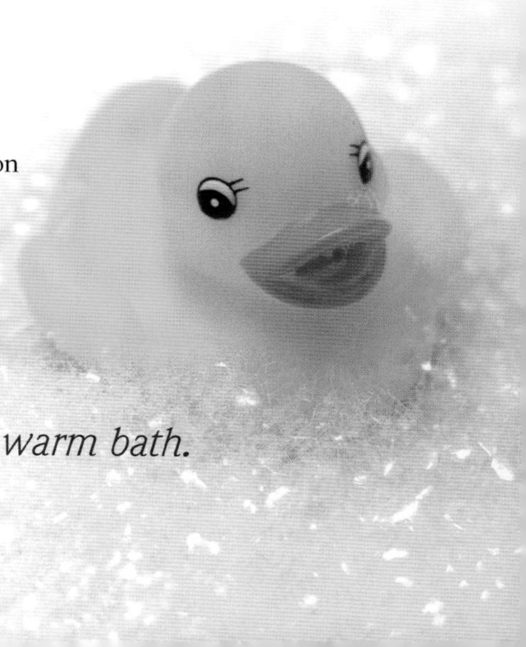

Wind down and relax before bed by having a warm bath.

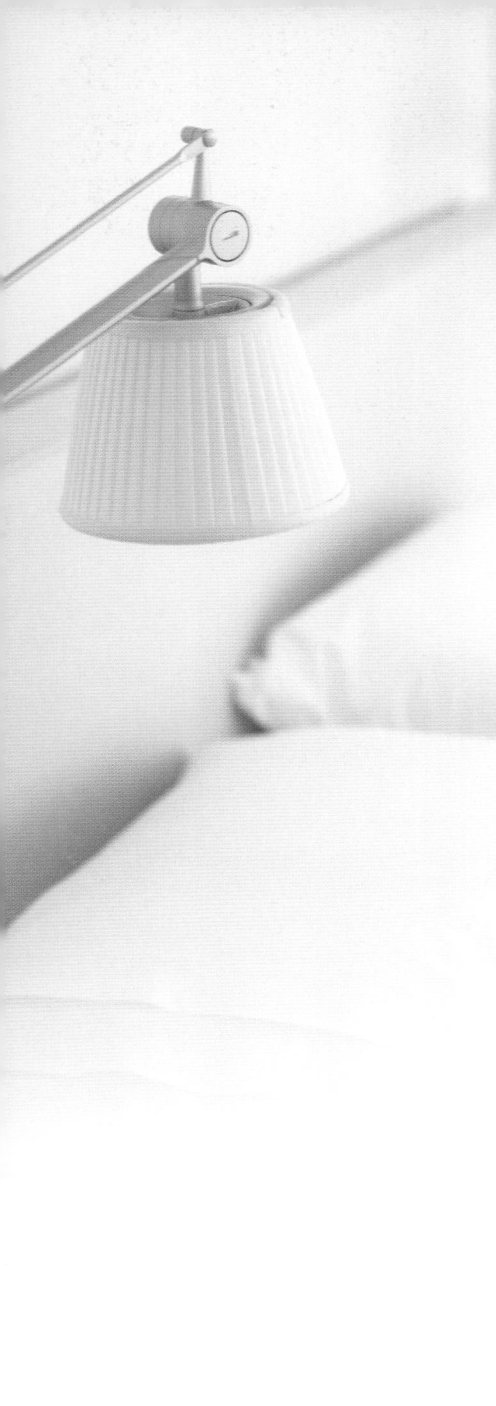

Use low-watt light bulbs in the bedroom.

A place to rest

Keep your bedroom for sleep and sex only – banish the television and laptop – to help make it a place that invites slumber:

1 **Block out noise** Wear earplugs, install double glazing or hang heavy curtains to reduce the volume. An air-conditioning unit or white-noise CD can also help, especially if you have tinnitus.

2 **Keep it dark** Use low-watt bulbs in the bedroom. When it is time to go to sleep, make sure it is really dark: have thick curtains or blackout blinds or wear an eye mask. When getting up at night, use a torch if it's safe to do so – this makes it easier to drop back off.

3 **Get the temperature right** Make sure your bedroom isn't too hot or cold. Open the window (if safe) or turn the heating down: a cooler room mirrors the natural drop in body temperature that occurs when you sleep; French researchers found that 16°C to 19°C was about right. But warmer hands and feet help you sleep, so wear bedsocks, gloves, thermal underwear or a nightcap if you feel the cold. Or use a hot-water bottle or heat pad (make sure it's not too hot, especially if you have poor circulation).

● **TAKE CARE** If you like an electric blanket to warm your bed, buy one with overheat protection for safety (look for a blanket that meets Australian standards) and use according to the manufacturer's instructions – some fires each year involve electric blankets. Never use an old, damaged or scorched blanket, and make sure it lies flat; the electrical cord and switch should hang outside the bed. Don't have it on all night. Some models can't be used on futons or water beds; check before use. Never use an electric blanket with a hot-water bottle. Have your blanket inspected at least every three years (by the makers or a qualified electrician) to check it's in good working order.

During the day

What you do during the day can be as important to good sleep as your night-time strategies. Here's what to aim for:

1 **Light up** Spend time sitting in light rooms, and get outside as much as possible. Sunshine will also boost your vitamin D levels,

5 tips on choosing a **NEW BED**

If you don't wake up feeling refreshed, the fault may lie with your bed or mattress. If they are showing signs of wear, or the mattress is more than seven years old, it may be time for a new one. Here are some tips to help you choose the best for you:

1 DO YOUR RESEARCH A firm mattress isn't necessarily better for your back. The best mattress is one designed to conform to your spine's natural curves and keep it in alignment. A memory-foam mattress (first used in the space industry) could be a good option, as it gives all-round support, moulding itself to your body contours and returning to its original shape when you get up. Ask your doctor for advice if you have back problems.

2 LOOKS DON'T MATTER You don't need a luxurious mattress edged with hand-stitched satin – it will be covered by a sheet. But check how the sides of the bed are finished; hand stitching here means the bed will keep its shape for longer.

3 TOP UP Consider buying a mattress topper to alter the level of support – some differ on each side – ideal for couples with different preferences.

4 CHECK NEW MEANS NEW If you buy a new bed that comes with a money-back guarantee, you may be splashing out on a mattress that someone else has tried for a few weeks then returned.

5 GET THE SET Make sure your bed base and mattress fit together well; this can prolong the life of the mattress as the base absorbs up to 50 per cent of the impact. Avoid box platforms – plain box supports covered with fabric – as these have no springs and can cause the mattress to wear out quicker.

which is good for your bone health as well as your immune system (*see* page 120). During short winter days, getting early-morning bright light or using a light-therapy box (available online – *see* Resources) can be helpful in setting your body clock.

2 Get active Scientists in Chicago found that aerobic exercise improves sleep, mood and quality of life in older people with insomnia. Go for a walk, swim, dance or cycle to prepare for good sleep. Ideally, exercise for 30 minutes a day – but not too close to bedtime – 5 to 6 hours before bed is ideal.

3 Try new interests Taking up a new activity you've never had time for before (such as painting, learning a foreign language or photography), social activities, spending time with grandchildren – all offer daytime stimulation that can enhance night-time relaxation and improve your sleep.

4 steps to GOOD naps

A daily nap is a great way to increase your sleep quota. Although 30 minutes is the usual recommended nap time, a 2011 study by researchers in New York found that healthy older people – with an average age of 70 – could benefit from a daily nap lasting 45 minutes: there was no negative effect on night-time sleep, and their daytime function was enhanced. But:

- **DON'T REST TOO LONG** Restrict napping time so that it doesn't interfere with your night's sleep.
- **HAVE IT AFTER LUNCH** A Greek study suggests that afternoon naps are linked to increased longevity and better cardiovascular health. But don't leave it too late or, again, it might affect your night's sleep.
- **MAKE IT COSY** Nap in a comfortable environment with limited light and noise.
- **COME TO SLOWLY** Don't plan anything too demanding (mentally or physically) straight after your nap when you may be a little groggy.

Eating for sleep

What you eat and drink – especially during the evening – may contribute to sleeping problems. To make sure you get optimum rest, try the following tips:

1 **Don't eat a big dinner** The cut-off time should be 3 hours before bed, according to experts. Avoid rich, fatty, spicy or acidic foods, which are harder for your stomach to digest and may keep you from sleeping, or wake you up in the night. This is especially important if you suffer from heartburn. Researchers at Walter Reed Army Medical Center in Washington DC measured the difference in acid levels in people who went to bed 2 hours after dinner and those who ate very early. Eating late resulted in significantly more reflux, as does sleeping on your back (*see* opposite).

2 **Avoid the nightcap** Having a wee dram to help you nod off may seem like a good idea. But though alcohol acts as a sedative when it first enters your bloodstream, several hours later it has the reverse effect and makes you wakeful. And a 2011 Japanese study at Akita University suggested that alcohol taken about 2 hours before bedtime actually interferes with the restorative powers of sleep. It's more sleep-friendly to go for a glass of warm, soothing milk instead (as long as it doesn't make you get up in the night).

3 **Cut back on caffeine** A coffee will invigorate you in the morning and, by the same token, it will keep you from sleeping at night. What's more, it can affect sleep for up to 12 hours after drinking it – so try to eliminate caffeine (in coffee, non-herbal teas, chocolate and soft drinks) altogether after lunchtime. (Caffeinated drinks also act as diuretics, so it's best to avoid them if you want to cut down on night-time visits to the bathroom.) Hidden caffeine in some medications can also make it more difficult to get to sleep, according to researchers at the National Institute on Aging in Maryland, USA. So always read the label on medications, and select medications that are caffeine-free, where possible.

focus ON ... YOUR SLEEP POSITION

What does your sleep position say about you – and how healthy is it? The way you lie in bed may indicate your personality type, says Professor Chris Idzikowski, director of the Sleep Assessment and Advisory Service in the UK. It may also have an effect – for good or ill – on some conditions that are common in the over-60s.

The most common sleeping position – adopted by 41 per cent of those monitored by Professor Idzikowski – is the **'foetus'**. If you curl up in the foetal position (pictured), you're apparently likely to be tough on the outside but sensitive at heart. This is also a good position for alleviating lower back pain, as it takes the strain off your spine.

Studies have shown that over-60s tend to sleep on their right side, and those who do so sleep longer than people who lie on their left side. A 2011 study conducted in Ankara, Turkey, concluded that lying on the right side reduced breathing problems in people with sleep apnoea, (*see* page 251). Sleeping on the right side is better for your heart and digestion, too, according to Australian researchers at James Cook University in Townsville.

'Freefall' is the name that Professor Idzikowski gives to the position in which you lie on your front, hands around the pillow, head turned to one side. This position is good for the digestion, and may also benefit blood pressure: new research from Japan confirmed that blood pressure dropped significantly when people turned over onto their front. Freefallers tend to be gregarious and brash, but nervy underneath.

Lying on your back is not necessarily a good idea – whether in Idzikowski's **'soldier'** (both arms pinned to the sides, indicating quiet and reserved people) or in the **'starfish'** (both arms up around the pillow). Both positions encourage gastric reflux, and can lead to snoring or shallow breathing. Other research has shown that people with sleep apnoea experience breathing pauses when they sleep on their back. On the plus side, soldiers and starfishes are supposed to make good friends.

Though a change of sleeping position may improve your sleep, it is a hard thing to alter. Idzikowski's research also found that most people stick to one position: a mere 5 per cent of us vary it each night.

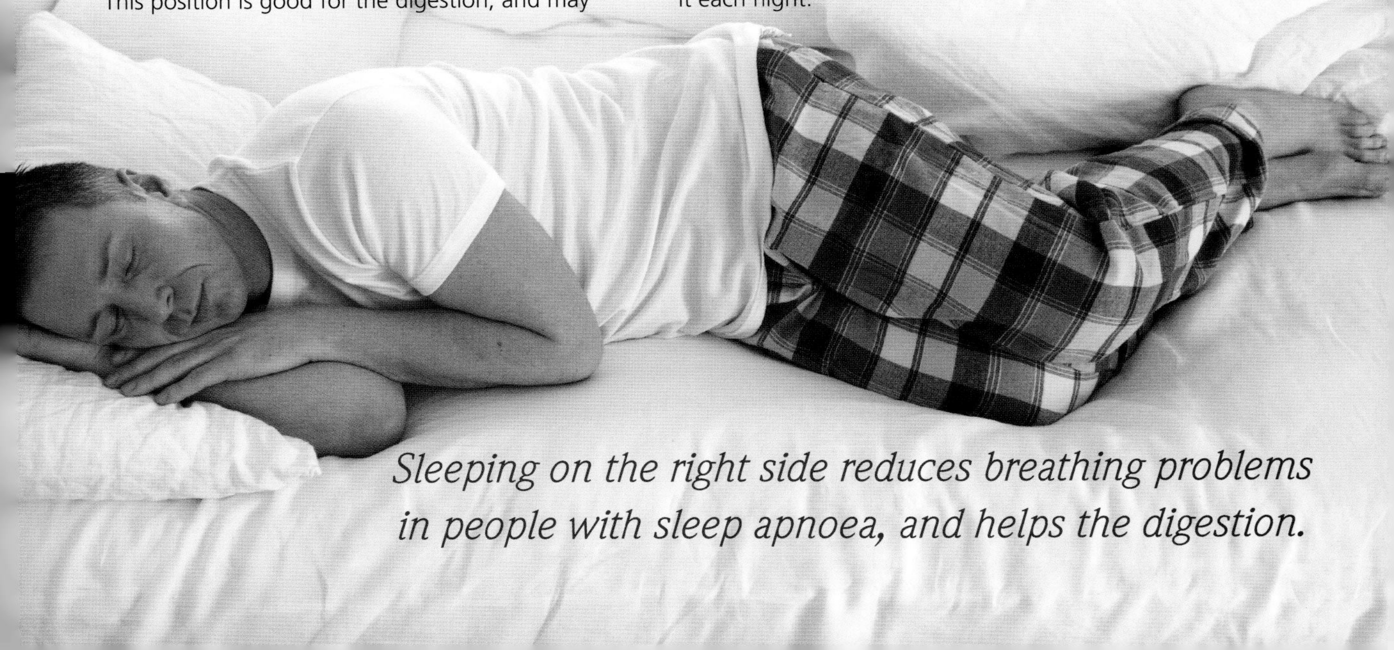

Sleeping on the right side reduces breathing problems in people with sleep apnoea, and helps the digestion.

Fifty per cent of people over 60 have their sleep interrupted by the need to use the bathroom.

RESTLESS NIGHTS
when sleep eludes you

If you lie awake at night, despite trying to improve your sleep hygiene, talk to your doctor. He or she can help you identify the causes of poor sleep and suggest ways to prevent them from jeopardising your health.

Sleep can be elusive as you get older for all sorts of reasons. Some illnesses associated with advancing years can also interrupt your sleep, especially those that cause pain or discomfort: arthritis, reflux, congestive heart failure, Parkinson's disease and asthma, for example. Depression can keep you awake in the small hours, but may also make it difficult to get to sleep. Medications may interfere with sleep, too.

Getting up in the night

One maddening sleep-interrupter, affecting more than half of over-60s, is the need to get up during the night to urinate. Nocturia, as this condition is known, was once thought to be caused principally by benign prostatic hyperplasia (BPH) – enlargement of the prostate. It's now known to have many causes, and is not confined to men, though a Danish study of 60- to 80-year-olds found that getting up more than twice a night was more common in men than women.

Why do we produce excess urine at night as we get older? There are many factors apart from BPH: variations in urine production by the kidneys, an overactive bladder, disease in the urinary tract or other parts of the body. Ankle swelling has an effect, too, because the fluid returns to the bloodstream when the legs are level with the body.

Here are some simple ways to help you avoid nocturia:

- Drink your normal liquid intake but have it earlier in the day.
- Avoid drinking late at night, particularly tea, coffee or beer.
- Keep a diary of how much you drink, what you drink and when. This will help you identify any triggers that make nocturia worse.
- Practise pelvic floor exercises to help you control your bladder.
- For ankle swelling, put your feet up for 2 to 3 hours in the early evening so you can pass some fluid as urine before going to bed.
- Don't smoke. Nicotine irritates the bladder.

HANDLING INSOMNIA

Insomnia becomes more common with age. More than half of over-65s have trouble sleeping, according to one recent study. Almost a quarter of over-65s admitted to having restless sleep on most nights, or even every night, in the previous two weeks (that's three times higher than in the 16 to 24 age group). It is more common in women than men. Insomnia is characterised by one or more of the following:

- Difficulty getting to sleep.
- Problems with staying asleep.
- Waking up too early in the morning.
- Having non-refreshing sleep.

Insomnia can be 'acute', where the problem is short term, lasting for anything from one night to a few weeks; or it can be 'chronic' – where sleep difficulty occurs for at least three nights a week for a month or more. Sometimes, temporary insomnia can be aggravated by anxiety: the belief that you won't be able to sleep becomes self-fulfilling; or you may worry about getting back to sleep, and clock-watch each time you wake. You may then have an impression that you've had a bad night's sleep, even if your total amount of sleep was normal.

'Lying in bed would be an altogether supreme experience if only one had a coloured pencil long enough to draw on the ceiling.'

G.K. Chesterton, English writer

Put your feet up for 2 to 3 hours in the early evening to help combat night-time urination.

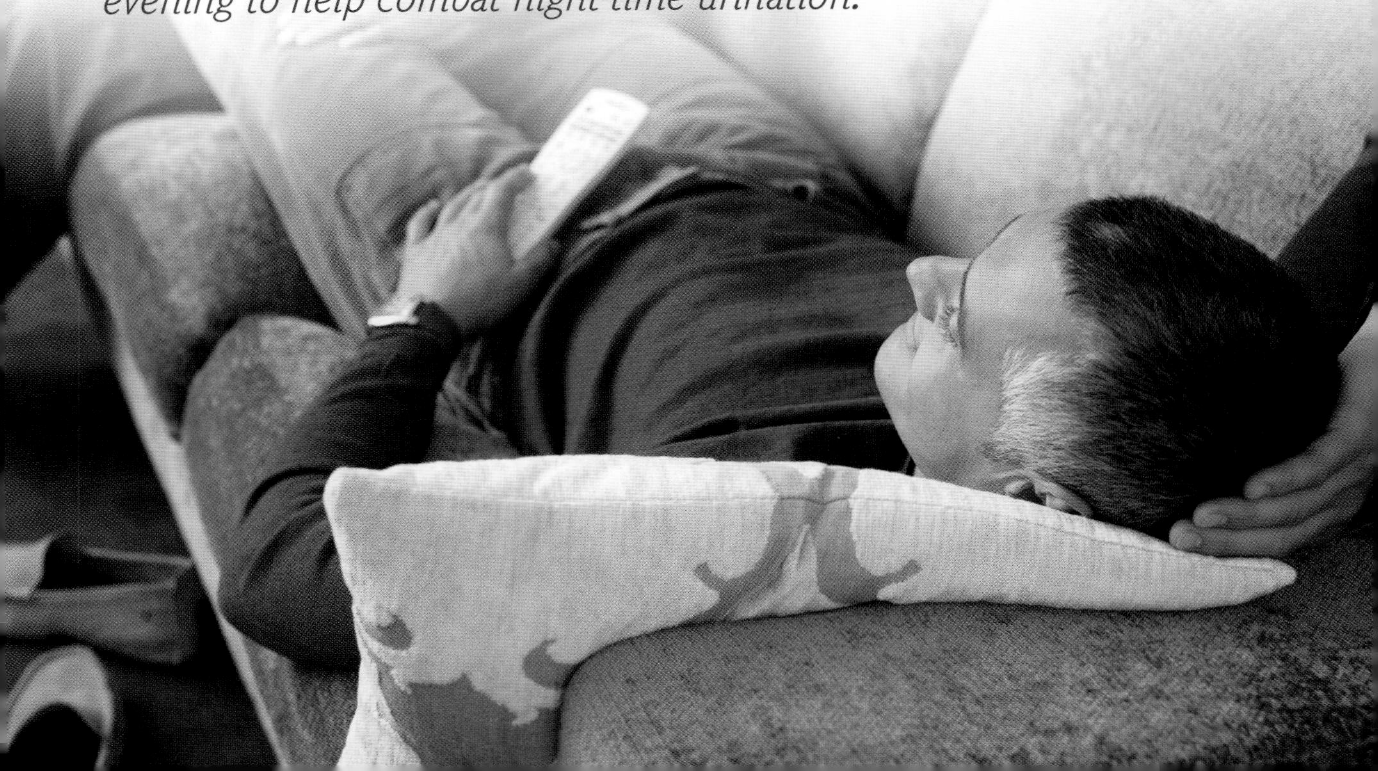

take CARE! SLEEPING TABLETS

Popping a pill may seem like an easy solution for insomnia. But especially as you get older, the risks of taking sedatives may outweigh the benefits. Researchers in Toronto examined the results of 24 studies on people with insomnia aged 60 and over. The subjects were people who took sedative hypnotics, including prescribed sleeping pills and over-the-counter medications such as antihistamines. Though participants' sleep time increased and was less interrupted, they had problems including drowsiness, dizziness and loss of balance – resulting in some serious accidents. To stay safe:

- Remember that any sedative can cause reactions such as rebound insomnia or even addiction if taken long term, and you'll end up feeling more sleep deprived, not less.
- Don't take over-the-counter medication or herbal products to treat insomnia. Always check with your doctor first.

A new option?

One alternative to sedatives may be slow-release melatonin tablets (*see* pages 238–239). They have been shown to improve sleep quality and morning alertness in people over 55 with insomnia. Talk to your doctor about whether these tablets could be suitable for you. They can't be taken by people with autoimmune disease (such as lupus, rheumatoid arthritis or multiple sclerosis) or reduced liver function. And you shouldn't smoke or drink alcohol while taking them since this may make them less effective. It can be used for up to three weeks.

Don't just live with insomnia. Talk to your doctor, describe the problem in detail and ask for advice. You may be offered medication or therapy. There are also simple steps you can take to help yourself:

- Try to identify the causes, and target underlying issues. Keep a sleep diary to help you understand the patterns.
- Establish a regular sleep routine (*see* page 241).
- Learn relaxation techniques to calm yourself before bed. Various therapies, such as biofeedback to control muscle tension, cognitive therapy to change unhelpful thoughts that may prevent sleep, and self-hypnosis, have been found to improve sleep in older people with insomnia (*see* Resources for advice on where to get help).

Tired all the time?

If you are permanently tired and low in energy, check with your doctor to eliminate any physical cause, such as diabetes, anaemia or thyroid problems. In over-60s, drowsiness and tiredness, coupled with an overwhelming need to sleep during the day, may well be a condition called excessive daytime sleepiness (EDS). While EDS is common in older people, it should always be investigated. A French study of more than 9000 older people with EDS found that it increases the risk of cardiovascular disease by 33 per cent. But whether EDS is a symptom or a trigger of cardiovascular disease is not known. It may help to:

- Take up a new activity to get you out and stimulate your mind.
- Experiment with taking a short afternoon nap (*see* page 244).

SHARED PROBLEMS

If you share a bed, you may be passing on a large portion of disturbed sleep. Loud snoring can affect your partner's sleep as well as your own. A 2011 UK survey found that over a third of people sleep in separate beds because of their partner's snoring. And things get worse with age: by 60, around 40 per cent of women and 60 per cent of men snore almost every night, an Italian study suggests.

Why is this? The muscles that hold open the throat relax during sleep, and the aperture becomes narrower. Air passing through this smaller opening can cause surrounding tissues to vibrate, producing the sounds of snoring. Snoring can occur during all stages of sleep, but it's most common during REM sleep, because you're likely to have looser muscle tone at this stage.

Help for snorers

Sporadic snoring occurs for many reasons, including sinus infections, colds and allergies that narrow the nasal passageways, or drinking alcohol late at night. Or it may be a nightly event if, for example, you're obese, have a broken nose, are a 'mouth breather', or sleep on your back – when gravity pulls your palate, tonsils and tongue backwards, narrowing the airways.

Loud snoring can affect your partner's sleep as well as your own.

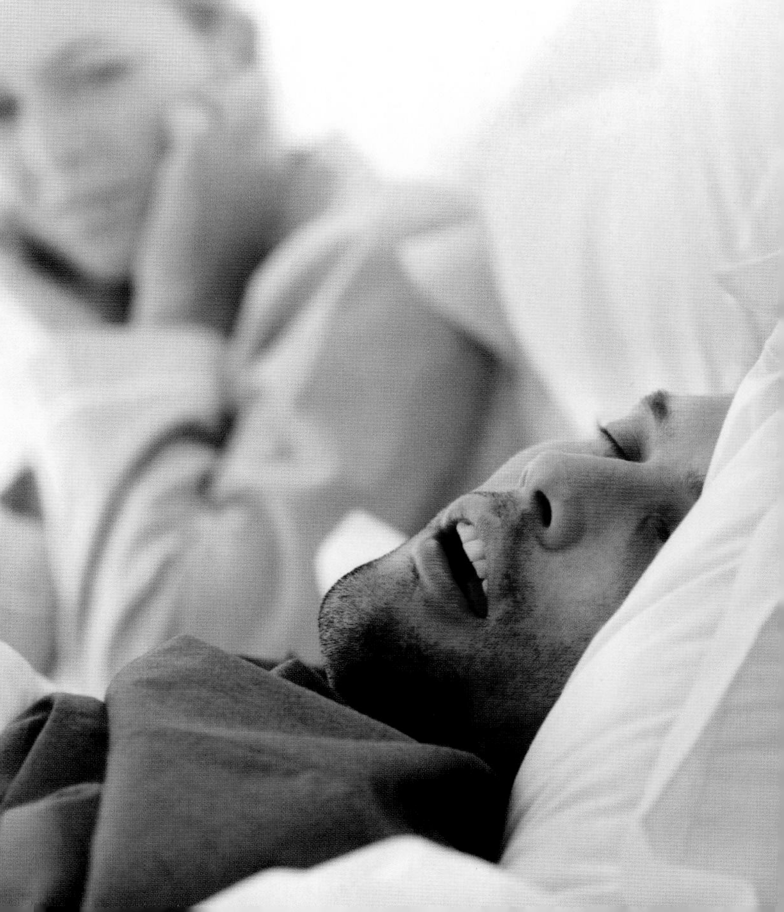

DID YOU KNOW?

US researchers found that a routine sleep history is taken in only 10 per cent of medical consultations. This seems strange when you consider that sleep disorders can be markers for various diseases, and the strong connection that exists between sleep and good health. Do mention any problems with sleep when you see your doctor about other health issues.

what's **NEW**

A WEIGHT-LOSS MEDICATION FOR SNORERS A one-a-day pill slashed snoring rates by almost 70 per cent in a small six-month US trial. The weight-loss medication combining the appetite suppressant phentermine and the anti-epilepsy medication topiramate was shown to have significant effects on snoring and sleep apnoea, reducing snoring by 70 per cent. The medication has not yet been approved, but large follow-up studies are planned.

Finding the best remedy is a question of trial and error, but the following can help:

- **Lifestyle changes** Avoid smoking, alcohol, caffeine, over-eating. Exercise more.
- **A new position** Sleep on your side, not your back. Or try a different pillow.
- **Extra help** You could try nasal and throat sprays from the chemist, nasal strips, drops of eucalyptus oil on the pillow or, in more severe cases, a continuous positive airway pressure (CPAP) device (*see* opposite).
- **Use your nose** Simply learning to breathe through your nose may also help – but you'll need to make a conscious effort to break the mouth-breathing habit and you may have to try a technique such as the Buteyko method (*see* Resources).

When you just can't stay still …

Sleep-related movement disorders also tend to surface more in the over-60s. The two most common are restless legs syndrome, which troubles 5 to 15 per cent of older people, and periodic limb movement disorder, affecting up to 45 per cent.

- **RESTLESS LEGS SYNDROME** This is characterised by creeping, crawling, burning, tingling or itchy sensations in the legs and feet, resulting in an irresistible urge to move – which is worse when you're drowsy. The cause is usually not known, but experts think it may be down to a lack of, or imbalance of, some brain chemicals, especially dopamine. See your doctor if it persists – restless leg can be a first sign of diabetes, Parkinson's disease and rheumatoid arthritis, while a 2011 Korean study found that patients with restless leg had higher levels of 'bad' LDL cholesterol than those without it. Treatment depends on the cause and severity but may include lifestyle changes – such as exercising, stopping smoking or avoiding alcohol or caffeine – or taking medication, for example, to regulate dopamine levels.

- **PERIODIC LIMB MOVEMENT DISORDER** The main symptom – repeated jerking in the lower leg muscles – can lead to fragmented sleep and daytime sleepiness. There is some evidence – illustrated by a 2009 study in São Paolo, Brazil – that exercising helps.

focus ON ... SLEEP APNOEA

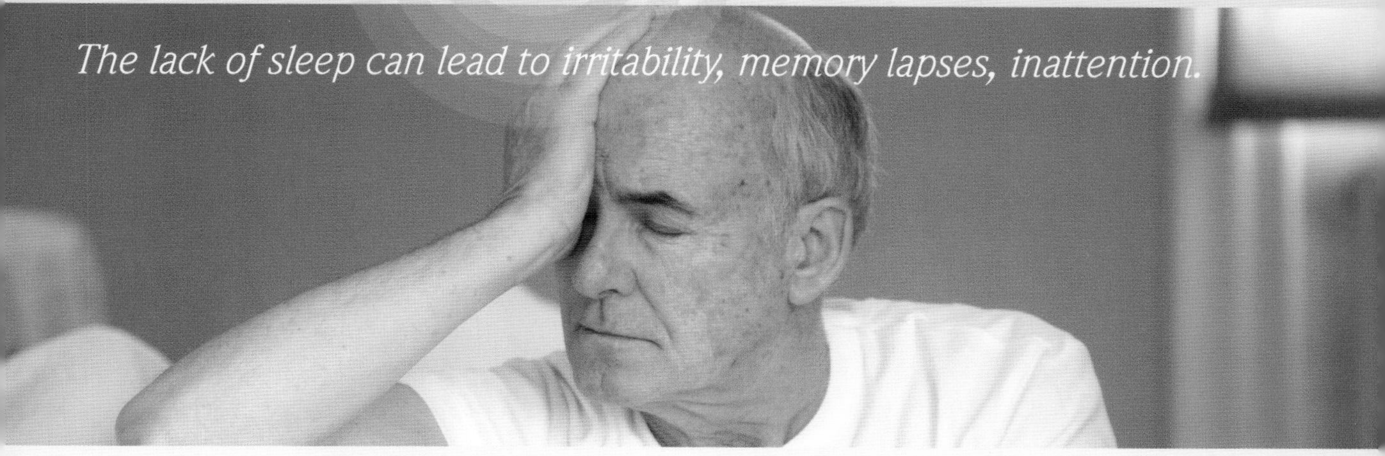

Sleep apnoea is a condition in which breathing is interrupted, or stops completely for short periods, during sleep. As many as one in five over-65s are affected.

The twin symptoms of sleep apnoea are snoring and excessive daytime sleepiness. See your doctor promptly if you have both – sleep apnoea can be serious if left untreated. Its effects can include:

- The lack of sleep can lead to irritability, memory lapses, inattention and personality changes.
- Low levels of oxygen can lead to depression, headaches and potential heart problems.
- Pressure changes in the throat can lead to an irregular heartbeat.

If your doctor suspects sleep apnoea, you may be referred to a sleep specialist. A sleep study (polysomnography) will monitor your oxygen levels, breathing and movements – and assess the quality of your sleep. In mild cases, simple steps can help:

- If you are overweight, try to lose weight.
- Avoid alcohol after 6 pm.
- Keep your nose as clear as possible; sleep on your side or half propped up.
- Try a dental device – such as a sports gumshield – which props open the jaw and the inside of the mouth to counteract muscle relaxation.

If the problem is more serious, the most efficient treatment may be a continuous positive airway pressure (CPAP) device. The narrowed inside of the throat is held open by slightly pressurised air delivered via a mask while you sleep. The mask fits over your nose and connects to a small, quiet pump beside the bed. With the air gently blowing through the nose, your breathing can return to normal during sleep. The result can be dramatic if used properly – greatly improved sleep and an end to daytime sleepiness. Surgery to remove the tonsils and adenoids may help some people.

And it is good news all round: a Mayo Clinic study in the USA found that when sleep apnoea and snoring were eliminated in their partners, the spouses gained an additional 62 minutes of sleep a night.

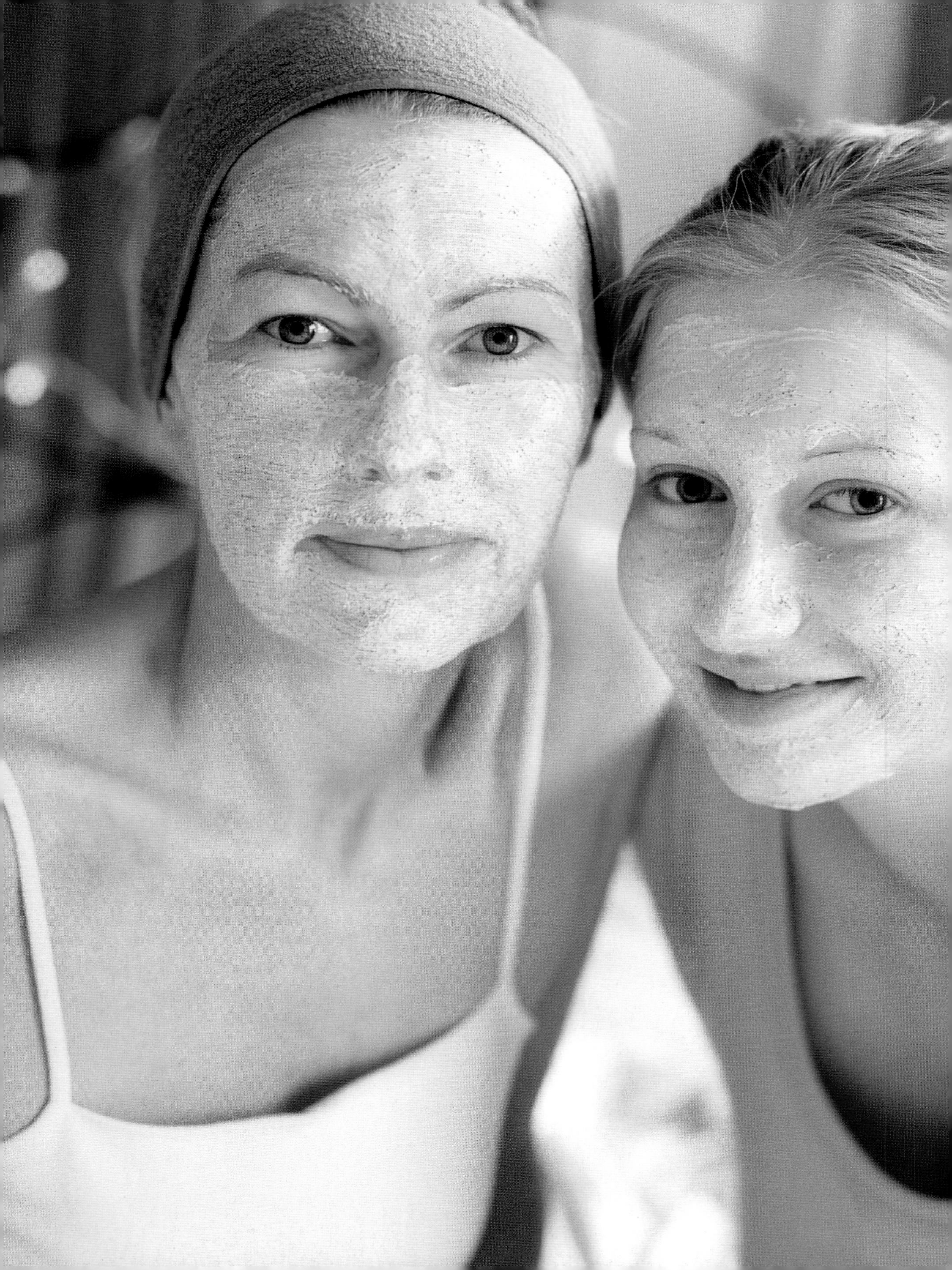

10

More than SKIN DEEP

Nature gives you the face you have at 20; at 50 you get the face you deserve – so Coco Chanel is said to have remarked. She may have meant it ruefully, but actually this is good news. There is much you can do to care for your skin and your general appearance as you grow older. It's not about making yourself look desperately or unnaturally youthful; it's about having a countenance that reflects clearly, as if in a mirror, your personality, your acquired wisdom, your rich inner life. A face that does that is by definition beautiful – at 50, 60 or any age at all.

Eat foods rich in vitamin A or beta-carotene to hold wrinkles at bay and aid skin healing, say US scientists.

HEALTHY SKIN
how it changes

Your skin will alter as you grow older. But the lifestyle choices you make, and the way you care for your skin, will have a big impact on the way it looks and feels.

As you age, the cells of the skin's outer layer (the epidermis) become visibly thinner and paler. The dermal layer beneath also thins. The dermis is the part of the skin that contains collagen, the protein that gives the skin strength; here, too, is the elastin that makes it stretchy. So with age, the skin has a reduced ability to snap back into shape after being stretched. This is what leads to wrinkling and sagging.

These skin changes are made more obvious because the fat cells in the subcutaneous layers of skin below shrink so there's less fat to plump out the loose skin. What's more, the blood vessels in these connective tissues become more fragile. Along with the loss of protective fat, this causes older skin to become more vulnerable to bruising and bleeding. And there's evidence that wounds take up to four times longer to heal in older people. So skin care isn't just about appearance – it's a vital part of health care as you get older.

THE CARE OF YOUR SKIN

Although changes to the skin are a natural part of ageing, lifestyle factors still play a big part. And there's a lot that you can do to keep older skin looking and feeling healthy. For a start, nothing ages your skin quicker than getting too much sun. That's why dermatologists say that the number-one product for mature skin is sunscreen. Shielding your skin from sunlight is also the best way to avoid age spots – mottled patches of discoloration due to melanin (skin pigment) accumulation; special skin-bleaching products can help to lighten these. To sun-proof older skin:

- Apply sunscreen daily whenever you go outdoors to prevent further damage from ultraviolet rays.
- Choose a product that blocks both UVA and UVB rays with SPF30 or higher on all exposed areas.

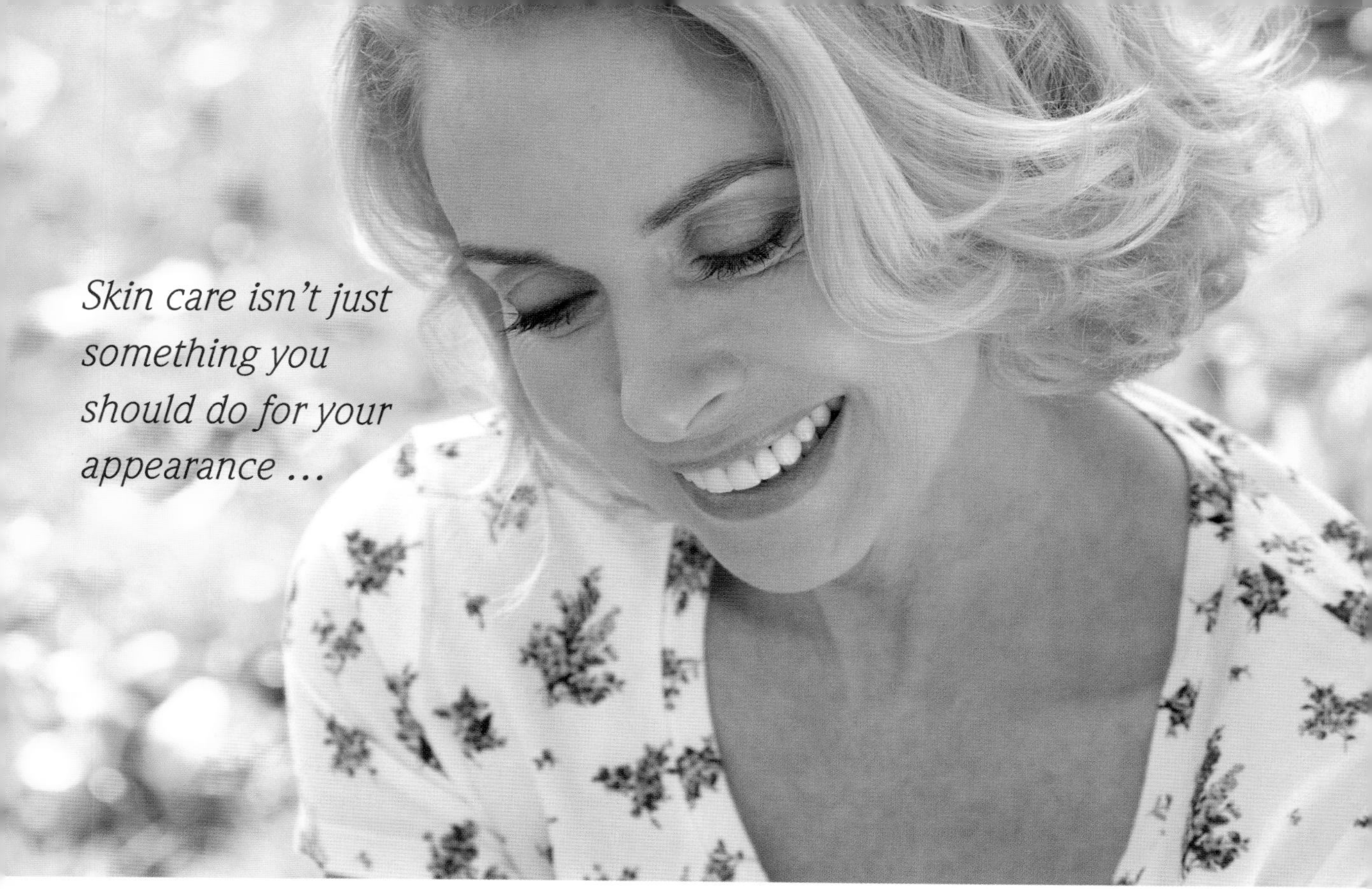

- For thinning hair, wear a hat; apply sunscreen to any bald patches.
- But don't slap on the sunscreen too soon: some exposure to sunlight is important for processing vitamin D (*see* page 120).

As well as using sunscreen, be kind to skin in the following ways:
- **Keep fit** Exercise nourishes your skin cells by increasing blood flow, helping to flush toxins out of the body, as well as improving tone in the muscles supporting the skin.
- **Become a non-smoker** Smoking reduces blood flow in the skin, damaging the connective tissue and causing wrinkling.
- **Get your beauty sleep** The skin repairs itself as you sleep, and too little sleep triggers the production of cortisol, a stress hormone that breaks down skin cells, increasing wrinkling and inflammation.
- **Eat a skin-friendly diet** Have lots of fresh fruit and vegetables and stay well hydrated. Avoiding alcohol at least two nights each week and cutting down on coffee and sugar helps clean up your liver – and thereby clears your skin of blemishes, say some dermatologists.
- **Beat stress** Stress disrupts your natural hormone balance, which in turn hinders your skin from healing itself. Taking daily exercise

DID **you** KNOW?

Your nose and ears often look bigger as you get older. This is not because they actually get bigger, but because weaker muscles make your skin less resistant to gravity and this elongates your ears and the tip of your nose, as well as pulling down the skin around your eyes and along your jaw. And if you lose fat underneath your skin, it can make your cheeks and eye sockets look hollow.

take CARE! Spot SKIN CANCER

Skin cancer is a growing problem in later life. People over 75 are five times more likely to have the most common form – basal cell carcinoma – than people aged 50 to 55.

Watch out for lumps, sores that don't heal or spots that ooze or crust – and get them checked and treated as quickly as possible, beginning with a biopsy, followed by a minor operation, usually carried out under local anaesthetic. They are rarely if ever a serious hazard. It's also vital to watch out for other skin cancers. In squamous cell carcinoma, most common in people over 40, thickened, scaly skin slowly turns into a hard, reddish brown lump, usually on the face. Malignant melanoma, the most dangerous kind of skin cancer, affects all ages but is most serious in people over 65. It normally appears as a quick-growing irregular, dark-coloured spot on previously normal skin or an existing mole that changes size and colour and becomes itchy and crusty and prone to bleeding. If you notice any of these changes in the skin, see your doctor straight away – prompt treatment is essential.

and treating yourself to regular body massages are both good for your skin – and your stress levels.

- **Avoid crash diets** Researchers in Ohio, who compared 200 pairs of identical twins aged 40-plus, found that being excessively thin was more ageing than 'bad' genes. 'These findings give scientific credence to what we always thought but couldn't prove,' says Dr Rajiv Grover, president of the British Association of Aesthetic Plastic Surgeons. 'It is not what your mother or father looks like but volume-loss that makes you look older.'

Combating dry skin

In women, the skin becomes drier and itchier from around 50 when the sebaceous glands start to work less well. Men tend to get dry skin, too, but it develops much later. To keep your skin well hydrated:

- Bathe or shower once a day at most. Use lukewarm rather than hot water. Avoid soap that dries your skin – and ban sponges, scrubbing brushes and flannels that might scratch it.
- Use a humidifier to help replenish humidity in the skin's outer layer.
- Applying unperfumed moisturiser while your skin is still damp seals in moisture. Men often find themselves buying a moisturiser, hand cream or body lotion for the first time later in life – there are now many unperfumed products available.

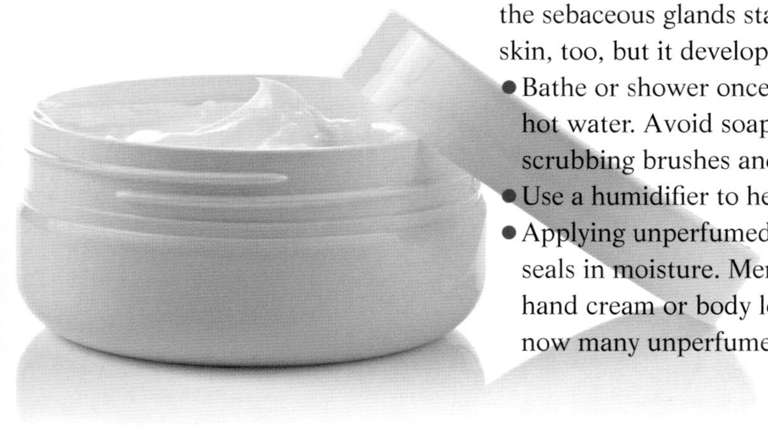

7 magical ways to nourish MATURE SKIN

Diet can be as important as lotions and potions in keeping your skin properly hydrated and as resilient as possible to bruising and wrinkling. Eating a variety of nutritious foods is the best way to nourish your skin from the inside. Here's the lowdown:

1 OIL FROM WITHIN Vitamin E in almonds, avocados, hazelnuts, pine nuts, and sunflower and corn oil is a powerful anti-oxidant that protects skin from sun damage and the harmful effects of toxic free radicals.

2 ENJOY GRAPES Sorbitol, which gives grapes, berries, plums and pears their sweetness, is a humectant, a substance that attracts water when applied to the skin, helping it to absorb and retain moisture.

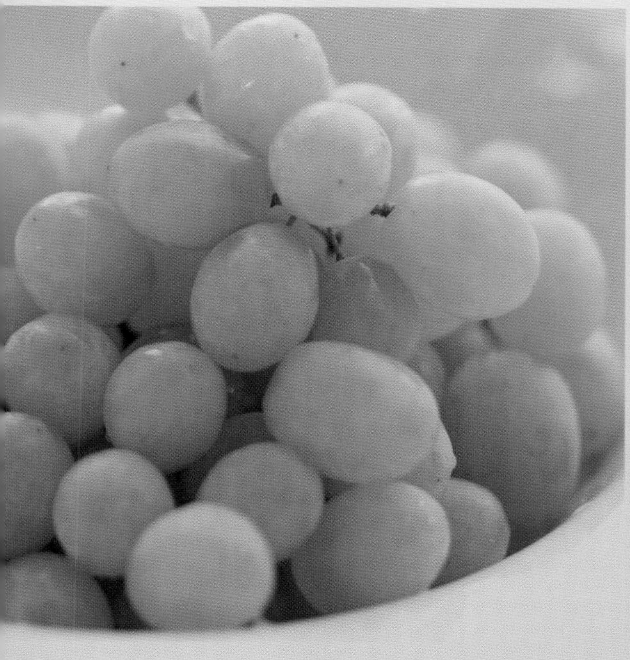

3 CHOOSE VITAMIN C–RICH FRUITS Vitamin C in fruits, especially blackcurrants, blueberries, kiwi fruit, oranges and strawberries, helps to make collagen, the structural fibres that speed wound-healing as well as strengthening your skin and helping to make it more elastic.

4 EAT OILY FISH Salmon and other oily fish are rich in DMAE (dimethylaminoethanol), a compound that boosts muscle tone and is one of the must-have ingredients in expensive 'mature' skin creams. Eating oily fish twice a week offers the same benefits.

5 GO GREEN Vitamin K – in kale and other green vegetables – helps your blood coagulate, reducing the impact of bruising. Avoid a sudden increase in vitamin K-containing foods if you're taking warfarin as it may alter its effectiveness.

6 GO RED Lycopene in tomatoes seems to give skin powerful protection against UV rays, according to a number of small studies.

7 ENLIST THE A TEAM Vitamin A in milk, eggs, liver and fish liver oil helps prevent further wrinkles as well as infections in injured skin, according to a study of 4025 women aged up to 74 years. Beta-carotene, which is transformed into vitamin A in your digestive tract, is found in orange, yellow, red and dark green fruit and vegetables.

Enjoy grapes ... they help to absorb and retain moisture in the skin.

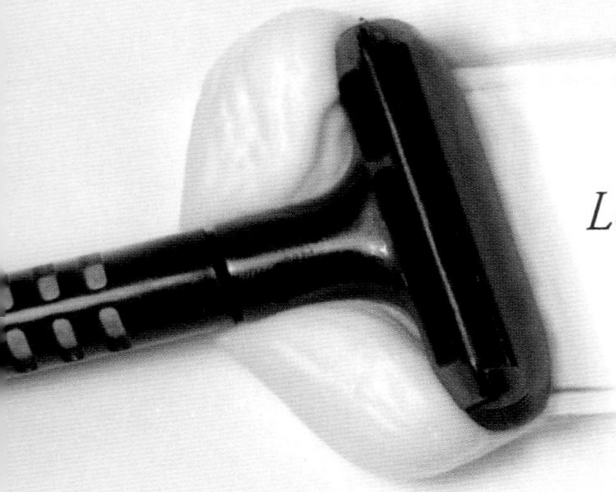

Leave your shaving cream or gel on your skin for several minutes before using the razor ...

- Never scratch an itch. It can lead to rashes and even bacterial infection. Use moisturiser or a cold pack to control itchiness.
- When shaving, use a shaving cream or gel and leave it on your skin for several minutes before applying the razor.

COMMON SKIN PROBLEMS

Nine out of ten older people have some kind of skin disorder. While symptoms such as dryness, a rash or discoloration can be part of ageing, they can also be a reaction to medication or a sign of nutritional deficiency (which can be rectified). Skin problems can also be associated with illnesses such as diabetes or heart disease, but it is unlikely that a serious problem would show only on the skin.

Bruising and wounds

As you age your ability to sense touch and pressure reduces – so you are more prone to injury. Your skin is also more likely to bruise: blood vessels are less robust in older people, so are more likely to rupture (the cause of bruising). In addition, some medications, including daily aspirin or warfarin, worsen bruising. There's good news if you keep fit, though: exercise may aid bruise and wound healing, according to researchers in Chicago.

- Speed healing by applying a cold compress and elevating the affected area. Many people swear by arnica cream, and some studies have shown positive results when it's used after cosmetic procedures.

Rosacea

This skin disorder, characterised by facial flushing and redness, is usually triggered by spicy food, alcohol and hot drinks, and possibly stress. It may be partly inherited and is most common in people with pale skin. It worsens with age if it's not managed, so:

- Avoid the food and drink that triggers it.
- Ask your doctor for an antibiotic cream – this appears to work by dampening down inflammation. Laser therapy may also help.

- Cover it up. Some experts advise against this on the grounds that cream will irritate facial redness, but a review of existing research, published in the *British Medical Journal* in 2012, shows that wearing appropriate camouflage cream (alone or under make-up) boosts morale in people of both sexes with rosacea.

Skin tags

These small flesh-coloured or brown growths, which grow in folds of skin, especially around the neck, armpits, groin, under the breasts, eyelids or buttocks, are more common with age. They are harmless and rarely cause pain unless they get caught in zips or jewellery. They don't usually need treatment, but you can get them removed if you dislike them – you may have to have this done privately.

HANDS, LEGS AND FEET

Your hands, like your face, tend to show your age. The skin on the backs is naturally thin and delicate, and made more so by frequent handwashing and sun damage (which also makes them prone to age spots). Hands tend to get bonier and more veiny with age, too, as muscle and fat tissue is lost or replaced more slowly, making them more at risk of bruising and injury.

- Use a good hand cream frequently. Slap on hand cream with added sunscreen whenever you go out.
- Brighten dull hands by exfoliating regularly: use sea salt mixed with lemon juice and gently scrub into your hands with an old toothbrush. Or go for a chemical peel that uses fruit acids or laser skin resurfacing from a qualified practitioner.
- Keep nails dry and clean to prevent bacteria or fungi growing underneath. Wear cotton-lined rubber gloves to do housework.
- Watch out for nail discolouration: it can be a sign of illness (though if you have dark skin, you may naturally have dark stripes on your nails). A dark, pigmented line on a nail can be an early sign of skin cancer – see a doctor if you spot this.

'Whatever you may look like, marry a man your own age – as your beauty fades, so will his eyesight.'

Phyllis Diller, American actress and comedian

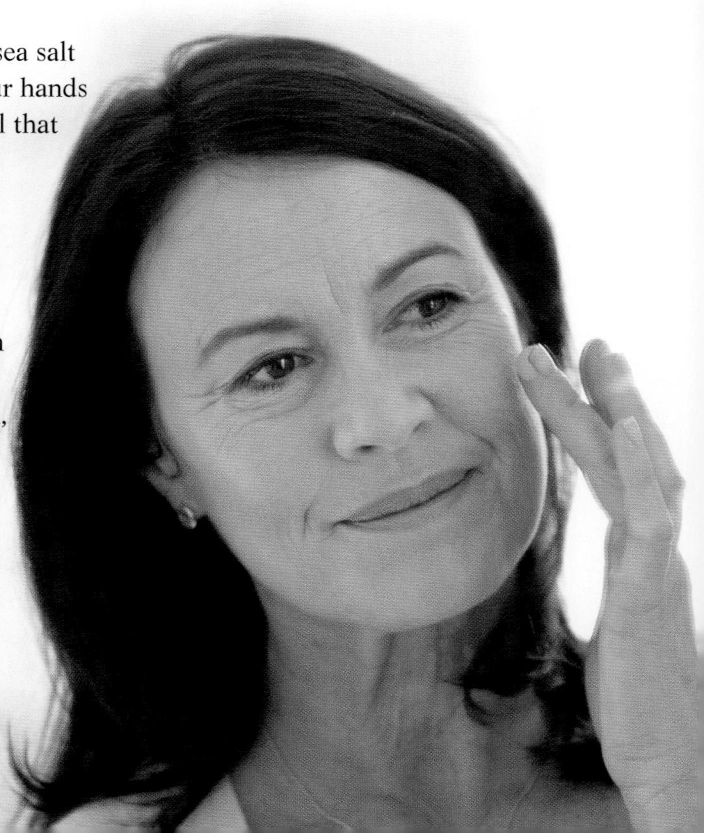

Rosacea – if the redness bothers you, cover it up ...

what's NEW

FOAM SCLEROTHERAPY The most effective treatment for varicose veins (*see* below) is also the cheapest, the least invasive and the one with fewest risks, less pain and a faster recovery, researchers at Imperial College London reported in 2011. Foam sclerotherapy, involving the injection of a chemical foam into the vein, has until recently been seen as only marginally helpful, appropriate solely for treating tiny spider veins. But the new study has given the thumbs-up to foam sclerotherapy for all types of varicose veins, which should save on time, money and suffering.

Pamper your feet

Healthy feet are crucial to your long-term independence and mobility, and it's important to examine your feet regularly, taking notice of any red patches, swelling, cracks or breaks in the skin, sores or very dry or hard skin.

Whatever you do, don't cover up problems with a slick of toenail polish or forgiving shoes and forget about them. Think about seeing a podiatrist, who can remove hard skin and give you a pedicure. Or treat yourself to a home pedicure (*see* right).

Beware toenail fungus, in which the nail becomes thickened and discoloured. It's more common in older people because of poor circulation. Cut the risk by keeping your feet clean and dry, wearing fresh cotton socks or tights daily, and using flip-flops at swimming pools. If you do get it, see your doctor for oral medications such as terbinafine or itraconazole.

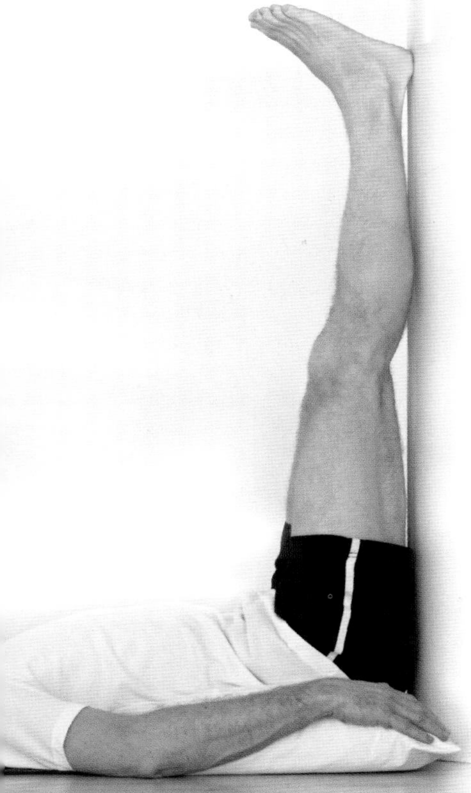

Varicose veins

Varicose veins occur when the valves in the veins stop working properly, so that blood flows back down and causes the veins to bulge. The problem worsens with age and is aggravated by prolonged standing, obesity or straining through constipation or a long-term cough. To keep leg veins healthy:

- **Keep walking** The pumping action pushes blood back to the heart.
- **Move about** Don't sit around for long periods – walk about, or do foot exercises when watching TV (*see* page 173).
- **Put your feet up** Raise your legs above the level of your heart for at least 15 minutes a day. Lie on your back with your bottom against a wall and legs raised; put a cushion under your hips.
- **Get support** Wear compression stockings to encourage good blood flow; ask your doctor what level of compression you need.

If your veins are painful or you dislike them, treatment options include sclerotherapy – in which a liquid chemical is injected into the vein – or simple surgery (ligation) in which the ends of the veins are tied off and removed; you will need a general anaesthetic if the veins are large and deep. Laser treatment is also sometimes used.

Raise your legs to ease the pressure on damaged veins and help strengthen valves.

Work it out An **AGE-BUSTING** pedicure

Bathe your feet in warm water to ease aches and pains the traditional way. A weekly home pedicure – for men and women – helps keep your feet in top condition.

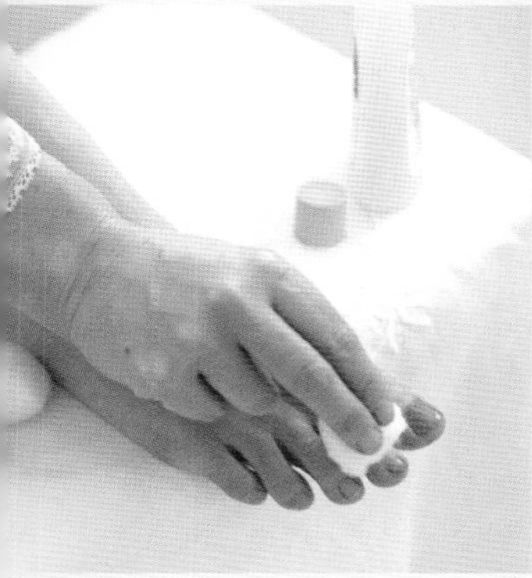

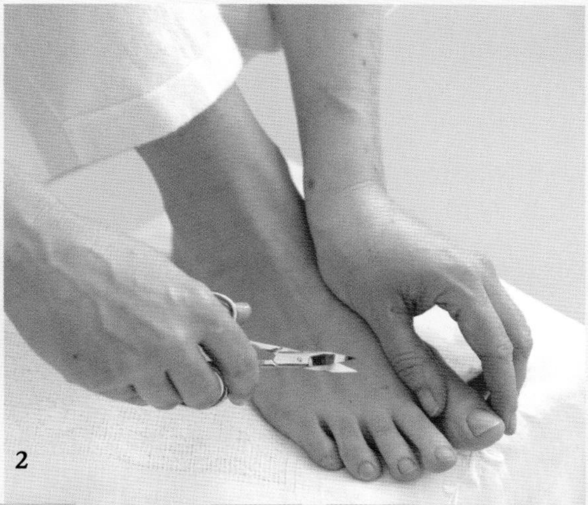

2

1 Wash your feet thoroughly using a good moisturising soap directly on your feet (women: remove any old nail varnish first).

2 Trim toenails straight across to avoid ingrown toenails (spikes of nail that can grow into the flesh around your toe and have to be surgically removed).

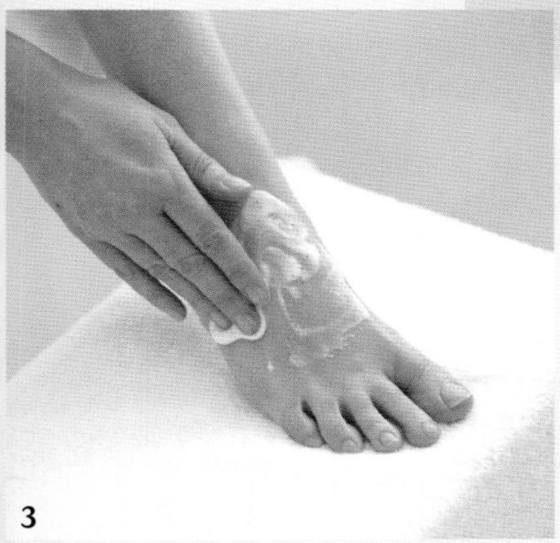

3

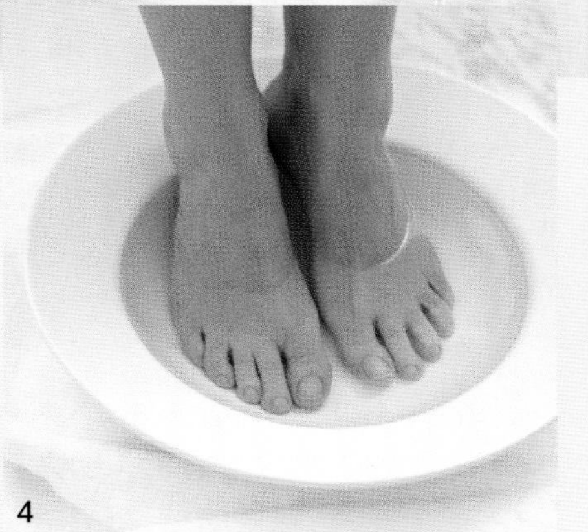

4

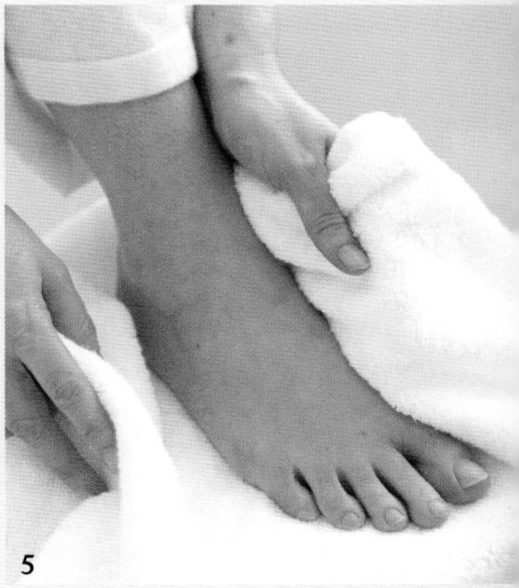

5

3 Massage your feet with an exfoliating foot scrub, using circular motions, then rinse it off afterwards. Gently rub with a foot file or rough washer to scrape away dead and dry skin on your heels and the bottom part of your foot.

4 Next, soak your feet for 20 minutes in a basin of warm water laced with Epsom salts and a few drops of tea tree or wild oregano oil. This remedy is believed to prevent toenail fungus and athlete's foot.

5 Pat your feet with a towel and apply petroleum jelly all over while your skin is still slightly damp to trap in moisture. The jelly helps to keep your nails hydrated and softens any dry, cracked skin. Put on cotton socks and keep them on for at least 20 minutes or overnight.

TEETH AND GUMS
keep them strong

Good dental care becomes even more important as you get older because your teeth are at greater risk of decay. And the latest research shows that problems in the mouth can trigger health conditions elsewhere in the body.

It's possible to have healthy teeth and gums into your 90s, if you practise good dental health care. But some changes are inevitable. The good news is that the nerves in your teeth become less sensitive to pain as you get older. But this could also mean that you don't detect a cavity or root problem until it is more advanced, so regular check-ups are even more important. And gums may recede more, exposing the roots and making them sensitive to hot or cold foods and more vulnerable to decay.

As you age, gum disease becomes more common and your saliva production diminishes (this happens naturally and can also be the result of medication and disease). All these changes can be counterbalanced by a good dental routine:

- **Brush up** Clean teeth at least twice, and floss at least once a day – crucial to avoid a build-up of tooth- and gum-rotting plaque.
- **Go electric** An electric toothbrush cleans efficiently and is easier to use if your joints are stiff. The small head is easy to manoeuvre, too.
- **All change** Get a new brush or head once the bristles start to splay.
- **Get checked** See your dentist at least once every six months. Your dentist doesn't just check your teeth but will also look for other oral problems including mouth cancer.
- **Limit sugar** Reduce your intake of sugary foods, which can erode dental enamel (though whole fresh fruit seems to reduce dental caries, according to researchers at the University of Newcastle).
- **Chew gum** Stimulate saliva flow by chewing sugar-free gum – very effective if you have a dry mouth – to help prevent dental decay.
- **Keep up calcium** Eat dairy foods for their calcium content. Cheese is good for teeth because it stimulates saliva flow and contains fats that stop bacteria sticking to tooth surfaces.

DID **you** KNOW?

Gum or periodontal disease is the most common cause of tooth loss in later life. Research conducted at Niigata University in Japan monitored the gum health of 4542 people aged 70. It found that when it comes to gum disease, the biggest risk factors are smoking, drinking and poor dental hygiene, but that it can be combated with simple measures such as regular brushing, flossing, using interdental brushes (small angled brushes to help you get between your teeth) and visiting a dental hygienist every six months.

A WHITER SMILE

Teeth get darker, yellower, and more stained with age, especially if you consume staining food and drinks or you smoke. Here are four of the best ways to give your mouth a natural-looking, youthful sparkle.

1 Use whitening toothpaste daily. It won't change the colour of your teeth, but will lift stains from coffee, red wine and spicy food.

2 If you want to improve your smile further, consult a dentist. You can swap amalgam fillings at the front of your mouth with white fillings – matched to your tooth colour.

3 Ask your dentist about getting a bleaching kit, the best-researched and most effective (not to mention cost-effective) way to whiten your teeth. A rubber mouth tray is prepared by your dentist to fit your teeth exactly – you then fill it with the bleaching gel provided and wear it during the night or over a period of hours each day for several weeks. It can whiten your teeth by up to 11 shades. Do a test first, to check that you are not sensitive to the bleach.

4 For damaged or chipped teeth, a range of treatments are available. The best are veneers – wafer-thin strips, normally made of porcelain, which are stuck to your existing teeth – or crowns that replace most of your tooth. Good dentists will recommend the most conservative and least invasive treatment. Putting in a single crown or a veneer to replace a damaged tooth, and matching it to the tooth on either side, requires immense expertise (beware dentists who suggest you invest in a strip of several veneers – especially at a reduced price per tooth). To replace missing teeth, a bridge or fixed partial denture is a joined set of artificial teeth. If there's not enough root to hold a bridge, an implant can be fixed directly into the jaw bone – provided the bone is healthy.

DID **you** KNOW?

An antiseptic mouthwash such as Listerine could save your life. How? There's increasing evidence that periodontal disease doesn't just affect your gums but causes body-wide inflammation that increases your risk of cardiovascular disease, diabetes and Alzheimer's. The mouthwash antiseptics help combat the bacteria involved in periodontal disease. A Taiwanese study found that people who regularly visited a dental hygienist (or had their teeth cleaned by a dentist) cut their risk of heart attack by 24 per cent and stroke by 13 per cent.

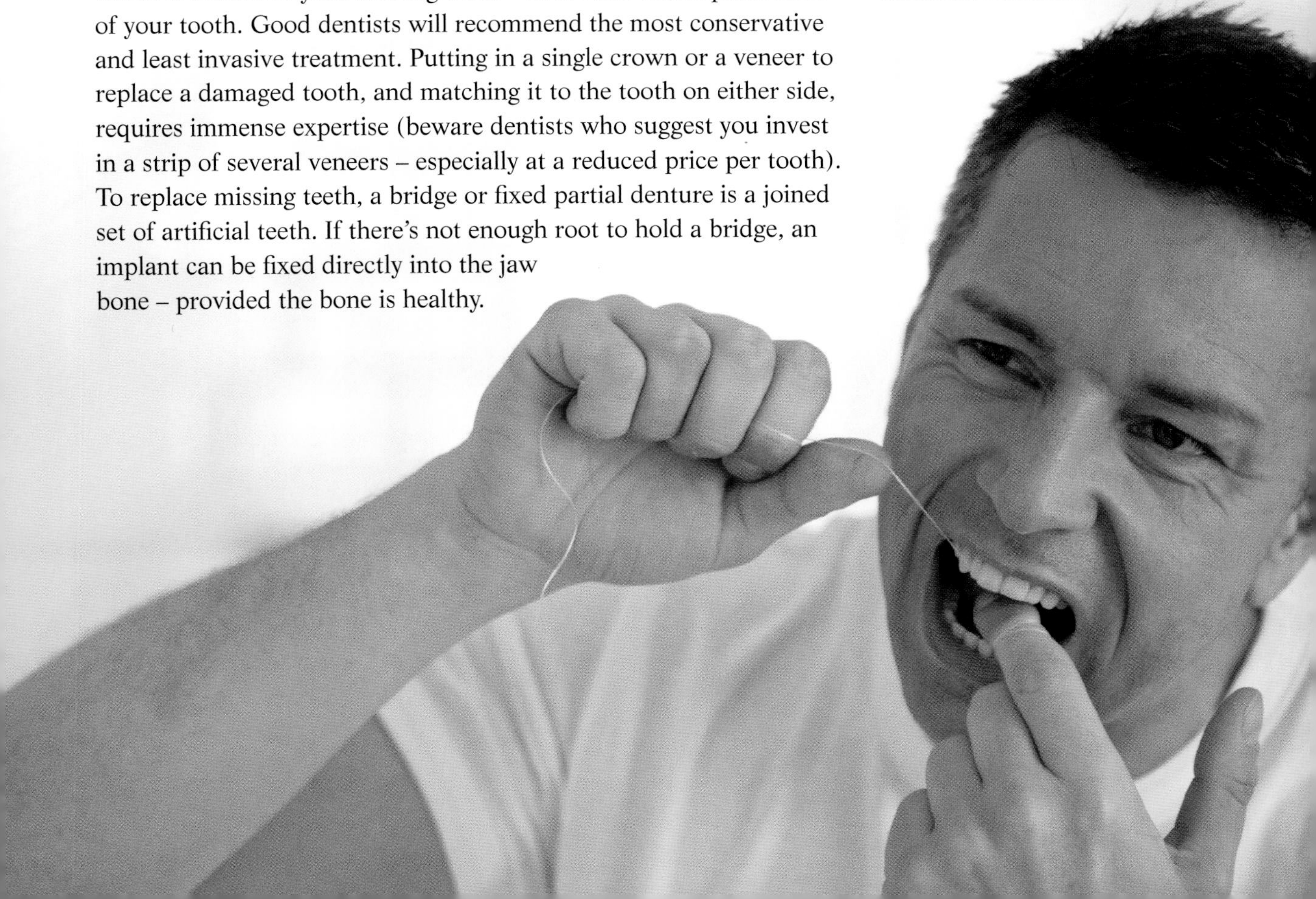

Disguise thinning hair with a good cut, a lighter colour, and by using volumising products.

CROWNING GLORY
you and your hair

Hairstyles for the over-60s used to be uniform: short permed iron-grey or white hair for women and a short back and sides or comb-over for men. The advent of non-messy, natural-looking hair dye and more adventurous barbers have changed all that.

You'll find you need to spend more time on your hair to keep it looking good as you get older. Most people find that their hair thins and the follicles produce less pigment, turning the hair grey. And a certain level of baldness becomes a fact for most men and a surprisingly large percentage of women: as many as three out of four women over the age of 65 are at least partly bald.

There are plenty of clever ways to disguise these changes. Volumising products can help with thinning hair – and a good cut can make all the difference to the way you look (*see* box, right). Grey hair can look very stylish, but dyeing hair is now so common – among men as well as women – that no one could call it vanity.

USING COLOUR

Many men and women dye their hair brown or black to help them look younger. But at some point, you may decide that dark hair no longer flatters your skin colour or fits your overall look. What then? Plan ahead, if possible with your hairdresser's help.

- Begin by going a shade or two lighter every couple of months, perhaps with lighter streaks. Hair that is dyed blond tends to look better than hair dyed dark.
- If you want to revert to your natural hair colour, expect the process to take 12 months or so.
- Add coloured streaks if you want a bit of a lift: perhaps dark blond or, if you want to make a dramatic statement, aubergine or red.
- If your natural colour doesn't now suit your skin tone, try a snowy white or silver. This can look sharp and attractive on both sexes while working well with an older complexion.

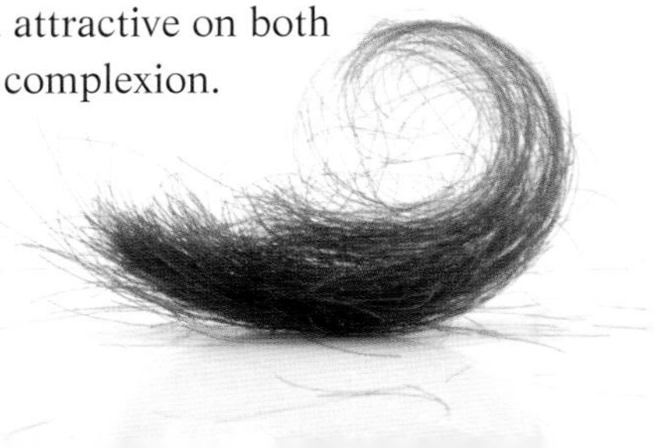

5 top styles to keep **HAIR LOOKING GOOD**

Men:

1 Keep your hair short: it gives it lift and makes it look as though you've got more of it.

2 If you've started to go bald, say no to a comb-over, which fools no one. If you have got a large bald spot, think about going completely clean-shaven, especially if you feel comfortable with exposing the shape of your head. The benefits include never having to worry about hairstyles again.

3 An alternative is the buzz cut: a very short haircut achieved with clippers all over the head – another low-maintenance option.

4 A slightly longer option is to have your hair cut to one inch all over your head, with longer layers on the crown and a fringe cut and combed forward.

5 A textured crop involves a series of layers cut into the hair on the top of the head and at the sides, giving a slightly more messy look that effectively disguises thinning or receding hair.

Women:

1 Long hair looks good pinned up or in a ponytail all the way through your 60s.

2 A short bob is a good way to disguise thinning hair, especially if it's fine and straight.

3 A short crop style, with lots of very short layers, looks fabulous on women who are happy with the shape of their head and have thick hair – and it can look great on greying hair.

4 A fringe or at least a half-fringe works to cover up wrinkles on the forehead, but it's not an inflexible rule: pulling your hair away from your face can be an attractive alternative, reflecting openness and confidence. Make sure you avoid pulling on the skin of your forehead too tightly – it looks unnatural and can give you a headache.

5 Use volumising styling products as your hair is likely to be thinner – and try a lighter colour as it can make thinning hair less obvious. Whether you have your hair washed at home or in a salon, use deep conditioning treatments regularly to combat dryness.

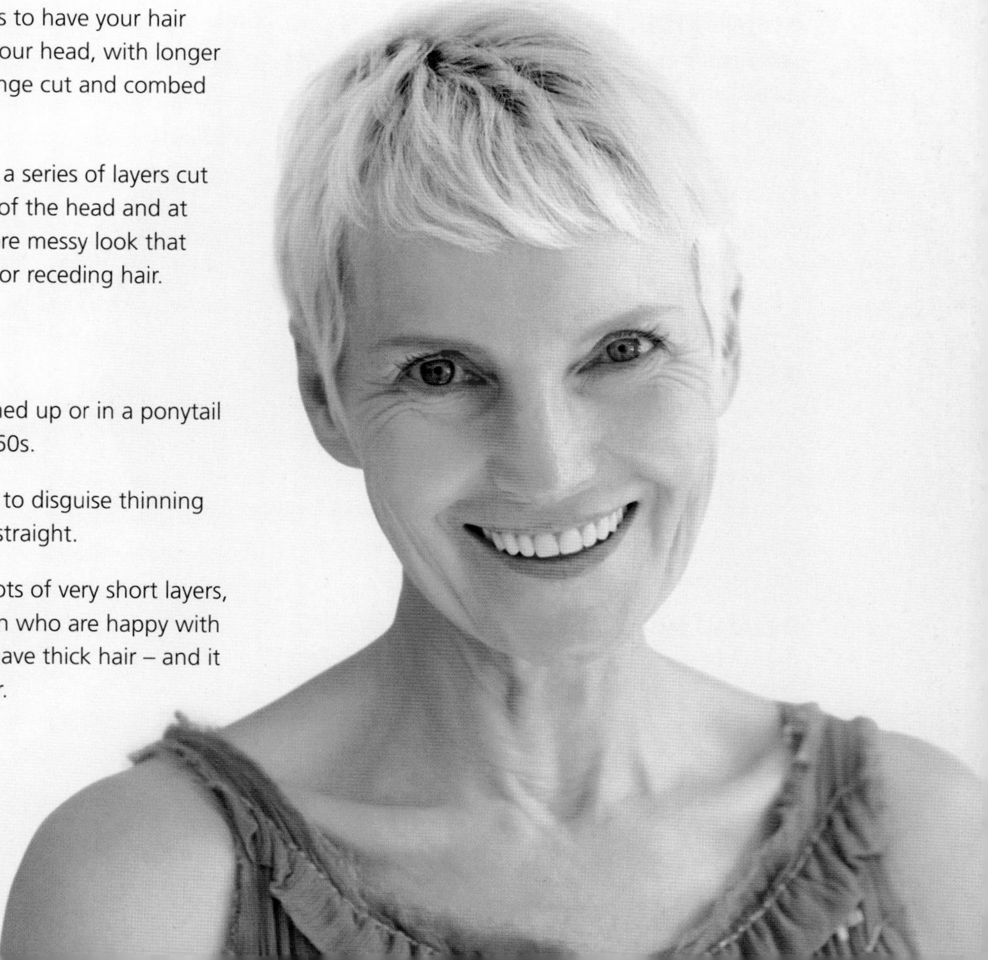

focus ON ... HAIR LOSS

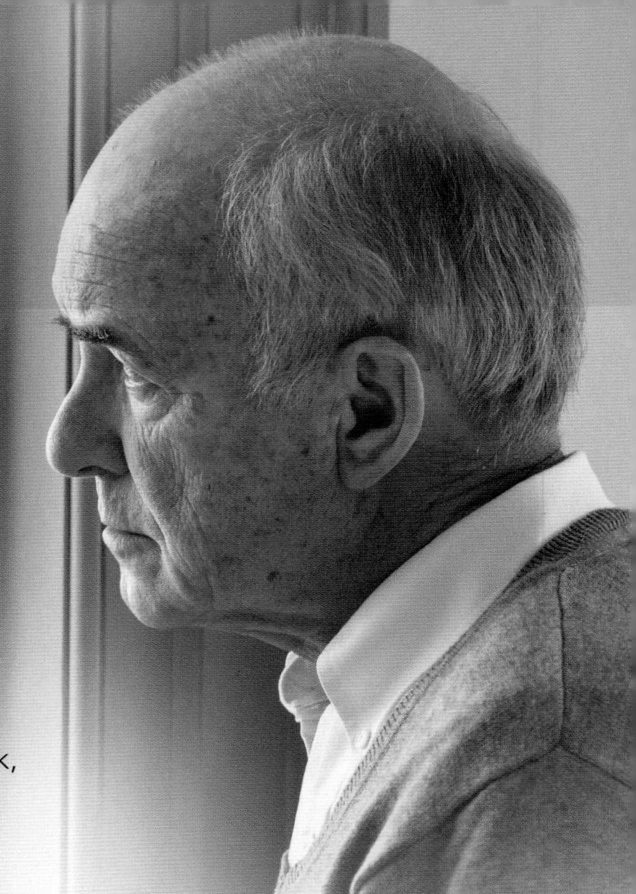

Is baldness irreversible? Many different products are available that promise to treat hair loss – some of them claiming impossible results. Here are five treatments that can work, at least for some people:

● **MINOXIDIL LOTION** First tested as an oral treatment for high blood pressure, minoxidil is now available as a lotion that you rub on your scalp. There is considerable evidence that it can stimulate new hair growth and strengthen existing hair. It doesn't work for everyone and it helps only for as long as you take the medication. Women seem to respond best – one in four has new hair growth, and others see hair loss slowed. You can get it from pharmacies without a prescription.

● **FINASTERIDE** This medication, used to treat prostate enlargement by inhibiting an enzyme involved in testosterone metabolism, can slow the progression of male-pattern baldness, and even promote hair regrowth. The effects last only as long as the tablets are taken; side effects may include erectile dysfunction.

● **HAND-HELD LASER THERAPY DEVICE** The science behind this device is exciting, the theory being that the laser delivers light therapy to the scalp, stimulating the mitochondria – the energy bundles within cells – to produce healthy, vibrant hair growth. The technology is still in its infancy, but it does offer new hope for the future.

● **HAIR TRANSPLANT** Scalp surgery involves transplanting your hair from one part of the scalp to another to fill in the balding areas. There's no need for stitches as the hair is held in place by the clotting action of the blood when the hairs are inserted. Within six months, the hair should settle and start to regrow. Hair transplants are normally carried out under local anaesthetic with several sessions usually required.

● **HAIR PIECES** The simplest way of addressing hair loss is with a wig or a hair piece. These used to be described as toupées – and were once seen as a bit of a joke. But hair pieces today can look very realistic. You can buy them in different sizes at department stores or over the internet. Acrylic versions are cheaper; if made from real hair, they can cost thousands of dollars.

LOOKING GOOD
your natural beauty

After the age of 60, your face may betray your years – no matter how fit and trim you are. But a regular skin-care routine and good grooming habits will help you to continue to look your best.

- **Cleanse with care** For men and women, cleansing and moisturising help to protect your skin and keep it healthy. Banish soap, which can be drying for older skin. Instead use a cleanser that gently washes without stripping skin of moisture. Avoid skin toners, especially those with a stringent or alcohol base. Use a good moisturiser day and night – and don't forget to apply sunscreen when you're out.
- **Close shave** Shaving can be harsh on the skin. Work glycerine-based 'skin food' into wet skin before you start, to avoid a rash. Then use a natural-based shaving soap (less drying than cream). Apply it with an old-fashioned shaving brush to lift the hairs away from the skin, allowing the razor to glide over your face. To shave your legs or under your arms efficiently, wet your skin with warm water (preferably in the shower). Massage the area with shaving cream or gel: this will make the hairs stand up and make shaving easier.
- **Frame your face** Keeping your eyebrows well groomed and shaped helps provide a frame for your face and draws attention to your eyes.
- **Remove excess hair** A good magnifying mirror and a pair of tweezers are essential for every bathroom. Facial hair is literally a growing problem as you age, so check your face regularly and remove excess hairs that sprout, or bushy eyebrow, nose and ear hair by tweezing, or get a barber to trim eyebrows, ears and nose hair (men) or see a qualified beauty therapist for threading (women).

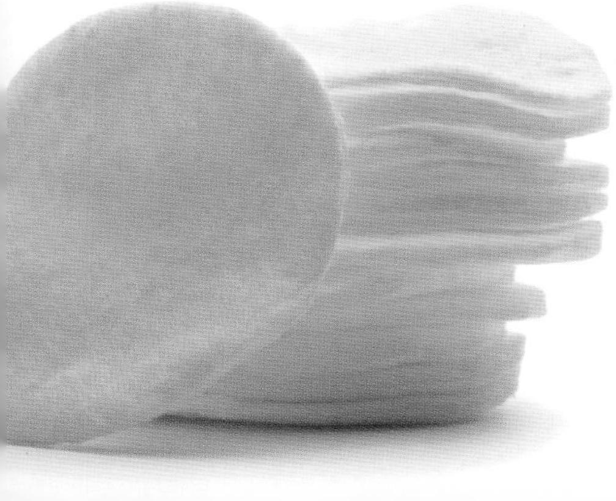

A good facial skin-care routine (for both men and women) will help to keep your skin healthy.

DID **you** KNOW?

Worrying about ageing is counterproductive according to a report published in the *Archives of General Psychiatry*. Scientists analysed the relationship between stress and wound healing and found that the stress hormone cortisol actually slows down the healing process in skin cells, thus promoting sagging, wrinkles and blemishes.

'By the time you hit 50, I reckon you've earned your wrinkles, so why not be proud of them?'

Twiggy, British model

- **Laser** A laser beam focuses on the area of hair growth to destroy the follicles beneath the skin surface, preventing hair from growing again. Laser treatment is expensive and should be provided only by trained practitioners – and perhaps reserved for very stubborn hair.

ANTI-AGEING PRODUCTS

Wrinkles are like scar tissue: once formed, they can be removed entirely only by surgery. Most of the products that claim to 'reduce the appearance of wrinkles' do so by filling in the cracks, like plaster on a wall. They have no actual effect on the skin.

So you shouldn't expect miracles, but a good anti-ageing cream can be a useful part of your skin-care regime, nevertheless. Creams containing active ingredients (dubbed 'cosmeceuticals') can be bought over the counter in department stores. You can also get stronger versions from cosmetic clinics – where they are individually selected by a dermatologist or qualified beauty therapist who will first conduct an examination of your skin. These tailored products are often no more expensive than over-the-counter versions.

Commercially available cosmeceuticals tend to contain one or more of the following active ingredients:

- Peptides: mini-proteins that stimulate the skin to make more collagen.
- Fruit acids or alpha-hydroxy acids (AHAs): that improve the smoothness and feel of the skin. To contain enough AHAs to be effective, they need to be dispensed by a doctor because they can cause irritation.
- Anti-oxidants: products containing vitamins C and E that help prevent wrinkles by soaking up harmful free radicals produced by the sun's rays on the skin.
- Coenzyme Q10: a vitamin-like substance thought to have anti-oxidant properties that may help protect skin.
- Tretinoin: a powerful Vitamin A derivative, used since the 1960s to treat acne, that can help to reverse wrinkles by increasing cell production, shedding dark pigment and increasing collagen formation.

what's **NEW**

EGF SERUMS AND ANTI-AGEING CREAMS are newly available from an Icelandic biotechnology company that has been able to reproduce naturally occurring Epidermal Growth Factor (EGF) from barley. In the human body, EGF works from the inside to speed up the rate of cell turnover within the skin, as well as maintaining and repairing skin cells. As we age, we naturally produce less EGF, which is why adding a drop or two of the biotechnologically produced EGF (which is genetically modified) is proving a successful formula – with research showing that it creates more radiance and reduces wrinkling.

8 new rules for MATURE MAKE-UP

'Be who you are' is the mantra for women who want cosmetics to look natural. That often means minimising the number of products you use – as well as finding make-up that suits your colouring today. Here's how to do it:

1 IDENTIFY STRONG POINTS Use make-up to emphasise your cheekbones, lips or eyes, thus drawing attention away from wrinkles and jowls. Find time for a free make-up lesson at your local department store to get ideas.

2 LESS IS MORE ON OLDER SKIN Heavy foundation creams and face powder can make dry older skin look flat and lifeless while also emphasising wrinkles and soft down on your face. Instead, use a light foundation that does not sit on wrinkles or, if your skin is good, a tinted oil-based moisturiser.

3 GO CREAMY A cream blusher can make a big difference to your skin tone by redressing the loss of vibrancy. Choose a colour that is slightly darker than your skin colour. Add a little dab of powder blusher to give staying power.

4 CONCEAL DARK SHADOWS If you use a concealer under your eyes, apply it from the inner corner to the midpoint, avoiding the outer corner, which will highlight wrinkles.

5 DITCH THE BLUE EYE SHADOW Avoid any kind of shiny or sparkly colour, too. Go for taupes and beiges, with the darker colour on the lid and a highlighting colour below the eyebrow, blended carefully.

6 CHOOSE THE RIGHT LIPSTICK This can add instant vibrancy to your appearance as well as making your lips look fuller. Experiment with pinks or reds that break new ground – and be prepared to ask for advice.

7 MATCH YOUR LIP LINER Make sure it is of similar colour to your lipstick – a darker liner will look harsh and ageing.

8 GET THE RIGHT MASCARA Choose one that doesn't smudge. Apply it to the top lashes and only lightly, if at all, to the lower lashes. Avoid eye liner in the daytime – and if you feel like using it in the evening, do so sparingly.

Choose the right lipstick – experiment with pinks or reds.

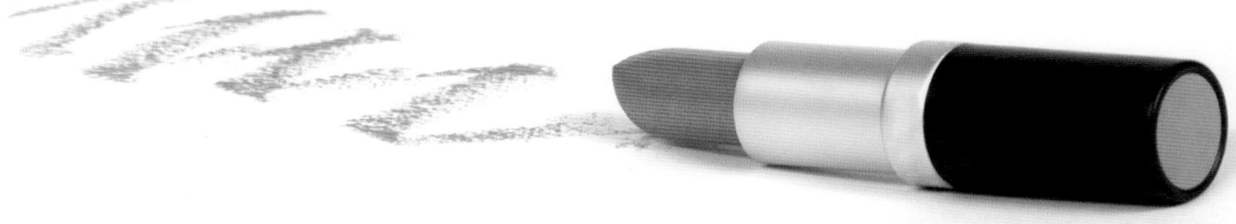

GET DRESSED UP
and feel fabulous

There are no hard and fast rules about looking stylish in your 60s and beyond. Instead, with the pressures of work and family taking less time, you can rethink your look, focusing on an honest assessment of what makes you look and feel great.

Some people find that with age they prefer to dress for comfort, while others want to take more chances, experimenting with looks that transcend their years. Whatever your basic style, one fundamental principle of good dressing is to avoid looking scruffy – this generally doesn't work for the older man or woman. Be ruthless with your wardrobe, getting rid of anything that you no longer wear or that doesn't suit you. Focus on what you do wear – and identify favourite shapes, fabrics and colours so that you can bear them in mind when you're next shopping for clothes.

Remember size is not important. If you're shy about revealing your shape, don't try to disguise it with loose, tent-like clothing. Instead, choose individual pieces with a good cut that accentuates your best features, whether these are your shoulders, chest/bust, a neat waist or long legs. Consider investing in some of the new shapewear garments that smooth and hold in the flesh. These come in the form of shirts, vests, pants and even suits for men, as well as leggings, swimwear and dresses for women, shaping tummies, bottoms and thighs that could do with a little firming.

Five rules for women

1 Great styling involves knowing what to show off and what to cover up. Three-quarter-length sleeves cover elbows and fleshy arms. Wear polo necks, high Mandarin-style collars, bright scarves or large chokers to hide a lined neck – while long skirts, well-cut trousers or flat boots will conceal varicose veins. New bolero-like arm stockings on sale in large stores are just the thing for covering up 'batwings' if you are self-conscious. Use hats to cover thinning hair or roots that need touching up.

DID you KNOW ?

Eighty-five per cent of women are wearing the wrong bra size, according to a Wollongong researcher. A common mistake is wearing a cup size that is too small and a back size that's too large. A good bra becomes even more important with age because breasts tend to droop after menopause due to reduced oestrogen. Get measured regularly and be prepared to pay more than you expect: modern well-made bras are small engineering triumphs, often comprising more than two dozen working parts.

One fundamental principle of good dressing: avoid looking scruffy ... this generally doesn't work for the older man or woman.

2 Limit the amount of beige and pastel colours in your wardrobe as it can be draining on pale skin and sends out a sartorial signal that says, 'Ignore me'. Many older people look better in bright, jewel-like colours: amethyst, turquoise, ruby. If that seems too strong for your colouring, try ice-blue, heathery greens and lilacs or silvery pale greys. Navy or clean, bright whites are flattering neutrals.
3 Use jewellery to add sparkle and to highlight your best features: a large ring or delicate bracelet emphasises beautiful hands or slender wrists, while bold sparkling earrings add warmth and colour to your face.
4 There's nothing wrong with keeping up with fashion, but bear in mind that classics have years of wear in them and properly fitting clothes look great on mature bodies. Invest in well-cut coats, suits, shirts and dresses and good-quality handbags or shoes.
5 Check your appearance in the mirror before you go out somewhere special. Use the time to fiddle with a scarf, make certain that your make-up is perfect, check you haven't overdone the jewellery.

Five rules for men

1 Know what to cover up. Keep shorts for the beach. Be aware that if you have a wrinkly neck and jowls, it's best to avoid tight-fitting polos or crew-neck jumpers, which squeeze the skin upwards. A shirt collar over a round-necked jersey is a good option. Wear a good dark-coloured shirt if you have a large stomach.
2 Get the details right: opt for well-cut classic lines and tailored clothes you can wear again and again – a dark suit, good jeans or cords, jumpers and a decent coat.
3 Choose richly coloured and patterned fabrics for shirts, ties, socks, hats and scarves. Joke ties and socks are best avoided.
4 Never leave the house with a broken zip or a missing button. If you find even a small hole in a jumper, stop wearing it and either get it darned or send it to a charity shop.
5 Don't skimp on your shoes. Cheap shoes can ruin a good outfit, and may even damage your feet. Ideally, buy one pair each of well-cut black and brown shoes and keep them polished. Keep your trainers for summer walks or for lazy days when you're wearing jeans.

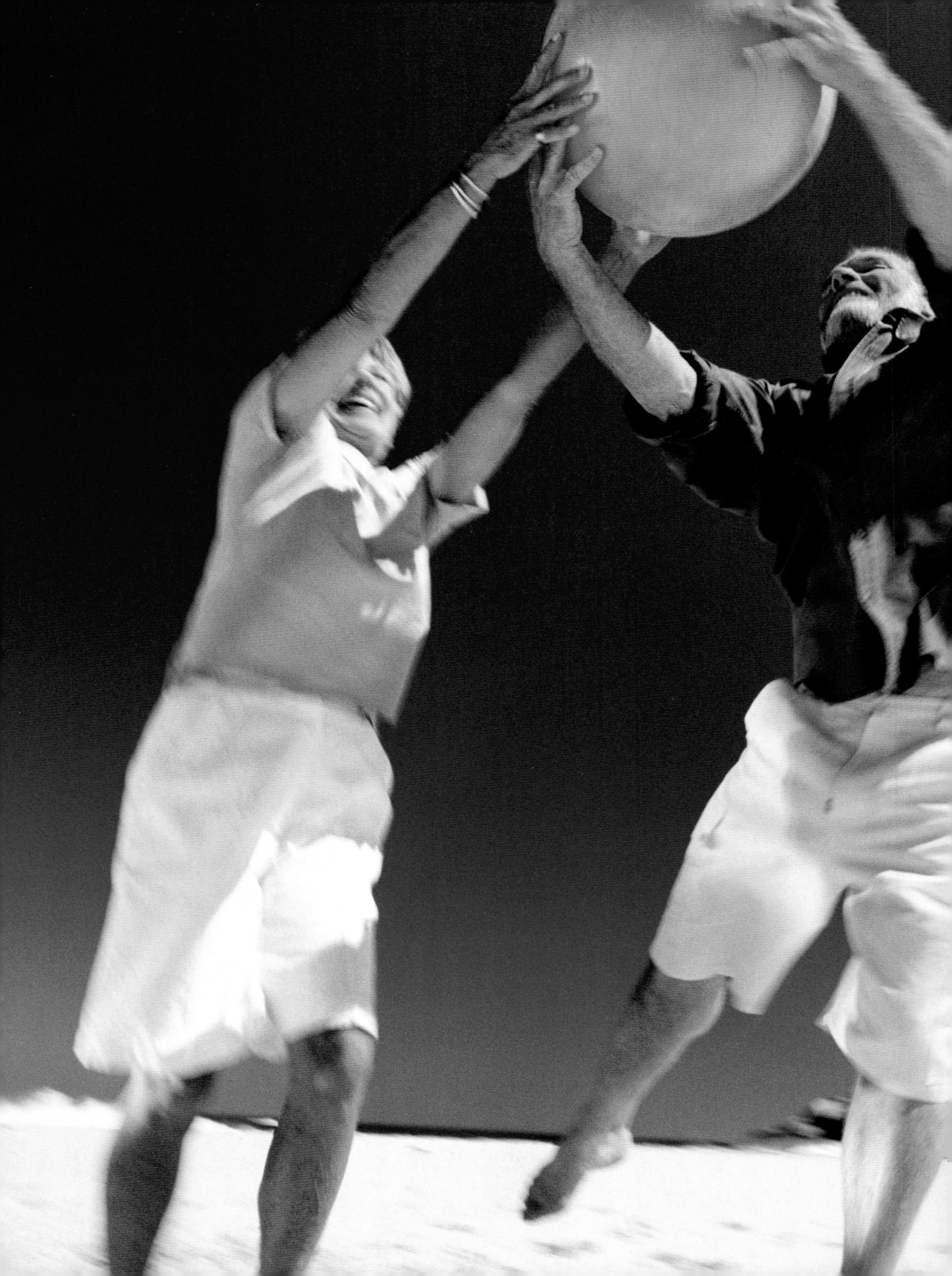

11

Loving LIFE

Most of us can hope to enjoy long years of retirement after our working lives come to an end – we have far more time to spend than any previous generation. It takes skill and planning to ensure that those post-work years are as healthy, happy and secure as can be. You may also have to put some effort into maintaining friendships and contacts – and there will be adjustments to be made in your relationship with your partner. But these years – your 60s, 70s, 80s and beyond – are above all a golden opportunity: a chance to enjoy new things, to fulfil long-nurtured ambitions, and to grow in ways that were not possible when your life was filled with workaday stresses and cares.

Age is a state of mind. Just 14 per cent of people over 60 feel their age, says a UK survey.

THE BEST IS NOW
living in the present

Our extended life spans mean greater possibilities in our later years than ever before. Not only are we living longer, we're staying 'younger' longer, in mind and body. It's up to you how you choose to spend your days: your 'golden years' are what you make of them.

The current generation of people in their 60s and beyond is surely the most active and adventurous ever. We're working, volunteering, travelling, writing blogs, running marathons, and learning to skydive and speak Italian. We may use our superannuation to start a business, sail around the world, or build the home we've always dreamed of. And we're enjoying having time to renew friendships and expand our horizons. In one British survey conducted in 2011, 62 per cent of over-60s said they had a better social life than their parents did at that age, and 73 per cent said they had more hobbies and interests.

EMBRACE YOUR AGE

What's so good about being old? Where do we start? Here are five great things to celebrate about the later years:

- **You can please yourself** Once you retire you can enjoy the freedom to focus your time and energies according to your own priorities, doing what motivates you, with the people you value and who enrich your life most. You know what you like and appreciate, but you stay open to new experiences, thoughts and challenges, too.
- **The concept of 'old' has changed** People in their 60s and 70s no longer accept being labelled as 'old'. According to a survey by one British insurer, only 14 per cent of over-60s said that they feel their actual age, with most believing that age is a state of mind.
- **Older people are a powerful force** Three-quarters of the over-60s say the 'old-age pensioner' label is out of date. And it is true. Older people are an increasingly powerful demographic group, influencing advertisers, politicians and the media. They also have the time, money and experience to play important roles in their communities.

- **There are benefits to an ageing population** Older people tend to be more law-abiding (it's predicted that crime rates will fall as a result of our ageing society). They read more and attend more theatre productions, concerts and art exhibitions, so demographic changes will benefit the arts. They volunteer more, helping to unite communities, and give considerable practical and financial support to the next generation.
- **Retiring is good for your health** You have no need to dread the health implications of ageing. In a UK study of people born in 1921, 78 per cent rated their health as good, very good or excellent. And a study of over 7000 British civil servants found that retiring was associated with better physical and mental health.

9 STEPS TO THE GOOD LIFE

There is no doubt that retirement can be a time of opportunity and independence, a chance to pursue your dreams and fill your days as you will. But you'll be able to take better advantage of your later years if you plan ahead. Surveys show that more than half of retirees, though happy with their lifestyle, wish they had done more to prepare, above all financially.

Not only are we living longer, we're staying 'younger' longer, in mind and body.

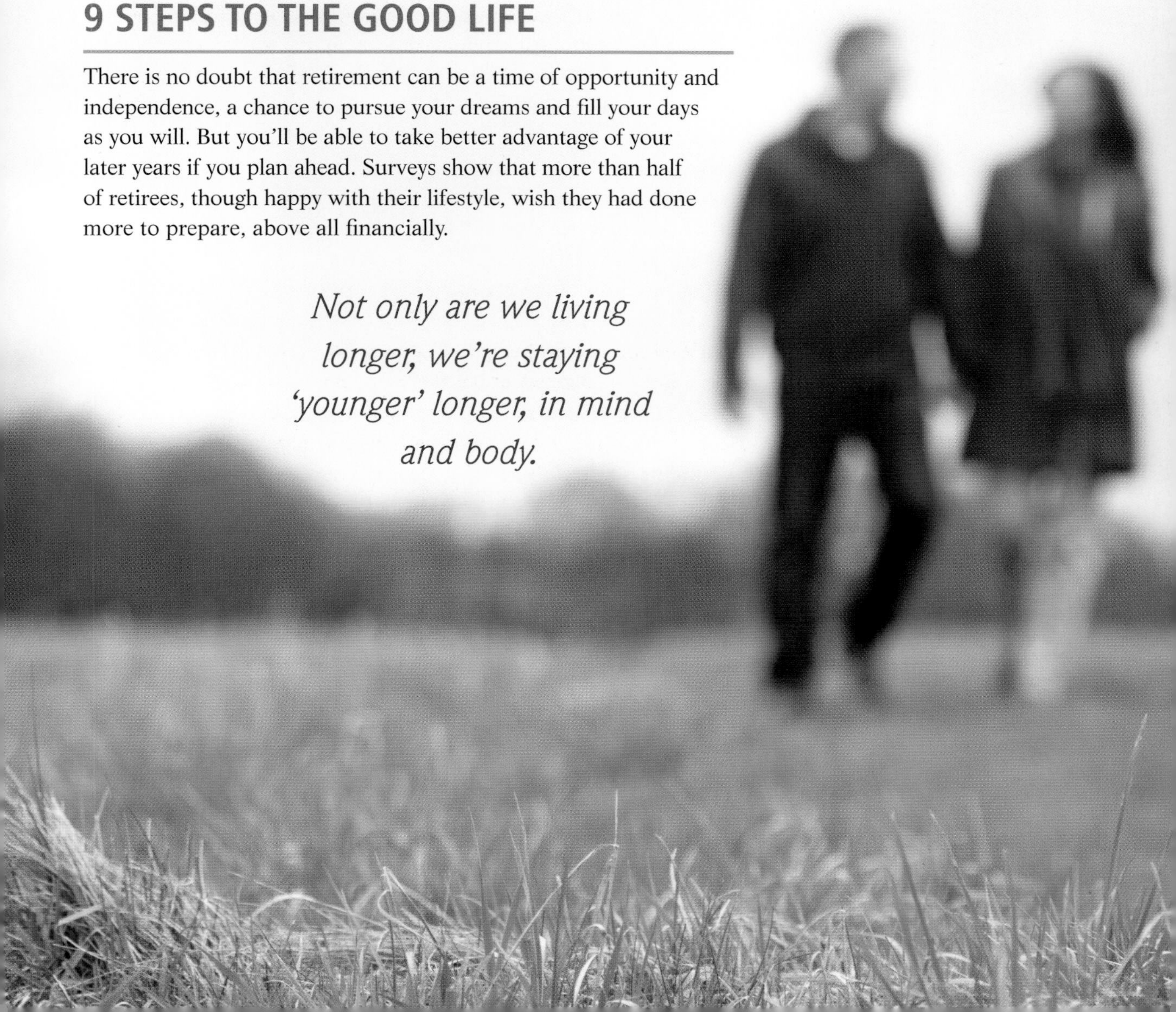

'Live your life and forget your age.'

Norman Vincent Peale,
American author

These are the key things to consider for a happy future – whether or not you have already retired:

- Think about the lifestyle you want – would you prefer to remain in work, stay in your current community, move to the sun or closer to your children, travel the world, return to education?
- Research the possibilities and think about the implications of your choice and how it affects your family and your finances.
- Consider whether you want to stop work abruptly, or would it suit you better to have a gentler transition through part-time or flexible working.
- Make sure your plans include productive activity, absorbing interests, nurturing relationships and an active social life. Whatever your age, it's important to have goals for the future.
- Conduct a thorough assessment of your current financial situation, superannuation, post-retirement budget and possible future financial needs (*see* pages 292–295).
- Look after yourself. Poor health is a major influence on wellbeing in retirement. If you have any concerns, see your doctor for prompt treatment.
- Get your weight within the healthy range (*see* pages 96–97). Obesity in later life is linked with chronic disease and a higher risk of falls and associated long-term disability.
- Make sure your preparations include provision for possible future ill health or care needs, as well as an emergency plan for support in a crisis.
- Get your house in order. Whether you stay where you are, downsize or relocate, your home should be a sanctuary, not a source of worry. Keep your house properly maintained, consider adaptations to make everyday life easier, and get rid of possessions that you no longer use or value.

WORK AND RETIREMENT

You may decide to stay on at work past the official retirement age, for personal fulfilment or for financial reasons. This is a more feasible option than ever before because our occupations tend to be less physically demanding than in the past, and anti-discrimination legislation has reduced age restrictions. And it has been shown that older workers compensate for any decline in their physical abilities, reaction times and information processing by using their superior

it's a **MYTH ...**

... that **OLDER PEOPLE** are more **MISERABLE**

After the stresses and strains of young adulthood and middle age, older people actually become happier and more contented again. In a survey of more than 340,000 Americans, people aged between 50 and 80 expressed the highest levels of contentment. Stress, anger and worry decreased, and happiness and enjoyment of life surged after middle age. This finding supports research using data on 2 million people from 80 countries: it revealed a U-shaped pattern for life happiness globally – meaning that people are generally least content in middle age, and happiest in their youth and old age.

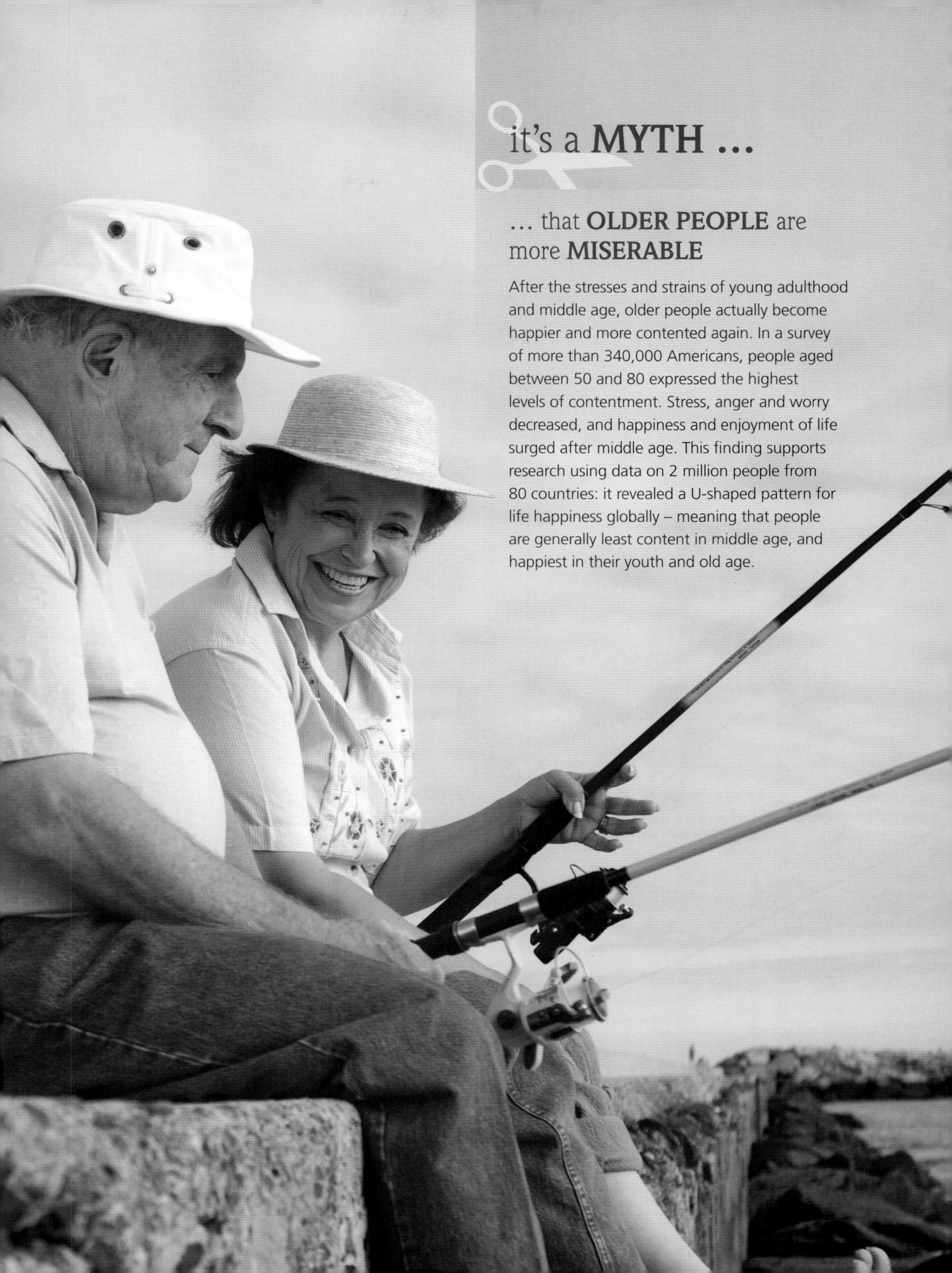

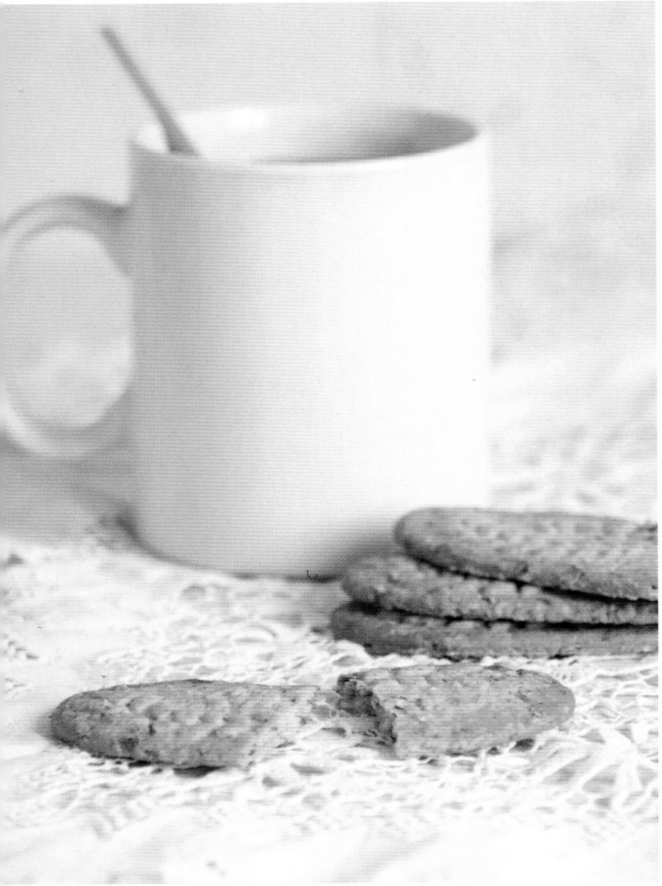

Share a drink and a chat with someone as often as you can.

experience, judgment, patience and foresight. Those are the findings of a report by the International Labour Office in Geneva. Employers are increasingly recognising that older employees actually add value. That's because they are statistically more likely to:

- Stay with the company longer than younger people.
- Have fewer accidents in the workplace.
- Experience greater work satisfaction.
- Have a more positive work ethic.

Of course, carrying on working doesn't have to mean keeping to the same job and routine. You may want to switch to a less demanding career, offer your skills and experience on a consultancy or freelance basis, or simply cut down your hours.

Easing the transition

When the familiar routines of work change, there's a big adjustment to make. You'll find it easier to make the transition if you:

- **Prioritise friendships** Strong social ties help to compensate for the loss of role, social status and routine contacts that affects many people after retirement. Try to share a friendly chat with someone every day, and meet up as often as you can. And while old friends can offer valuable support, it's important to keep creating new, wider social circles (*see* pages 286–288).
- **Pursue other interests** Hobbies or activities keep you enjoyably occupied, and fill the gap that work can leave. Ideally have something to do outside the home most days.
- **Help others** There's ample scope to find a fulfilling role as a volunteer. Studies in the USA have shown that volunteering offers people over 65 a strong sense of personal accomplishment. Two hours of voluntary work a week can lead to better health, lower levels of depression and longer life expectancy. There are plenty of organisations looking for people to offer time and skills – whether you want to walk a dog for someone who is housebound, do conservation work, run an arts group or offer your services as a handyman (*see* Resources for details).

BE prepared ... RETIRING as a COUPLE

If you are part of a couple, you will need to plan the transition to retirement to take account of both your needs. Here are some questions to consider:

- Have you discussed your expectations and aims for retirement? Are they compatible? If not, how will you compromise?
- Do you have the same views on living arrangements? How about climate, location, housing and proximity to family, friends, social amenities and health care?
- Do you have similar attitudes to financial priorities, savings, budgeting, debt and financial planning? Are your finances sufficient? How will you cope with a lower retirement income or different spending habits?
- Unless you plan to retire at the same time, how will you deal with one partner being in work and the other retired?
- How might your respective roles change after retirement, especially in terms of earning, managing household expenses and domestic chores?
- Once you are both retired, how much time do you expect to spend together? Is this enough, or too much? Are you compatible enough not to irritate each other if you're together more?
- Do you have shared interests, or new activities that appeal to you both? Do you each have enough interests and friends away from work and home to have a life of your own as well?
- Have you considered the probability that one of you will eventually spend some retirement time alone? Often women form stronger social links, but men are better placed financially. Do your plans take account of this?

Thinking about and discussing these issues help you avoid potential problems.

Plan the transition to retirement together.

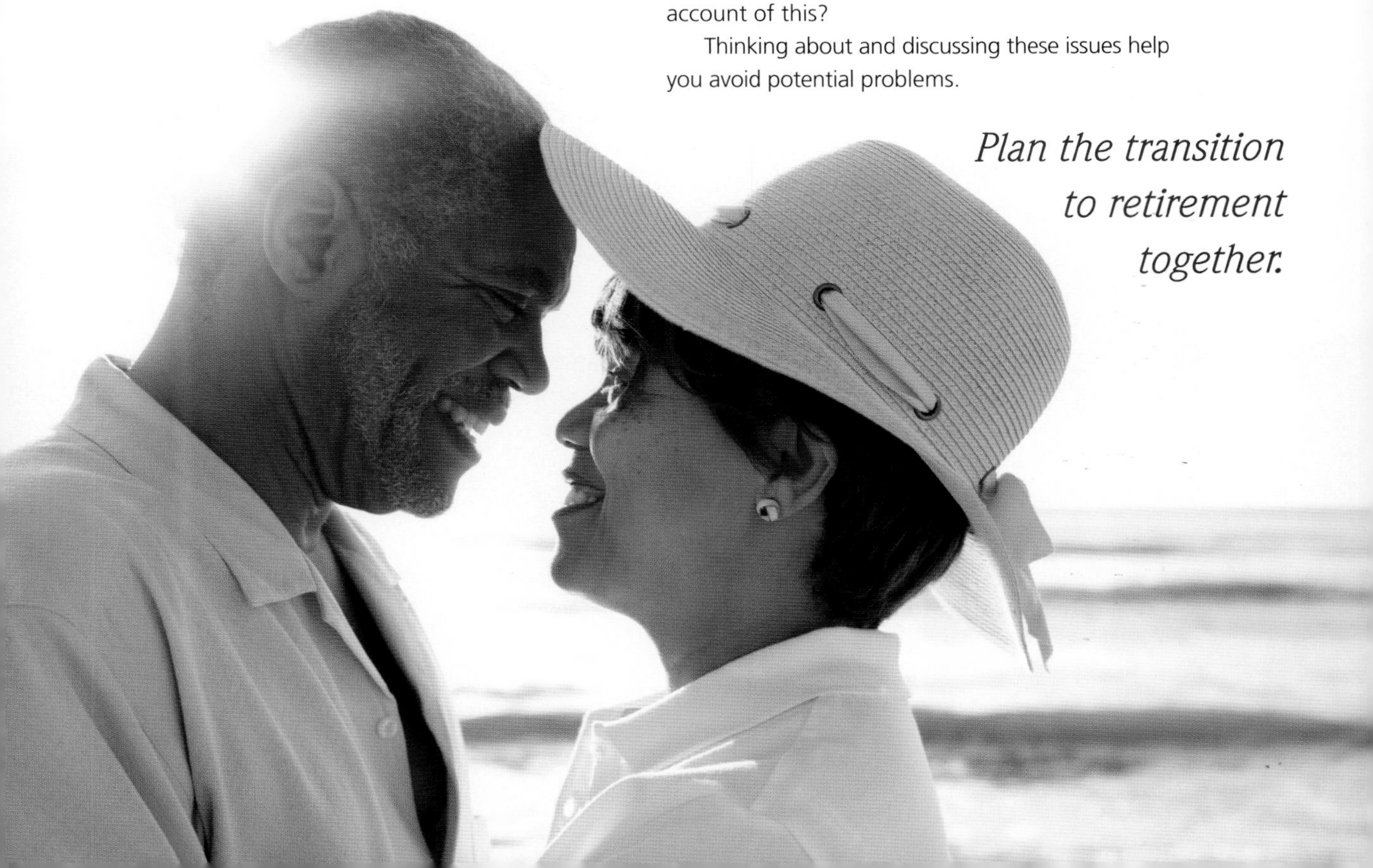

Quiz Are you **ready** for **later life?**

Work your way through the sections below then tot up your scores to find out how well prepared you are for the future. Tick all that apply then check the scoring section at the end.

A Which of the following do you do in a typical day?

- ☐ Walk half a kilometre or more.
- ☐ Perform a mentally challenging activity such as learning a language, doing a crossword or playing chess.
- ☐ Read a newspaper, or check an internet news site.
- ☐ Exercise sufficiently to get out of breath.
- ☐ Read a book.
- ☐ Brush and floss your teeth.
- ☐ Eat seven portions of fruit and vegetables.
- ☐ Get a good night's sleep.

B Which of these have you done in the past week?

- ☐ Telephoned or emailed a friend or had someone to visit.
- ☐ Hugged somebody.
- ☐ Engaged in a productive activity outside the house (for example, work, volunteering).
- ☐ Taken part in something purely for fun or excitement (TV doesn't count).
- ☐ Chatted to a neighbour.
- ☐ Helped someone.
- ☐ Eaten at least one portion of oily fish.
- ☐ Gone to a social gathering or visited friends.
- ☐ Attended a cultural event (such as a concert, play, exhibition, museum, historic home).
- ☐ Practised a muscle-building activity or strength training.
- ☐ Kept active for at least 90 minutes at a stretch (perhaps walking, playing golf, gardening).
- ☐ Attended a regular class or interest group (for instance, bridge club, religious service, band practice).

C In the past six months, have you?

- ☐ Had your blood pressure checked.
- ☐ Seen the dentist.
- ☐ Made a new friend.
- ☐ Travelled to somewhere you have never been before.
- ☐ Learned something new or acquired a new skill.

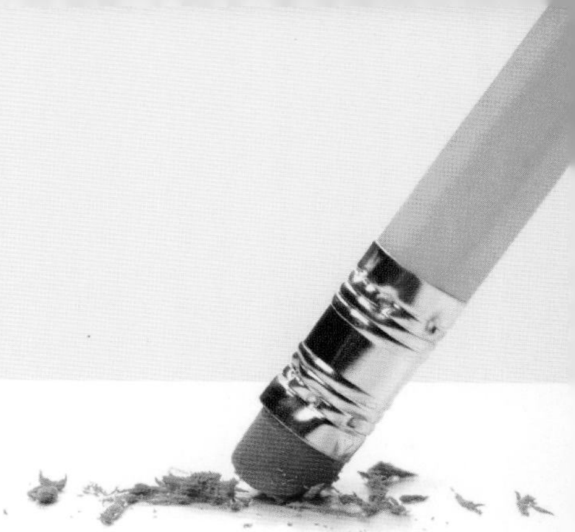

D Answer yes or no to the following:

☐ **Yes** ☐ **No** Have you made a will?

☐ **Yes** ☐ **No** Are you reasonably clear about the current state of your finances?

☐ **Yes** ☐ **No** Do you have sufficient superannuation to manage comfortably in the future?

☐ **Yes** ☐ **No** Do you have a 'rainy day fund' to cover unexpected major expenses such as car or household repairs?

☐ **Yes** ☐ **No** Do you have at least one good friend outside work and family circles?

☐ **Yes** ☐ **No** Have you talked to your family or made advance decisions about the health care you would want if you became incapacitated?

☐ **Yes** ☐ **No** Have you talked to your family about what you want to happen when you die (for example, legacies, cremation or burial, funeral service)?

☐ **Yes** ☐ **No** Do you have a hobby or interest that you find absorbing?

☐ **Yes** ☐ **No** Do you have a neighbour, friend or family member you could telephone at 4 am for help in a crisis (if you live with others, assume for some reason they're not around)?

☐ **Yes** ☐ **No** Can you get up from a chair without pushing with your arms?

☐ **Yes** ☐ **No** Is your BMI within the normal range (*see* page 96)?

☐ **Yes** ☐ **No** Have you thought about how you could adapt your home (*see* page 293) if you became frail or incapacitated (taking into account factors such as size, stairs, garden)?

☐ **Yes** ☐ **No** Do you have at least one major goal or plan for the next year?

☐ **Yes** ☐ **No** Do you know your vital financial details and the location of your important documents (for example, wills, insurance policies, bank accounts and passwords)?

☐ **Yes** ☐ **No** Could you deal unaided with an immediate household problem, such as finding the fuse box or turning off the water mains?

SCORE YOUR ANSWERS

A and B – one point for each tick.

C and D – two points for each tick or yes answer.

0–20 You may already feel dissatisfied with your life, or you may be so involved with day-to-day issues that you haven't stopped to look at the big picture. Pick one new action from A or B, and one item from C or D to which you answered no, and do something about it as soon as possible. Gradually add more items to keep on building your happy and healthy future.

21–39 You're moving towards a positive and productive later life, but it's worth taking a little time now to make sure that all the major aspects of a balanced lifestyle are in place.

40–60 Congratulations. You seem to be managing the transition to later life well. Keep it up, but also look out for any areas that might still need a little attention.

LOVE AND PASSION getting closer

A loving relationship can be one of the greatest strengths and joys in life. Retirement can offer you the opportunity to spend more quality time with your partner, but changing routines can also bring challenges.

Sometimes, retirement forces you to realise that as a couple you've grown apart, and once children have left home, you may have less incentive to stay together. Unlike in other age groups, divorce among the over-50s is increasing. There are no tricks to turn basic incompatibility into loving harmony, but there are ways to help heal and strengthen a fundamentally solid connection, and also to give a new attraction the best chance to grow into a lasting partnership.

- **Be a best friend** Be kind, considerate and respectful to your partner. Show you're happy to see him or her. Listen to what they have to say, and offer help and support.
- **Make time** Set aside at least a few minutes each day to focus on each other and share a chat. Have a regular weekly 'date' doing something you enjoy together.
- **Focus on positives** Think about your partner's good points rather than the things that irritate you – and let him or her know what you appreciate. Research shows that for strong relationships you need five positives (such as affectionate statements or gestures) to counteract each negative (for instance, complaints or quarrels).
- **Develop a shared interest** Is there an activity you both enjoyed when you were younger but haven't had time or money to pursue since? Now is your opportunity to rekindle your interest.

DID **you** KNOW?

If you're single there are more opportunities to find new love than ever before – whether you've been on your own for years, are recently divorced or have been bereaved. In the USA, the over-55s visit more internet dating sites than any other group, and many sites now cater specifically for older people (*see* Resources).

SEX AT SIXTY

If you're in a long-term relationship, you may find that your love life improves in your 60s. You experience the heightened intimacy that comes from knowing the other person well, or there may be a chance to recharge a passion submerged by years of work and child-care stresses.

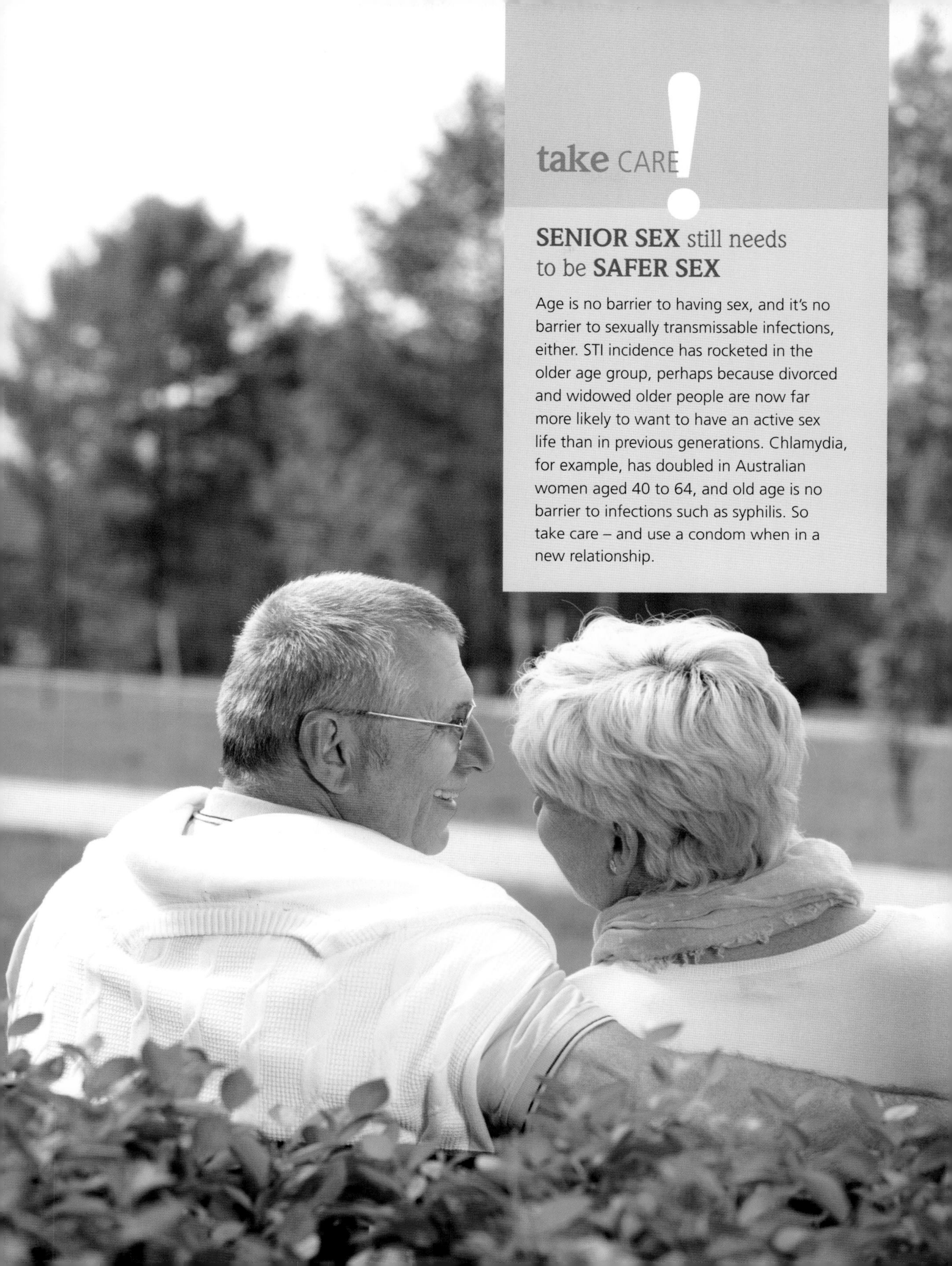

take CARE!

SENIOR SEX still needs to be **SAFER SEX**

Age is no barrier to having sex, and it's no barrier to sexually transmissable infections, either. STI incidence has rocketed in the older age group, perhaps because divorced and widowed older people are now far more likely to want to have an active sex life than in previous generations. Chlamydia, for example, has doubled in Australian women aged 40 to 64, and old age is no barrier to infections such as syphilis. So take care – and use a condom when in a new relationship.

The sex can be better, too. With age, you can relax and explore not just physical sensations but other aspects of your emotions and sensuality, free from the constraints and distractions of family and the pressures of youthful expectations. Here are some great ways to enhance your sex life:

- Be playful – sex need not be serious.
- Encourage spontaneity – when you're in the mood, go for it. Experiment and be creative – try different locations, times of day.
- Communicate – be open about your desires and ask about your partner's. In long-term relationships, assumptions about each other's needs and fantasies may be decades out of date. Just talking about sex can be, well, sexy.
- Focus on intimacy not intercourse. Cuddling, kissing and touching can be satisfying if physical problems preclude penetration.
- Remember romance – set the scene, walk hand in hand, arrange candlelit dinners or weekends away.
- Build touching, affection and sensuality into your everyday life – hug, kiss, cuddle, massage each other or bathe together.

'Grow old with me, The best is yet to come.'

Robert Browning, English writer

Why sex is good for you

Sex isn't just about sex. It benefits your health and wellbeing in many different ways. For instance, it:

- **Gives you a great cardiovascular workout** – in other words, sex is excellent exercise. You can burn around 1260kJ per hour during sex, so it helps to keep your weight down, too.
- **Reduces blood pressure and protects against heart disease.** Among 914 middle-aged men followed for ten years by University of Bristol researchers, those having sex less than once a month were 2.8 times more likely to have a fatal heart attack than those having sex at least twice a week.
- **Enhances intimacy and strengthens your relationship.** The more often older couples have sex, the more likely they are to be happy in their relationship, and with life in general, according to an American survey of 238 married people aged 65 or over.
- **Releases feel-good hormones** Endorphins, the body's natural pleasure-promoting and pain-killing hormones, relieve anxiety, boost mood and promote relaxation and sleep. Oxytocin, known as the 'love hormone', is released at orgasm. It promotes wellbeing and calmness, lowers blood pressure and promotes bonding in relationships.

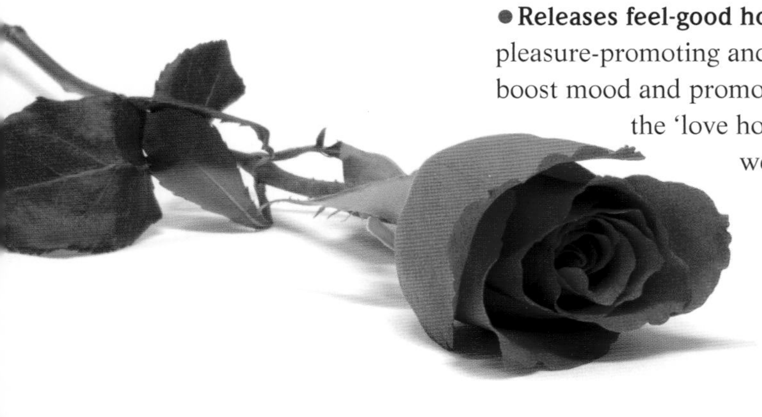

focus ON ... Later life SEX PROBLEMS

Both men and women may encounter problems having sex in later life. Often the difficulties have more to do with health than with age. Be patient and understanding with your partner (and yourself); in many instances there are things you can do to improve matters.

Whatever your problem, don't be afraid or embarrassed to talk to your doctor. Underlying conditions such as diabetes, atherosclerosis or prostate problems may be treatable.

Medication for high blood pressure or depression can cause erectile dysfunction (impotence), and many medications can lower desire, arousal or sexual response in both men and women. If it's medication that's causing the problem, it may be possible to change it. Your doctor may also offer erection-promoting devices or medications: pellets, creams, injections or oral tablets such as Sildenafil.

Pain or limited mobility resulting from arthritis and other conditions can make intercourse more difficult or reduce enjoyment. Trying different positions often helps.

After the menopause, women's vaginal tissues may grow thin and their secretions dry up, making intercourse uncomfortable. If foreplay doesn't do the trick, this is easily resolved with a lubricant, or your doctor may prescribe vaginal oestrogen.

Exercise for sexual health

Simple exercises to strengthen the pelvic-floor muscles (Kegel exercises) can enhance sex for both men and women; they also help with health problems such as vaginal prolapse (which becomes more common with age) and urinary incontinence. Start by identifying the muscles you would use to stop your urine flow midstream. Gently squeeze for a count of ten, then release, and repeat ten times. Do this as many times a day as you can.

- **Boosts immunity** In one study conducted in Pennsylvania, USA, people who had sex once or twice a week had better immunity than those who had intercourse less – or more – often.
- **Preserves your looks** According to a Scottish study of more than 3500 people, those having sex at least three times a week can look ten years younger than their peers who have sex less often.
- **Strengthens pelvic-floor muscles and protects against erectile dysfunction** In a Finnish study of 989 men aged 55 to 75, those having intercourse at least once a week were half as likely to experience erectile dysfunction as those having it less frequently.
- **Prolongs life** In a study of 918 men at the University of Bristol, those who had the fewest orgasms were twice as likely to die over the subsequent ten years as those having the most orgasms.

Make friends. Having a wide social network can prolong your life, says an American survey.

KEEP CONNECTED family and community

Strong family and social connections boost your health and longevity as well as your enjoyment of life, whereas loneliness and isolation are linked to shorter life spans. So it is in your own interest to make the most of your family circle, and the wider circle outside.

Modern life is less community-oriented than ever. Most of us no longer live in extended families; we often relocate for employment so live far from our relatives. We delay marriage, have fewer children, and are more likely to divorce. And our social networks have progressively shrunk. Many of us scarcely know our neighbours. One 2011 US survey showed that most adults have only two close friends – 25 years ago the average was three. Another American review, by psychologists at Brigham Young University, Utah, which looked at 14 separate studies of older people, found that those with the most extensive social networks were 50 per cent more likely still to be alive an average of 7.5 years later than those with fewer connections.

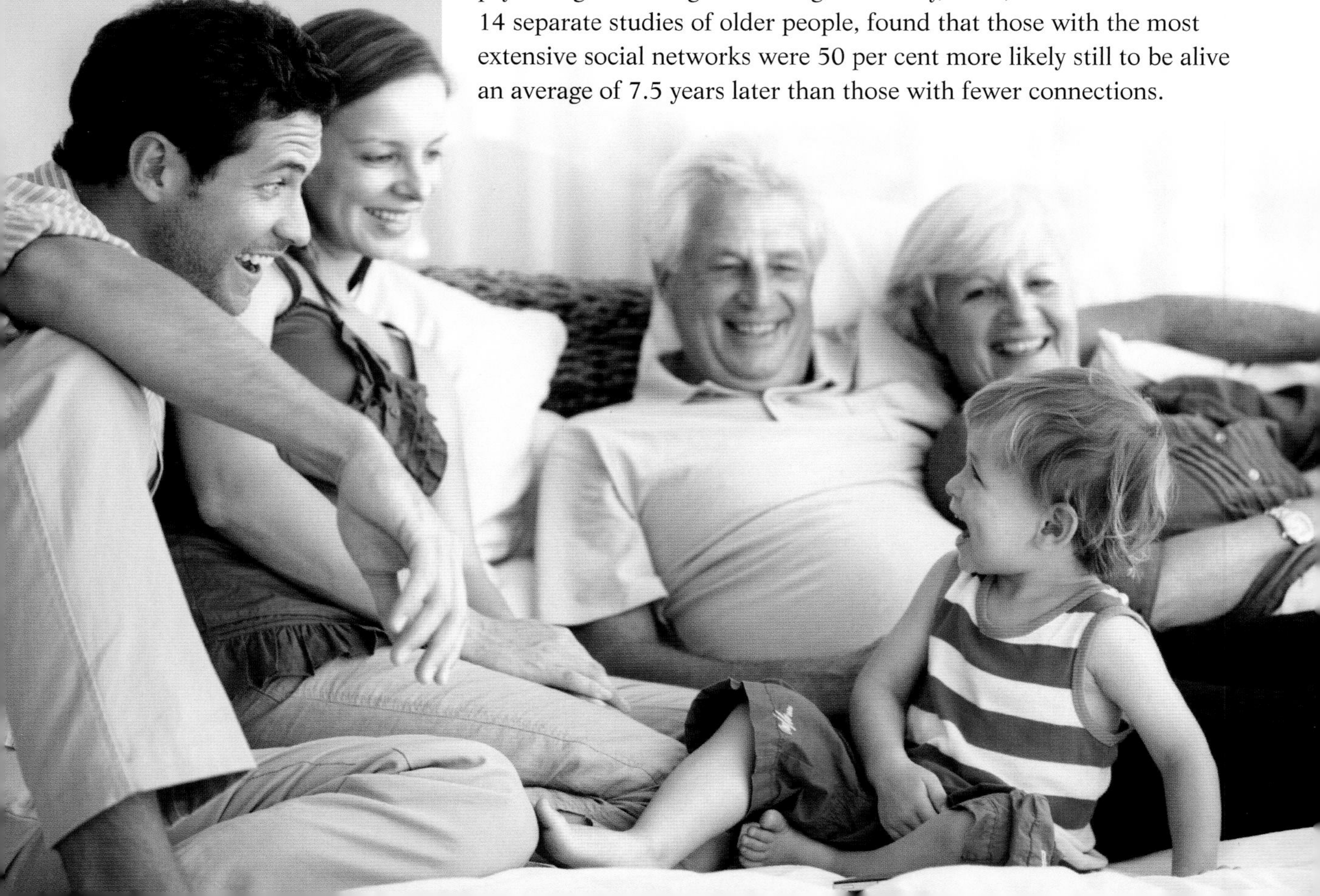

It is a fact that one in three over-65s lives alone. But the good news is that single people can fare just as well as those who are married – provided that they have good emotional support from friends. Researchers in the Utah study review mentioned opposite found that people who lived with someone else had 19 per cent better survival rates than those who lived alone, but this was much lower than the staggering 91 per cent increased survival rate for those with the strongest social networks and community ties.

A ZEST FOR LIFE

So how do you go about keeping in contact with the wider world, once your work no longer provides that connection automatically? It's vital to develop interests and maintain your zest for living, and not to become isolated or spend your days alone in front of the television. How you pass your time in your later years really matters. A Swedish study that tracked people's participation in leisure activities for 34 years found that over-65s with low levels of participation had twice the mortality risk of people with the highest.

And data from the Einstein Aging Study in New York showed that the more time you spend enjoying different hobbies, the lower your dementia risk, too. Specifically protective interests include reading, enjoying board games, playing musical instruments and dancing. Another American study found that frequent social or productive activities – such as preparing meals or gardening – increased both length and quality of life and, remarkably, were as effective in enhancing survival as activities involving physical fitness.

> *'Never have children, only grandchildren.'*
>
> Gore Vidal, American writer

Busy, busy, busy ...

The good news is that more entertaining pastimes are accessible to older people than ever before: you've just got to find something that suits you. Step outside your 'comfort zone' if necessary, and you'll find a host of like-minded people and a vast range of stimulating activities, places to go and absorbing interests. If you're having difficulty finding something that attracts you, ask yourself:

- What activities have I done in the past – however long ago – that I really enjoyed?
- Are there any subjects I might find intriguing to study?
- Does anyone I know have a hobby or belong to a group that sounds interesting?

DID **you** KNOW?

Pets improve health, boost mood, reduce anxiety and promote social contact according to the US National Institutes of Health (NIH).

- A three-year NIH study of people aged 71 to 82 found those who regularly walked a dog got more exercise, walked faster and had better mobility than those who didn't.

- Dog-walking encourages conversation and increases the frequency of social interactions, concluded a study at the University of Warwick.

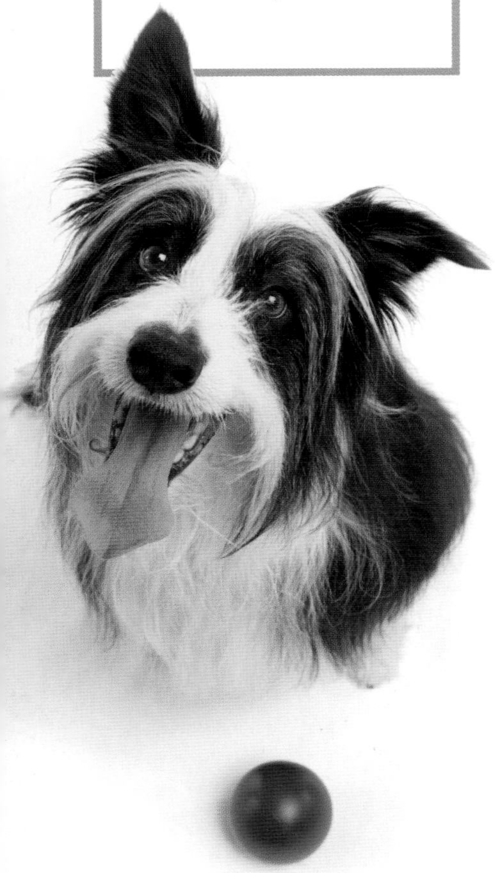

- Which places am I curious to visit?
- Could I be more physically active than I am at present?
- Do I have any useful skills? Perhaps I could use them to do some volunteer work, or get involved in campaigning on political issues.

Ten health-boosting hobbies

When it comes to taking up a new interest, the possibilities are endless. Here are ten suggestions with proven benefits for your health and wellbeing:

- **Take an evening class** Learning new things keeps your brain connections active (*see* pages 178–180). In one study conducted by the National Institute of Adult Continuing Education (England and Wales), 87 per cent of adult learners reported improved physical health, including feeling less tired or managing pain more effectively.
- **Sing it loud** Singing in a choir – but not just listening to choral music – boosts immunity and mood, according to a German study.
- **Go to yoga** In a study led by neurologists at Oregon Health and Science University in Portland, USA, 135 people aged 65 to 85 were allocated at random to a yoga class, a walking exercise class or a control group. After six months the yoga group had better balance and flexibility, enhanced energy, less fatigue and better overall quality of life compared with the control groups.
- **Volunteer** A review of 16 studies at the University of Jyväskylä, Finland, showed that older volunteers rated their own health, functioning, physical activity and life satisfaction as better, and had less depression and longer lives than non-volunteers.
- **Become a culture vulture** In a study at the University of Umeå in Sweden, 10,609 people aged 25 to 74 were interviewed about their cultural habits and followed for 14 years. People who most often visited the cinema, museums or art exhibitions, or who went to concerts lived longer than those who did so rarely.
- **Join a walking group** Walking with other people is an easy way to socialise, and a brisk constitutional is one of the best ways to boost your longevity. Researchers from University College London reviewed 18 studies including nearly 460,000 people in total and found that those who walked the most were 31 per cent less likely to have developed cardiovascular disease and they were 32 per cent less likely to have died after various follow-up periods than those who walked the least.

focus ON ... Being a top GRANDPARENT

Grandparenting is in many ways more fun and less stressful than parenting: you're not really responsible for dull stuff such as discipline, and you're not on duty full-time, so you can see your grandchildren whenever it suits you and their parents.

As a grandparent, you have the chance to play an important role in your grandchildren's lives. You can offer undivided attention, unconditional love and security, and be a positive role model. You can contribute to their development by playing, reading, teaching skills such as sewing, cooking or woodwork, sharing activities – and just by listening. You can also give your grandchildren a sense of family history.

Children with a close connection to a grandparent develop higher self-esteem, are better able to withstand peer pressure, have better emotional and social skills and do better in school. Research at Oxford University involving more than 1500 children aged 11 to 16 showed that those with an involved grandparent were kinder, more considerate, more sociable and coped better with adverse life events such as parental separation.

And of course you can, if you want to, be an immense help to your own children by babysitting, picking up from school and so forth. As a result, you may find that grandparenting strengthens your relationship with your own children.

There are, however, tricky areas to negotiate, and it's important to help without judging or interfering. Here are some pointers:

- Find out and respect parents' rules on eating, sleeping and TV.
- Ask parents about their rules and practices and follow them – even if they are not what you did, or would choose to do now.
- Be aware of modern safety and child-proofing requirements and gadgets. Never take children out in the car without appropriate car seats, and make sure they're safely strapped in. Collaborate with their parents in childproofing your house and ensuring that sharp objects, potential electric, choking and strangulation hazards, medicines and household chemicals are safely out of reach. If you have a pond or pool, make it safe.
- Find out how much supervision parents expect – whether children are allowed out to play alone, say – and stick to it.
- Know what to do in case of illness, and keep emergency numbers close to hand.
- Maintain limits. Don't be an unpaid childminder unless you want to.

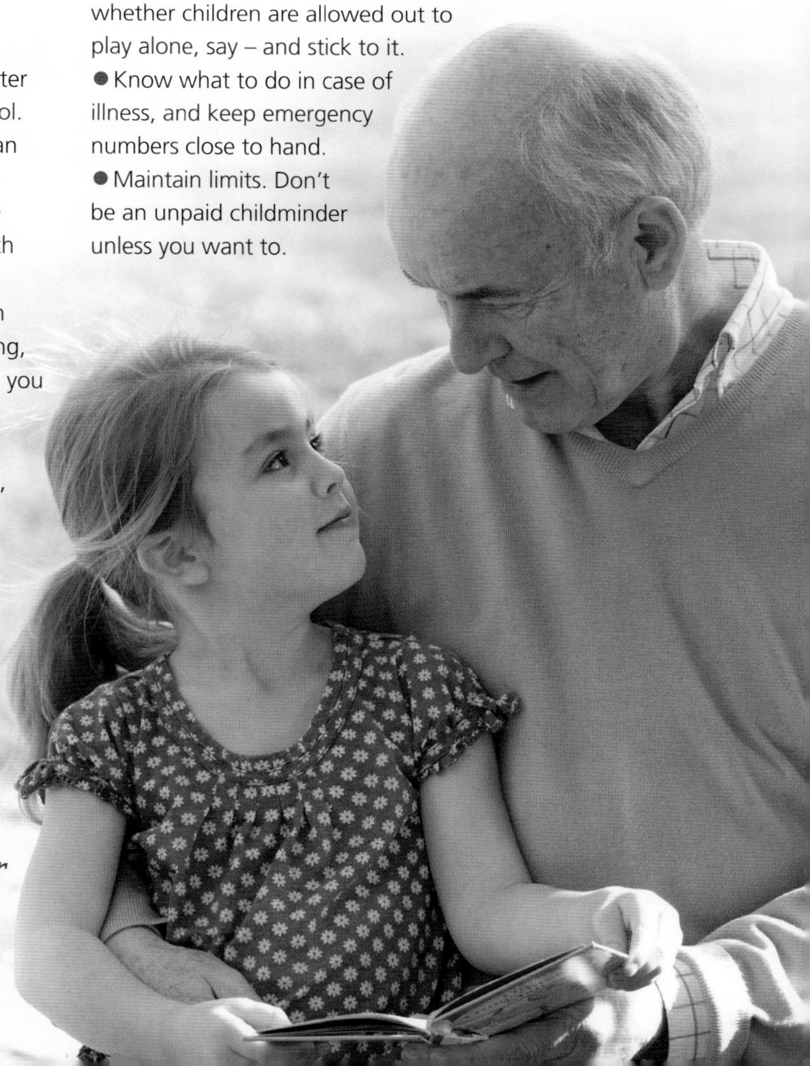

As a grandparent, you can offer undivided attention ...

DID you KNOW?

One in five holidaymakers travels alone, either completely unaccompanied or as part of a singles group. Many companies cater specifically for solo travellers, including breaks especially for the over-50s, so there's no need to give up travelling if you're single, recently divorced or bereaved (*see* Resources).

- **Play bridge** A study from the University of California, Berkeley, of 12 female bridge club members in their 70s and 80s showed significant increases in immune cells after a 90-minute game.
- **Go to a wine tasting** Know and enjoy good wines. Red wine particularly – in moderate quantities – has numerous health benefits, especially for your heart (*see* page 32).
- **Join a dance class** Any sort of dancing offers good exercise, fun and a chance to meet new people. In a German study conducted at Friedrich Schiller University of Jena, an eight-week salsa program helped the 28 subjects, with an average age of 71, increase their stride speed and length dramatically.
- **Do some gardening** In one Dutch study, allotment gardeners aged 62 or over had significantly better physical health than their neighbours without allotments. And research at the University of South Florida on over 3000 people aged 65 or over showed that those who spent an hour or more gardening every week had better balance and walking speed, fewer chronic health conditions or limitations than non-gardeners, and significantly fewer had sustained a fall in the previous two years.

GET ON THE NET

One 21st-century innovation has made keeping in touch with the wider world a possibility for everyone – no matter your age or how housebound or immobile you are, and whatever your interests. It is the miraculous internet: a priceless technological gift to the older generation. More and more over-60s are getting online. If you're still not confident, many introductory courses are geared towards 'silver surfers' (*see* Resources for details).

Keep in touch – with family, old friends and your grandchildren – through email, free phone services such as Skype, or social networking sites. More than one in ten Australians over 50 regularly use social networking sites, which allow them to connect with family and friends, and start new friendships.

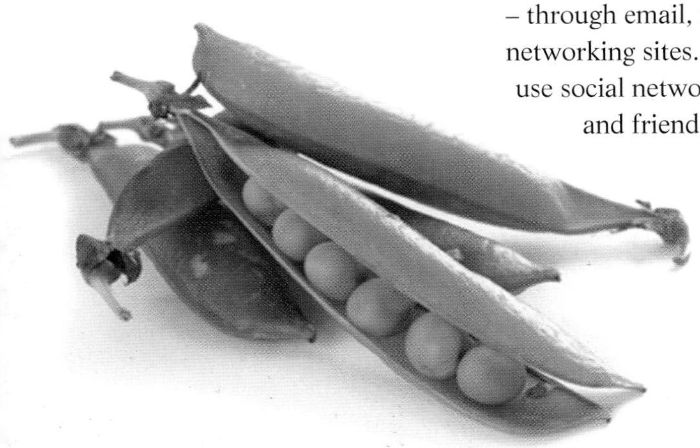

Do some gardening ...

focus ON ... TRAVEL planning

Older people are travelling more than ever, especially after retirement. Many holiday companies arrange trips just for older travellers, or offer special-interest breaks – such as vineyard, battlefield or archaeology tours, art cruises and spa or golfing holidays.

Good planning is essential and helps ensure a smooth trip. Factors to consider include:

Travel insurance

- As you get older it may be harder to arrange cover, especially with pre-existing medical conditions. Check before you book. An annual policy is often cheaper if you travel more than once a year.
- Make sure your policy covers medical evacuation, to fly you home if you fall ill or have an accident abroad.

Medical needs

- Get your doctor's OK to travel if you are unwell.
- Take supplies of any medication to last at least a week longer than your stay, to allow for any circumstances that might delay your return.
- Carry prescriptions for your medicines with you, and check your medication is legal at your destination.
- Carry medication in your hand luggage, not in check-in baggage – in case it goes missing.
- Arrange in advance with your airline if you'll need oxygen during the flight or if you use syringes.
- For a long stay, check that your medicines are available at your destination; find out about local treatment facilities if you have serious health problems.

Sensible precautions

- If you're going to an unfamiliar country, find out well in advance about any vaccinations needed.
- Research your destination. It's helpful to know if the beach is accessible only via steep steps, for example.
- Photocopy documents such as passport and insurance details, and note travellers' cheque and credit card numbers in case they are lost or stolen.
- Leave details of your travel itinerary with friends or family and a note of where you'll be staying.
- If you're facing long travel times, take precautions to avoid deep vein thrombosis.

Making the most of your trip

- Stay as long as you can. The cost difference of an extra week or two is often relatively small.
- Travel can be more tiring for older people. Give yourself time to adapt at your destination, especially when crossing multiple time zones. Combat jet lag by staying well hydrated, eating meals at the appropriate time for your destination and getting early-morning sunlight as soon as you can after arriving.

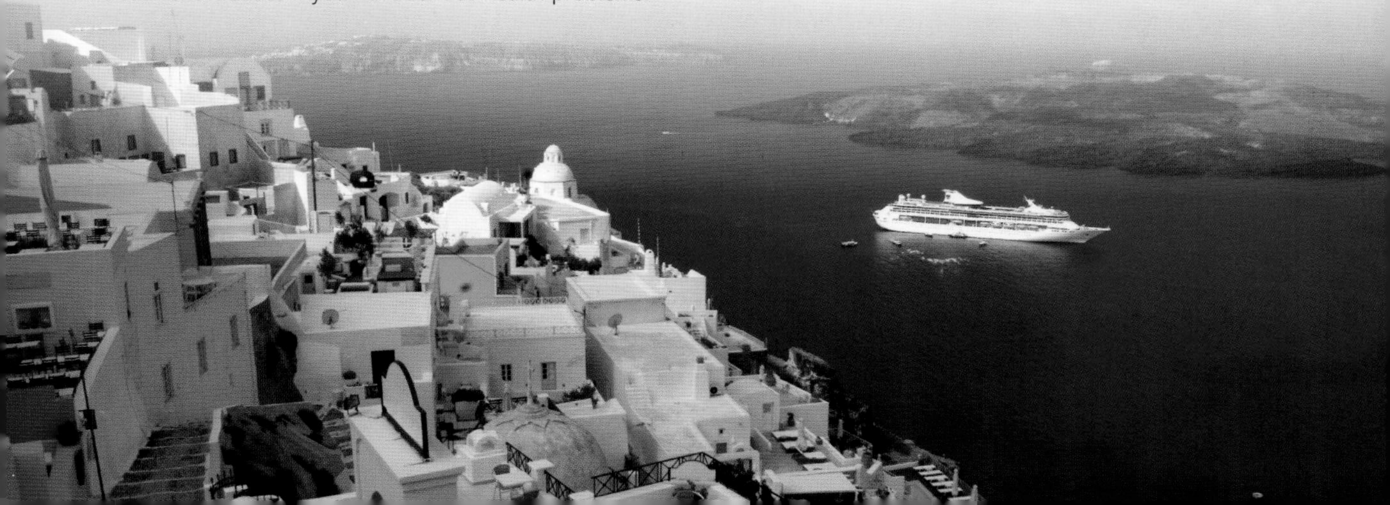

Age-proof your home. Four out of five people still live independently in their 80s.

YOUR HOUSE IN ORDER
home and finances

The first years of retirement are a good time to arrange your home in a way that will suit your needs for the next ten, 20 or even 30 years. It will pay to give some thought at this time to your financial wellbeing, and also to your legacy.

If you reach the age of 65 as a couple and in good health, there's a 50 per cent chance that one of you will still be alive at the age of 95, and there's a 25 per cent chance that the woman will survive to be 100. This rather startling statistic has important implications. It means you ought to consider whether the home you have will continue to be suitable for you in the years to come. You might like to think about adapting your home while you have the strength and energy for the task, or about moving to somewhere smaller that is cheaper and easier to run.

To move or not to move

Some people leap at the chance to move house once they retire. You might, after years of working in a big city, yearn for the peace and quiet of the countryside or a seaside town. If that's your dream, then pursue it. But whether you plan to stay put or to relocate, consider these things:

- Is the home you plan to live in manageable and secure, now and in the future (*see* box, opposite)?
- Is there a welcoming community that you can join? If you are moving to a new area, will you miss friends and family?
- Will you be comfortable in the home and the neighbourhood?
- Can you afford the house, and all its running costs? Or is it worth downsizing in order to release some capital?
- What is the local area like? Friendly? Walkable?
- Who lives near you?
- What local facilities are available? Where will you do your shopping? Is there a doctor's surgery? Are there the leisure facilities that matter to you – a shopping centre, say, or a cinema?

BE prepared ... ADAPTING YOUR HOME

If you start to find your house awkward to live in, there are many simple adaptations that can alleviate problems without major upheaval or expense.

Most commonly, older people need help with stairs and bathrooms. A bath or shower seat, free-standing frames or fitted handrails and grab rails may be sufficient, or you may need a stairlift, level-access shower, bath lift or a high-level lavatory. You can set the height of some sinks to give you better access for washing, and you can have taps fitted so that they're not at the back of the sink.

Simple steps

A small amount of household help, even just a few hours' gardening or cleaning every fortnight, can make a home more manageable. And arranging direct debits or standing orders to pay bills automatically helps if you develop eyesight, memory or concentration problems. There are also many helpful gadgets, including:

- A grabber – to pick things up without bending.
- Risers under chairs and bed feet, or a powered riser-recliner chair – to make getting up easier.
- Kettle-tippers, tap-turners, wide-handled cutlery, two-handled cups, high-rimmed plates, jar and bottle openers, non-slip mats – to help with preparing food.
- A door-release intercom – to enable you to check callers and let them in by pressing a button.

If you live alone, a careline or community alarm can keep you independent but safe. Modern systems, known as 'assistive technology' or telecare, can incorporate sensors that detect power and phone outages, and monitor you or someone you're caring for in case of falls. A key safe can hold door keys in a secure box outside, to be accessed with a code in an emergency.

MAKING ENDS MEET

Growing numbers of people reaching retirement make the alarming discovery that their financial provision may not be enough to see them through to later life. More than two out of five Australians have inadequate savings for a comfortable retirement.

Here's how to make sure you stay on top of financial matters:

- Note any major expenditures or gains involved in retirement (buying a boat, selling your house, paying off the mortgage).
- Calculate your net worth – assets minus debts. Include any lump-sum payment you'll receive on retirement.
- Work out how much you expect to receive from superannuation. Factor in any continuing income, state benefits, insurance or

endowment payouts, and likely savings or investment income, allowing for interest rate changes.

- If you still have time to save, or have significant funds already, take independent advice on how best to invest your money.
- Now calculate your income minus expenditure. Assess possible future variations with changes in your living situation, income fluctuations and increases in the cost of living. Make allowances for eventualities such as major household repairs or needing a new car, bereavement and associated loss of work or superannuation income, having to move or adapt your house, or needing long-term care. Do you have sufficient to meet your needs?
- If you have a shortfall, think how you might increase your income, for example, by delaying retirement, taking part-time work, cutting back expenditure, moving to a smaller house. Often it's not big outlays that cause ongoing hardship but the steady drip-drip of day-to-day expenses – but these are easy to trim. If a setback could tip you over the financial edge, how can you build up an emergency fund?
- Once you have a complete picture of your aims and financial situation, seek professional advice. Review your situation annually, to be sure you're still on track.

'A man is not old until regrets take the place of dreams.'

John Barrymore, American actor

WHERE THERE'S A WILL

You must make a will: it is foolish not to. If you die intestate (with no will), dealing with your estate takes longer and is more complex. This could cause financial hardship and friction in your family. Without a will, you have no control over your estate, which may then not benefit those you expect, and could go to people you wouldn't choose. Your partner could be left with few assets, or your house sold to distribute your estate. There are other very good reasons for making a will:

- You can appoint executors of your choosing to handle your estate, and you can specify your choices about the funeral ceremony.
- If you have no family, you can leave your estate to a friend or organisation. Without a will, everything goes to the state.
- You can set up stipulations such as ensuring that children or grandchildren gain access to money only at a responsible age.

4 ways to provide for your **LOVED ONES**

- **MAKE A WILL** and review it every ten years or whenever your circumstances change (for instance, as the result of an inheritance, divorce, a child's marriage, or a new grandchild, say). Tell your next-of-kin where your will is, and make it easy to find. For security, leave a copy with your solicitor or bank.

- **LEAVE A LETTER OF INSTRUCTION** with your will. It could contain important information such as the location of important documents, your bank account numbers and computer passwords. It might say what should happen with pets or personal items, or contain messages to be passed on to your descendants. A letter of instruction is not legally binding, but it's simple to update and it can make things easier for your executors.

- **CONSIDER MAKING AN ADVANCED DECLARATION** (a 'living will') to specify medical care that you would like or, more importantly, that you would refuse, if you became incapacitated. You cannot compel medical staff to provide particular treatment, but you are entitled to refuse intervention in advance as long as you're mentally competent when making the decision. Talk to your loved ones about your healthcare wishes should you become incapacitated, so that they're aware of your attitude. Consider appointing someone to take financial and/or medical decisions if you become unable to do so.

- **OPEN A JOINT ACCOUNT** with your heirs. Make sure it contains enough money to provide for financial dependents, funeral expenses and taxes. Funds in joint accounts usually pass automatically to the survivor. Otherwise, the deceased's accounts are frozen until legal formalities are completed, which can take months – even years if there's no will.

Are you covered?

As well as a will, think about insurance – to cover mortgage or other payments if you lose your job, or to protect your family should you fall ill or die unexpectedly. Single people may have less need for life cover, but disability or long-term care insurance is more important if you are dependent on your own resources.

Women may have particular difficulties because they are more likely to find themselves alone in old age. It's important that both partners in a couple can manage joint finances and practical matters (from paying bills and accessing bank accounts to working the air-conditioner) and know the wishes of the other in case of incapacity or sudden death.

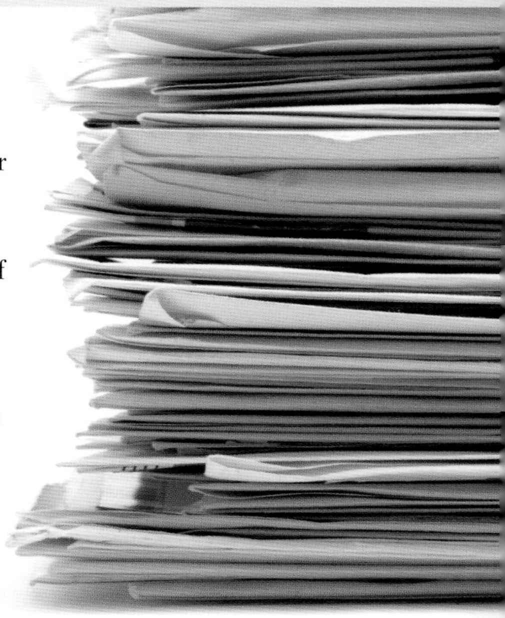

it's a MYTH ...

... that GROWING OLD means you'll end up in a CARE HOME

Most older people live in their own homes. Only about three in 50 Australians over 65 live in residential aged care and the overwhelming majority of residents are over seventy-five.

ILLNESS AND CARING

As you get older, there's an increased chance that you'll be diagnosed with a serious disease or will need to care for a loved one who is ill. Such events may be life-changing. Almost any continuing health problem affects everyone in the family – because day-to-day care and support is needed or because responsibilities and domestic or financial arrangements change.

Caregiving can cause stress, exhaustion, depression and marital disharmony. The key to coping is to have the right strategies in place.

- Take regular breaks. Look into day centres or respite care. Use the time to do something rewarding for yourself.
- Share information, whether about your own or someone else's health, or practical challenges – don't keep things to yourself.
- Talk – vent negative feelings with a friend who's not involved, and find a support group for carers or people with the condition.
- Recognise when you need help. Accept offers from friends.
- If you're caring for someone, don't do more than is necessary – it can make the person feel more vulnerable and powerless.
- Make your relationship a priority and try to sustain intimacy.
- If caring starts to feel overwhelming, seek help at once.

The sandwich generation

If you're caring for elderly parents while supporting adult children, then you are part of the so-called sandwich generation – meaning you're squeezed financially and perhaps emotionally by the generations above and below. A century ago, only 4 to 7 per cent of people in their 60s had at least one parent still living; today it's nearly 50 per cent. And compared with 20 years ago, more children in their mid-20s and early 30s still live with parents, or return home after university.

If you find yourself in this position, it's important not to sabotage your own retirement fund. As well as loans, investigate scholarships, bursaries and grants for your children. Use your parents' own funds to pay for their care. If there's time, save separately for your children's education, and investigate long-term care insurance for your parents.

BE prepared ... BEREAVEMENT

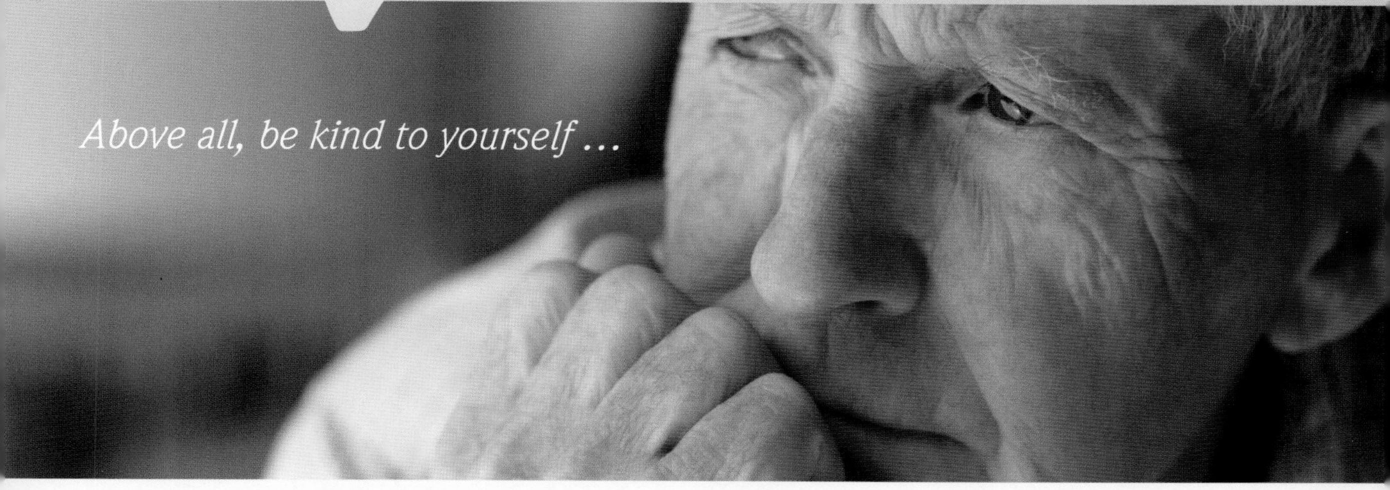

Grief is a fact of life. At some point you are sure to face the death of a parent, spouse or friend. People want to help at such times, but often don't know how. Tell them what you need to get you through, and be open to any act of kindness.

If someone for whom you are responsible dies, you must attend to certain matters straight away.

- Register the death and find out what other legal formalities are necessary.
- Locate any will, and contact the executors.
- Arrange for burial or cremation, and a funeral service, if desired.
- Look for any insurance policies or schemes that pay out on death.
- Cancel ongoing financial commitments of the person who has died, and inform banks and pension providers.
- Make a list of everyone who should be notified.

If your spouse or someone living with you dies:

- Check how your finances are affected, including pensions and benefits. Reassess your budget.
- Arrange for bills to be put in your name.
- Make a list of the domestic duties that you need to take on – renewing insurance policies, say.

Coping with grief

Allow yourself a period of mourning and adjustment – expect the grief to last at least 18 months. This is, among other things, a period of adjustment. Being bereaved often means considerable changes, but you can help yourself in many ways:

- Talk about your feelings, or write them down. Most people have a range of emotions and you may experience all or some of the following at any time: shock, denial or numbness; anger or anxiety; regret or guilt; emptiness, sadness or despair; acceptance and sometimes relief. See your doctor if your emotions become overwhelming or you're not sleeping or eating at any stage.
- Anticipate good days and bad days. There will be times when you feel you're moving on, and others when you slip back into sadness. This is natural and part of the healing process.
- Keep busy, but if possible don't commit to major life decisions for at least a year.

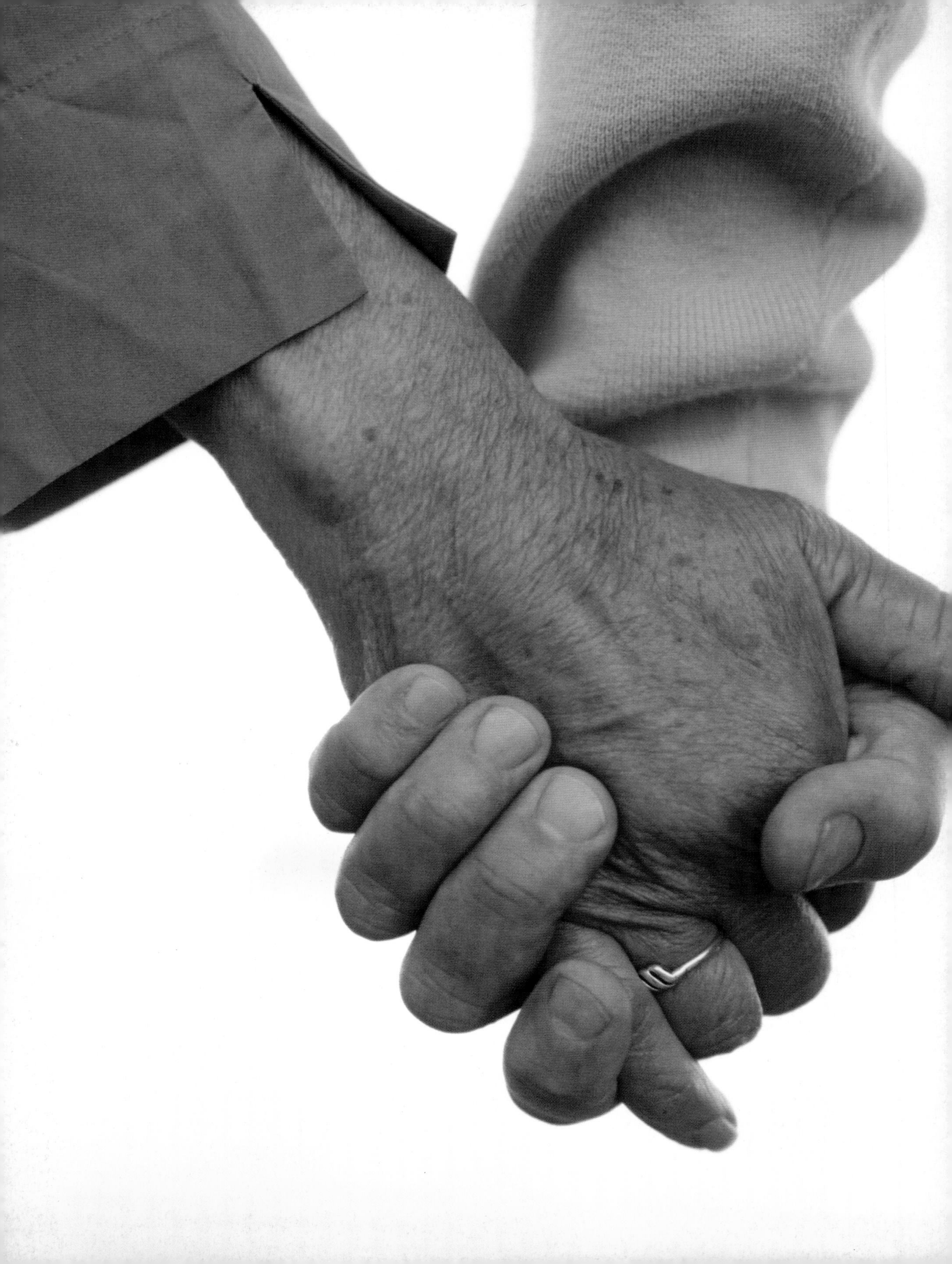

12

RESOURCES

Here are some organisations that will help you uncover a world of exciting new possibilities or provide a helping hand when you need it most. If you have a problem, whatever it concerns – from health or financial worries to travel issues or finding the best ways to keep active or meet new people – assistance is just a phone call or a mouse click away.

ACTIVITIES

One of the most liberating aspects of getting older is that you can please yourself, and do what you want when you want. Below are contact details of organisations that can help you develop your interests and meet new people. Also check your council's website or ring your family doctor or church for local suggestions. Then Google 'sport and recreation' to find your state's department and browse for activities for seniors.

Leisure interests

Bridge To find a local club, go to **www.abf.com.au**

Cake decorating Find a course via **www.cakedecoratingcourses-au.com** or try an online course from **www.cakedecoratingcourses.co.uk**

Dance Ever wanted to learn to dance? Try DanceSport Australia. Go to **www.dancesport.org.au** and click on 'getting started'. What about folk dancing? There's a website for you: **www.folkdanceaustralia.org.au/default.aspx**

Exergaming, using video technology to exercise via devices such as Xbox Kinect and Wii, is a new way for older people to get fit. Ask your local gaming store for advice.

Life Be In It Look for Life Be In It programs and events in your state via the parent website **www.lifebeinit.org**

Lifeball Lifeball is a team sport for all ages. See **www.lifeball.com.au** to find a team.

Meditation Learn to meditate – online – with the Meditation Society of Australia. See **http://meditation.org.au/index.asp** for details.

Physical activity programs The YMCA runs an Active Ageing Network in some states, providing a range of physical activity programs for people over fifty: **www.ymca.org.au, http://ymca.org.nz/**

Pilates Find a Pilates instructor at **www.australianpilates.asn.au** or **www.thewellnessdirectory.co.nz/therapy/pilates**

Rotary Make friends and help your community: **www.rotaryaustralia.org.au** or **www.rotary.org.nz**

Tai chi You can find a list of classes from the Taoist Tai Chi Society of Australia: **www.taoist.org.au/content/standard.asp?name=Classes**. Videos are available from **www.taichiacademy.com.au/products.php**

Walking For a range of walking options, contact your state's national parks department.

Wine The Wine Society offers courses and events: **www.winesociety.com.au**

Yoga There are many styles and many teachers to choose from. Yoga Australia offers a search engine to help: go to **www.yogaaustralia.org.au** and click on 'Courses and events'. In New Zealand, go to **www.thewellnessdirectory.co.nz/search_directory/yoga**

Socialising

Country Women's Association This is the largest women's association in Australia. Their website is **www.cwaa.org.au**

Dating Online dating organisations for older people include Older Dating Online (**www.olderdatingonline.com/australia** and **www.olderdatingonline.com.nz**) and 50and (**50and.com.au**)

Men's shed Men's sheds provide a safe, friendly space for men to work on projects at their own pace in the company of other men. Go to **www.mensshed.org** and click on 'Find a shed'.

The New Zealand Federation of Women's Institutes The largest women's organisation in New Zealand. Go to **www.wi.org.nz**

Old friends Track down people with whom you have lost touch via **www.facebook.com**

TeleCross The Red Cross offers a daily phone call to isolated older people from volunteers. Call **1300 885 698** to find out more about getting a call or volunteering yourself.

Travel

Organised tours For a company that arranges travel for seniors, go to **http://seniorsholidaytravel.com.au/info/home/** or **www.funoverfifty.com.au/**

DID YOU KNOW?

The Australian Government has a one-stop shop for information for Australians over fifty. **www.seniors.gov.au** covers both Government and non-Government information and services.

Seniors cards To find out if you're eligible for a seniors card, YOURLifeChoices can help: **www.yourlifechoices.com.au/news/seniors-card-who-can-get-one**. In New Zealand, go to **www.supergold.govt.nz/**

Smart Traveller This Australian Government website provides all sorts of advice for people travelling overseas. **www.smartraveller.gov.au**

Staying on the road

Older drivers must pass a medical examination and an eyesight test each year (you are posted a certificate of fitness to drive to take to your GP to complete) and must pass a practical driving test each year. However, the age at which these requirements take effect varies from state to state.

Want to review your own fitness to drive? Try the NRMA's self-assessment, available from **www.mynrma.com.au/images/Motoring-PDF/Senior-drivers-driving-self-assessment.pdf**. Or try the NSW Government's Road & Maritime Service's self-assessment quiz: **www.rta.nsw.gov.au/licensing/downloads/olderdriverguide_dl1.html**

Some specially trained occupational therapists can assess older drivers and make recommendations for car modifications. You can find out more at **www.otaus.com.au**. The Commonwealth Rehabilitation Service offers driver assessments in many locations as part of their rehabilitation programs: see **www.crsaustralia.gov.au**

EMPLOYMENT and LEARNING

Learning new skills isn't just for the young. Get online and become a 'silver surfer'. Or join an organisation keen to benefit from older people's skills and experience.

Learning

University Take a course at U3A, the University of the Third Age, online or in person: **www.u3aonline.org.au**. There are Community Colleges throughout Australia and you can find out more via Community Colleges Australia through their website **www.cca.edu.au**. Or visit the homepage of a university near you and to find a fee-paying, non-degree course that interests you.

Getting online For courses designed to help seniors learn to use the computer and get online, go to **www.silversurf.com.au**

Jobs and volunteering

Jobs There are organisations specialising in finding jobs for older Australians, such as **www.olderworkers.com.au** and **http://adage.com.au**. The Australian Government is starting a Mature Age Participation – Job Seeker Assistance Program. See **www.deewr.gov.au/Employment/Programs/ExpPlus/Pages/MatureAgeParticipation.aspx** for more information.

Volunteering To find out more about volunteering, contact organisations such as Volunteering Australia (**www.volunteeringaustralia.org**) or Volunteering New Zealand (**www.volunteeringnz.org.nz**).

FINANCIAL and LEGAL

Whether or not you're now retired, it makes sense to take charge of your finances, address legal concerns and keep abreast of the latest developments.

Benefits

Centrelink To find out what benefits you might be entitled to, visit Centrelink at **www.humanservices.gov.au/customer/information/centrelink-website** and click on 'Older Australians'.

Financial planning Find a financial planner through the Financial Planning Association of Australia: **www.fpa.asn.au**, or through the Institute of Financial Advisers in New Zealand: **www.ifa.org.nz**

Financial planning

Centrelink The Centrelink Financial Information Service provides a free education service and expert information: **www.humanservices.gov.au/customer/services/centrelink/financial-information-service**

Legal

Legal advice For a directory of free legal advice, see **www.freelegal.com.au** in Australia or **www.communitylaw.org.nz** in New Zealand.

Wills For information on wills, go to **www.lawsociety.com.au/community/publicationsandfaqs/legalquestions/ShouldImakeawill/index.htm**

HEALTH CARE

Making sure you know how to access the wealth of healthcare advice available, and which are the best sources of information, is key to staying well in later life.

General

Aged Care Australia is the Australian Government Department of Health and Ageing's online source of information about aged care: **www.agedcareaustralia.gov.au** or **1800 200 422**

Better Health Channel Sponsored by the Victorian Government, this excellent website provides up-to-date healthcare information: **www.betterhealth.vic.gov.au**

CPR Take a lifesaving course through the Royal Lifesaving Society (**www.royallifesaving.com.au**) or St John Ambulance (**www.stjohn.org.au**).

myDr This website offers practical information about a large range of health conditions, including healthy living in older life: **www.mydr.com.au**

Staying healthy

Diet Read the latest National Health and Medical Research Council Dietary Guidelines For Older Australians at **www.nhmrc.gov.au/guidelines/publications/n23**

Exercise Get expert advice from the National Health and Medical Research Council National Physical Activity Recommendations For Older Australians via **www.health.gov.au/internet/main/publishing.nsf/content/phd-physical-rec-older-guidelines**

Sexual health For the latest advice, visit your state's Family Planning Association website or find a clinic by going to **www.shfpa.org.au** and clicking on 'Find a clinic'.

Smoking See the Quitnow Website **www.quitnow.gov.au** or call the Quitline on **13 78 48**.

Specialised health advice

Alcohol Alcoholics Anonymous supports people with a drinking problem (**www.aa.org.au**) while Al-Anon supports their families and friends (**www.al-anon.org/australia**).

Arthritis Arthritis Australia provides a wide range of services: **www.arthritisaustralia.com.au.** In New Zealand, go to Arthritis New Zealand: **www.arthritis.org.nz**

Asthma Expert guidance is available from Asthma Australia: **asthmaaustralia.org.au**

Cancer Visit Cancer Council Australia **www.cancer.org.au** or call their helpline on **13 11 20**.

COPD Find out more about smoker's lung from the Australian Lung Foundation: **www.lungfoundation.com.au**

Counselling Lifeline offers a 24-hour Telephone Crisis Support Service on **13 11 14**. The website is **www.lifeline.org.au**. The Veterans and Veterans Families Counselling Service is a free counselling service for veterans and their families, and the number is **1800 011 046**.

Dementia Information is available from Alzheimer's Australia through their website **www.fightdementia.org.au** or the National Dementia Helpline **1800 100 500**. In New Zealand, go to **www.alzheimers.org.nz**

Depression Visit beyondblue: the national depression initiative **www.beyondblue.org.au** or the Black Dog Institute **www.blackdoginstitute.org.au**

Diabetes For all the latest information, see Diabetes Australia. **www.diabetesaustralia.com.au** or call them on **1300 136 588**. In New Zealand, go to **www.diabetes.org.nz**

Hearing problems Useful organisations include the Australian Government Hearing Services Program **www.health.gov.au/hear** and Deaf Australia **www.deafau.org.au**

Heart health Get the latest advice on everything from blood pressure to good cholesterol levels from the Heart Foundation: **www.heartfoundation.org.au.** In New Zealand, **go to www.heartfoundation.org.nz**

Incontinence The Continence Foundation of Australia provides top tips via **www.continence.org.au/site/index.cfm** or the National Continence Helpline **1800 330 066**.

Insomnia For information on light-therapy boxes to help reset the body clock in winter, go to **www.mcsaustralia.com.au/light_therapy.html**. For information and advice concerning other issues around insomnia, go to **www.sleeptherapy.com.au/** or **www.helpguide.org/life/insomnia_treatment.htm**. To learn the buteyko method of mouth-breathing, go to **www.buteyko.info**

Kidney disease Contact Kidney Health Australia: **www.kidney.org.au**

Macular Degeneration The Macular Degeneration Foundation has a website at **www.mdfoundation.com.au**. In New Zealand, go to **www.mdnz.co.nz**

Menopause For reliable information, see Jean Hailes for Women's Health **www.jeanhailes.org.au** or call **1800 532 642**.

Mobility For help with mobility aids, go to **www.independentliving.com.au**. For tips on information for people with mobility issues wanting to exercise, go to **www.helpguide.org/life/workouts_exercise_overweight_disabled.htm**. For exercise classes for seniors, contact your local fitness club.

Osteoporosis Osteoporosis Australia can provide vital information at **www.osteoporosis.org.au.** In New Zealand, go to **www.bones.org.nz**

Palliative care See Palliative Care Australia **www.palliativecare.org.au/**

Parkinson's disease Parkinson's Australia has a website at **www.parkinsons.org.au.** Parkinson's New Zealand has a website at **www.parkinsons.org.nz**

Stroke Patients and carers can visit the National Stroke Foundation: **strokefoundation.com.au** or call **1800 787 653**. In New Zealand, go to **www.stroke.org.nz**

Vision problems Visit Vision Australia: **www.visionaustralia.org.au**

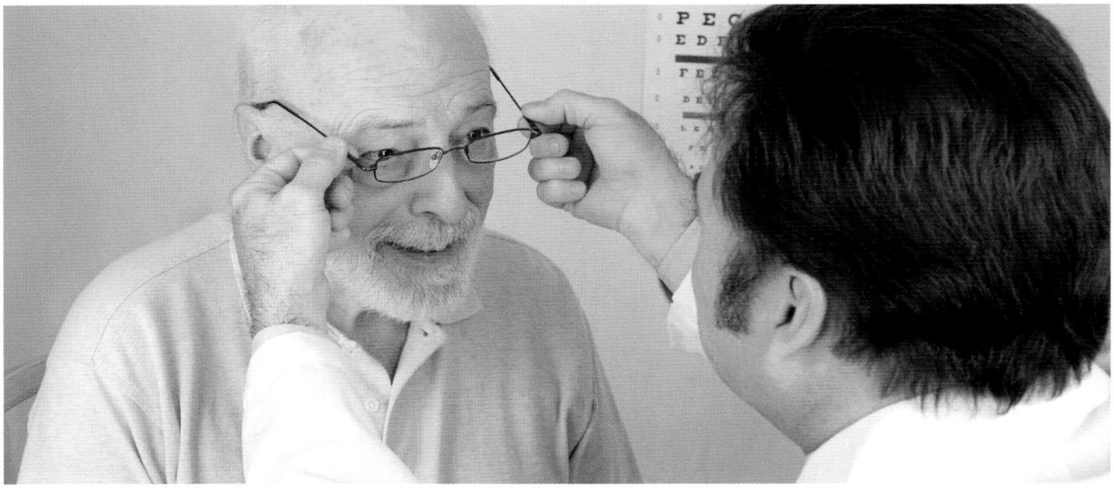

HELP at HOME

Community care The Australian Government can steer you through the various types of community care services, including home modifications, that are available and how to arrange them: **www.agedcareaustralia.gov.au/internet%5Cagedcare%5Cpublishing.nsf/Content/help+staying+at+home**

Personal alarms A number of organisations provide personal alarms, including the Independent Living Centre **www.ilcaustralia.org** and VitalCall **www.vitalcall.com.au**

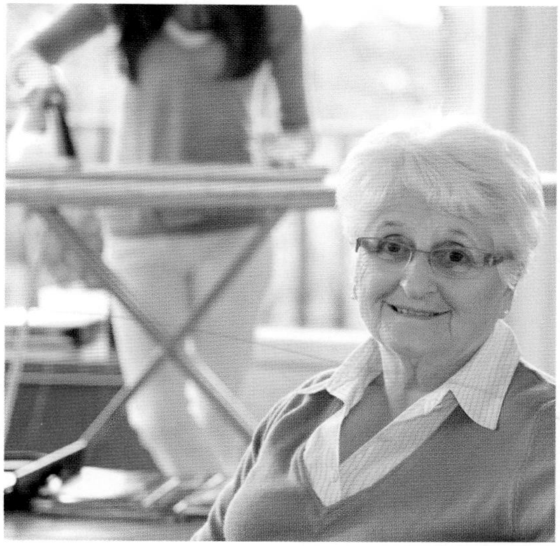

SUPPORT and CARE

If you're caring for someone else, you still need to care for yourself. Thanks to many organisations that provide support and care, you never have to go it alone.

Counselling

Cognitive behavioural therapy Moodgym is a free self-help program teaching valuable skills to people vulnerable to depression and anxiety: **www.moodgym.anu.edu.au**

Relationships For relationship problems, contact Relationships Australia in your state via their website **www.relationships.org.au** or by calling **1300 364 277**.

Disabilities

Disability support pension For Australia, see **www.humanservices.gov.au/customer/services/centrelink/disability-support-pension**. For New Zealand, go to **www.workandincome.govt.nz/individuals/a-z-benefits/disability-allowance.html**

Help with caring

Carers Australia is the peak body championing carers in Australia: **www.carersaustralia.com.au**. **Carers New Zealand** is the equivalent body in New Zealand: **www.carers.net.nz**

The Australian Government provides resources for grandparent carers through **www.seniors.gov.au/internet/seniors/publishing.nsf/Content/Resources+for+grandparent+carers** or contact Grandparents Australia through their website **http://grandparentsaustralia.org/Home_Page.html**

INDEX

Picture acknowledgments

The following abbreviations are used: t top; b bottom; l left; r right

FRONT COVER all Shutterstock; 2 Fuse/Getty Images; 4 top row l–r Henrik Sorensen/Getty Images, Brand X/Thinkstock, Shutterstock, Ruth Jenkinson; centre row l–r Getty Images, Tetra Images/Getty Images, James Woodson/Getty Images, Image Source/Getty Images; bottom row l–r Zoomphotographics/ Getty Images, Nick White/Getty Images, Laurence Monneret/Getty Images, Pixland/Thinkstock; 5 Fuse/ Getty Images; 6–7 John Lund/Getty Images; 8 Henrik Sorensen/Getty Images; 11 Suzanne Marshall/Getty Images; 12 Troels Graugaard/Getty Images; 13 Jamie Grill/Getty Images; 14 Shutterstock; 15 Thinkstock; 17 Ralf Nau/Thinkstock; 18 Shutterstock; 19 Shutterstock; 21 Shutterstock; 22 iStockphoto; 24 Brand X/ Thinkstock; 27 Helena Inkeri/Getty Images; 28 Taxi/Getty Images; 29 iStockphoto; 34 Thinkstock; 36 Shutterstock; 39 t STOCK4, b Creative/Getty Images; 40 Ben Richardson/Getty Images; 45 Thinkstock; 47 iStockphoto; 49 iStockphoto; 53 M Nader/Getty Images; 54 iStockphoto; 56 Shutterstock; 59 Shutterstock; 63 Shutterstock; 64 iStockphoto; 65 iStockphoto; 67 iStockphoto; 69 Shutterstock; 70 B2M Productions/Getty Images; 78 Jean Cazals/Getty Images; 79 Paul Bradbury/Getty Images; 81 Shutterstock; 86 Steve Baxter/Getty Images; 93 Maria Kallin/Getty Images; 98 Wade/Getty Images; 99 Thinkstock; 101 Images of Africa/Getty Images; 102 Comstock Images/Thinkstock; 106 Shutterstock; 108 Getty Images; 114 Thinkstock; 122 melh/Getty Images; 125 Squaredpixels/iStockphoto; 127 Thinkstock; 129 iStockphoto; 130 Tetra Images/Getty Images; 133 Shutterstock; 134 Vincent Hazat/Getty Images; 137 iStockphoto; 139 Shutterstock; 140 Jamie Grill/Getty Images; 163 Laurence Monneret/Getty Images; 164 Marc Romanelli/Getty Images; 174 James Woodson/Getty Images; 177 Ghislain & Marie David de Lossy/Getty Images; 181 Andersen Ross/Getty Images; 182 Image Source/Getty Images; 184 Kristin Duvall/Getty Images; 187 Thinkstock; 190 t iStockphoto, b Hemera/Thinkstock; 191 Robert Daly/Getty Images; 193 Thinkstock; 194 Jamie Grill/Corbis; 198 Wavebreak Media/Thinkstock; 202 iStockphoto; 203 Datacraft/Getty Images; 204 Dougal Waters/Getty Images; 206 Image Source/Getty Images; 208 iStockphoto; 210 Shutterstock; 213 Stockbyte/Thinkstock; 214 Shutterstock; 215 Shutterstock; 216 iStockphoto; 222 iStockphoto; 225 Shutterstock; 226 Shutterstock; 230 BLOOMimage/Getty Images; 233 Image Source/Getty Images; 235 Brand X Pictures/Thinkstock; 236 Zoomphotographics/ Getty Images; 241 Shutterstock; 242 Thinkstock; 247 Shutterstock; 249 Thinkstock; 250 iStockphoto; 252 Nick White/Getty Images; 256 Shutterstock; 258 Shutterstock; 260 iStockphoto; 264 Shutterstock; 265 Shutterstock; 267 Shutterstock; 268 iStockphoto; 269 Thinkstock; 271 Shutterstock; 272 Laurence Monneret/Getty Images; 277 Shutterstock; 283 Shutterstock; 278 iStockphoto; 279 Fuse/Thinkstock; 280 Shutterstock; 281 Shutterstock; 284 Hemera/Thinkstock; 286 Shutterstock; 288 BananaStock/ Thinkstock; 291 Shutterstock; 295 Shutterstock; 297 Thinkstock; 298 Pixland/Thinkstock

As young as you feel

Consultants
Sheena Meredith MB BS MPhil
Professor Ian Grierson PhD, CBiol, FB, FRCPath
Michele Harms PhD MSc MCSP
Fiona Hunter BSc Nutrition Dip. Dietetics
Dr Graham Jackson FRCP FESC FACC
Professor Robert Logie PhD FRSE FBPsS FRSA
Dr Kathy Kramer GP, BA/MBBS, BSc(Med) (Hons) (USyd)

Writers Elizabeth Adlam, Jane Feinmann, Jane Garton, Michele Harms, Sheena Meredith, Patsy Westcott
Editor Samantha Kent
Proofreader Susan McCreery
Indexer Diane Harriman

READER'S DIGEST GENERAL BOOKS
Editorial Director Lynn Lewis
Managing Editor Rosemary McDonald
Art Director Carole Orbell

As Young As You Feel was edited and produced by Reader's Digest (Australia) Pty Limited, 80 Bay Street, Ultimo, NSW 2007
www.readersdigest.com.au
www.readersdigest.co.nz
www.readersdigest.co.za
www.rdasia.com

Therefore Publishing would like to thank the following for their help in the preparation of this book: Action on Hearing Loss, Ame Verso, Rosie Taylor, Sarah Jane Green, Jo Winch and Julie Stewart.

Many thanks also to the John Lewis Partnership, www.physiosupplies.com and www.thera-band.co.uk for the kind loan of equipment for photography.

Models: Barry Ashton, Naomi Bastable, Craig Bryce, Alistair Hallam, Resi Harris, Kathy Hill, Debra Matthews, Samantha Ovens and Rupert Shelbourne.

This book is adapted from *As Young As You Feel* published by Vivat Direct Limited (t/a Reader's Digest), London, in 2012, using the services of Therefore Publishing Limited for The Reader's Digest Association, Inc.

National Library of Australia Cataloguing-in-publication data:

Title: As young as you feel: the essential guide for the over 60s.
ISBN: 978-1-922083-33-3 (hardback)
978-1-922083-34-0 (paperback)
Notes: Includes index.
Subjects: Older people–Health. Older people–Mental health.
Dewey Number: 305.26

If you have any comments or suggestions about the content of this book. Write to: The Editor, General Books Editorial, Reader's Digest (Australia) Pty Limited, GPO Box 4353, Sydney, NSW 2001, or email us at bookeditors.au@readersdigest.com.

To order additional copies of this book, please contact us at:
www.readersdigest.com.au or phone 1300 300 030 (Australia)
www.readersdigest.co.nz or phone 0800 400 060 (New Zealand)
www.readersdigest.co.za or phone 0800 980 572 (South Africa)
or email us at customerservice@au.readersdigest.com.

Pre-press by Sinnott Bros., Sydney
Printed in China by Leo Paper Products

Concept code: US6507/
Book Codes: 041-4902 (hb
041-4903 (pb